An Introduction to Nephroprotective Plants

Authored by

T. Pullaiah

Department of Botany
Sri Krishadevaraya University
Anantapur 515003
Andhra Pradesh
India

&

M. Ramaiah
Department of Pharmacognosy
Hindu college of Pharmacy
Amaravathi Road
Guntur 522002
Andhra Pradesh
India

An Introduction to Nephroprotective Plants

Authors: T. Pullaiah and M. Ramaiah

ISBN (Online): 978-981-5036-60-2

ISBN (Print): 978-981-5036-61-9

ISBN (Paperback): 978-981-5036-62-6

need for a court order if at any point you breach any terms of this License Agreement. In no event will any delay or failure by Bentham Science Publishers in enforcing your compliance with this License Agreement constitute a waiver of any of its rights.

3. You acknowledge that you have read this License Agreement, and agree to be bound by its terms and conditions. To the extent that any other terms and conditions presented on any website of Bentham Science Publishers conflict with, or are inconsistent with, the terms and conditions set out in this License Agreement, you acknowledge that the terms and conditions set out in this License Agreement shall prevail.

Bentham Science Publishers Pte. Ltd.
80 Robinson Road #02-00
Singapore 068898
Singapore
Email: subscriptions@benthamscience.net

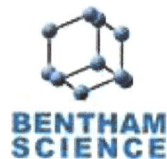

BENTHAM SCIENCE

CONTENTS

PREFACE

The kidney is a vital organ present in humans and vertebrate animals. Various toxic chemicals being used in food and water are causing toxicity to the kidney. There is a necessity to know about the methods of protecting this vital organ and the medicinal plants that are being used to protect it. The book An Introduction to Nephroprotective Plants gives an overview of nephrotoxicity and medicinal plants used for protecting the kidney and curing kidney toxicity and related diseases. Plants and plant-derived compounds have been a major source for the treatment and cure of diseases since ancient times. Even today, 25% of prescription drugs are sourced from plants. There is no comprehensive information on the plants that are used, both in traditional medicine and in modern medicine, for nephroprotection and curing kidney diseases. This book is an answer to this. It gives information on medicinal plants used in traditional medicine (both codified and noncodified) and ethnomedicine. Plant parts used, method of use and dosage, and references are given. Phytochemicals extracted from medicinal plants, screened and used in modern medicine for nephroprotection, and curing kidney problems are given in detail. Description of medicinal plants screened for nephroprotection and methods of screening are given. Methods of the assay for screening the medicinal plants for kidney protection and kidney toxicity cure are also given.

This book is a single point of reference for all researchers who require complete information on nephroprotective plants. It also gives information on phytochemicals used for kidney protection. Simply it will be a desk reference on herbal kidney protection.

The book will be useful for researchers working on kidney disorders and diseases, physicians treating patients with kidney problems, hospitals, pharmacy institutions, pharmacy students, pharmacy researchers, and ethnobotanists or people working on traditional medicine.

Since it is a voluminous subject, we might have missed some references. Readers are requested to bring such omissions to our notice so that the same can be included in future editions.

CONSENT FOR PUBLICATION

Not applicable.

CONFLICT OF INTEREST

The author declares no conflict of interest, financial or otherwise.

ACKNOWLEDGEMENTS

Declared none.

T. Pullaiah
Department of Botany
Sri Krishadevaraya University
Anantapur 515003
Andhra Pradesh
India

M. Ramaiah
Department of Pharmacognosy
Hindu college of Pharmacy
Amaravathi Road
Guntur 522002
Andhra Pradesh
India

CHAPTER 1

Urinary System, Its Functions and Disorders

Abstract: Kidneys (2), ureters (2), urinary bladder (1), and urethra (1) constitute the urinary system. Man is exposed to in the form of medicines, industrial and environmental chemicals, and a variety of naturally occurring substances and kidney is adversely affected by these chemicals. An acute injury is the result of this exposure that may lead to renal failure and renal malignancies. In this chapter, kidney functions, urinary system disorders, nephrotoxicity, nephrotoxic chemical substances, diabetic nephropathy, and urolithiasis are given.

Keywords: Cisplatin, Diabetic nephropathy, Gentamicin, Nephrotoxicity, Kidney, Kidney stones, Urolithiasis, Urinary system.

INTRODUCTION

A pair of fist-sized organs, called kidneys, are located outside the peritoneal cavity on each side of the spine. A kidney of an adult human is 10-12.5 x 5-7.5 x 3 cm in size (length x breadth x thick) and weighs 135-150 g. The functional unit of kidneys is nephrons and each human kidney contains about $0.8\text{-}1.2 \times 10^{-6}$ nephrons. Extra water and wastes from the blood are removed by the kidney and converted to urine. Kidneys also keep a stable balance of salts and other substances in the blood. Kidneys (2), ureters (2), urinary bladder (1), and urethra (1) constitute the urinary system. Ureters carry urine from the kidneys a triangle-shaped to the bladder in the lower abdomen. The bladder's elastic walls stretch and expand like a balloon to store urine. Urine is emptied through the urethra to outside the body when the walls of the bladder flatten together. By selectively excreting or retaining various substances according to specific body needs, the kidneys maintain the body's homeostasis.

FUNCTIONS OF THE KIDNEYS

Jayasudha [1], has given a detailed account of the functions and urinary system disorders.

1. The kidneys help regulate the blood levels of sodium ions, potassium ions, calcium ions, chloride ions and phosphate ions.
2. A variable amount of hydrogen ions (H^-) are excreted by the kidneys into the urine and conserve bicarbonate ions (HCO_3^-). These two activities help regulate blood pH.
3. Kidneys adjust blood volume by conserving or eliminating water in the urine.
4. By secreting the enzyme rennin, the kidneys help regulate blood pressure which activates the rennin-angiotensin-aldosterone pathway. Increased rennin causes an increase in blood pressure.
5. The kidneys help excrete waste substances by forming urine.
6. The kidneys maintain a relatively constant blood osmolarity close to 300 millimoles per litre by separately regulating loss of water and loss of solutes in the urine.
7. Two hormones, calcitriol, the active form of vitamin D and erythropoietin are produced by the kidneys. Calcitrol helps regulate calcium homeostasis and erythropoietin stimulates the production of red blood cells.
8. The kidney can use the amino acid glutamine in the synthesis of new glucose molecules. The kidneys then release glucose into the blood to help maintain a normal blood glucose level.

DISORDERS OF URINARY SYSTEM

Urinary system disorders range from easy to treat, to life-threatening in severity. These include Renal calculi or kidney stones (calcium oxalate, uric acid or calcium phosphate crystals), Cessation of glomerular filtration or renal failure [2], acute renal failure (ARF), chronic renal failure (CRF) [3], Glomerulonephritis, polycystic kidney disease (PKD), hydronephrosis, nocturnal enuresis, painful bladder syndrome/interstitial cystitis, urinary retention or bladder-emptying problems and urinary incontinence.

Nephrotoxicity

Toxic chemicals and medication may be poisonous to the kidney, which result in renal dysfunction or nephrotoxicity (Greek: *nephros*=kidney). Nephropathy is one of the progressive complications that arise due to the detrimental effects of metabolites created due to various metabolic and physiological reactions.

Because of high blood supply and the presence of cellular transport systems that cause accumulation of toxic compounds within the nephron epithelial cells, kidney becomes susceptible. Many drugs have been shown to induce significant nephrotoxicity. Aminoglycoside antibiotics have been widely used for gram-negative infections. However, their nephrotoxicity is a major limitation in clinical use. Among aminoglycosides, the grade of nephrotoxicity is in the following order, neomycin > GM > tobramycin.

The kidney is adversely affected by an array of chemicals that man is exposed to in the form of medicines, industrial and environmental chemicals, and a variety of naturally occurring substances. The level of exposure varies from minute quantities to very high doses. Exposure may be over a long period of time or limited to a single event, and it may be due to a single substance or to multiple chemicals. The circumstances of exposure may be an inadvertent, accidental, or intentional overdose or therapeutic necessity. Some chemicals cause an acute injury, while others produce chronic renal changes that may lead to end-stage renal failure and renal malignancies [4].

The kidney has several features that allow nephrotoxicants to accumulate [5]. It is highly vascular, receiving about 25% of the resting cardiac output (CO). The proximal renal tubule presents a large area for nephrotoxicant binding and transport into the renal epithelium. Reabsorption of the glomerular filtrate progressively increases intraluminal nephrotoxicant concentrations. It is the major organ of excretion and homeostasis for water-soluble molecules; because it is a metabolically active organ, it can concentrate certain substances actively [6]. In addition, its cells have the potential to convert chemicals and metabolically activate a variety of compounds [4].

GM mainly causes tubular toxicity, both lethal and sub-lethal alterations in tubular cells handicap reabsorption and, in severe cases, may lead to significant tubular obstruction [7]. Tubular cytotoxicity is the consequence of many interconnected actions triggered by drug accumulation in epithelial cells. An excessive concentration of the drug over an undetermined threshold destabilizes intracellular membranes and the drug redistributes throughout the cytosol. It then acts on mitochondria to unleash the intrinsic pathway of apoptosis [8].

A large number of chemicals in common usage nowadays are renal toxins. Administration of such toxins into the body may cause mechanical trauma to the kidneys and selectively interfere with certain functions of the renal tubules. Proximal renal tubular cells are particularly susceptible to acute injury by these substances and the exposure may be followed by acute tubular necrosis [9 - 11]. Certain food dyes are known to cause renal toxicity [12].

Some of the chemical nephrotoxicants and their activities are given below:

1. Cyclophosphamide (CP) is one of the most popular alkylating anticancer drugs despite its toxic side effects, including nephrotoxicity, hematotoxicity, mutagenicity, and immunotoxicity.
2. Deltamethrin, a pyrethroid insecticide, showed toxicity in mammalian animals.
3. GM-induced nephrotoxicity is a major contributor to Acute Kidney Injury (AKI) resulting from free radicals induced oxidative stress. GM nephrotoxicity, which occurs in about 15-30% of treated subjects, is manifested clinically as nonoliguric renal failure, with a slow rise in serum creatinine and hypoosmolar urinary output developing after several days of treatment.
4. Cisplatin (cis-diamminedichloroplatinum (II)) is an effective agent against various solid tumours. Despite its effectiveness, the dose of cisplatin that can be administered is limited by its nephrotoxicity. Hundreds of platinum compounds (*e.gl.*, carboplatin, oxaliplatin, nedaplatin and the liposomal form lipoplatin) have been tested over the last two decades in order to improve the effectiveness and to lessen the toxicity of cisplatin.
5. Overdose of Paracetamol (PCM) can cause nephrotoxicity.
6. Aminoglycosides, commonly used antibiotics against Gram negative bacteria, are nephrotoxic.
7. Amikacin, a valuable aminoglycoside, is associated with undesirable renal toxicity.
8. Cadmium, a known industrial pollutant, accumulates in the kidney and leads to nephrotoxicity.

Acute kidney injury (AKI) has become increasingly prevalent in both developed and developing countries, and is associated with severe morbidity and mortality, especially in children. Cerda *et al.* [13] have reviewed recent literature on AKI, identified differences and similarities in the condition between developed and developing areas, analyzed the practical implications of the identified differences, and made evidence-based recommendations for study and management.

Diabetic Nephropathy

Das *et al.* [14] have given a detailed account of Diabetic Nephropathy (DN). DN is characterized by an increase in various things *viz.* kidney size, urinary albumin excretion, glomerular volume and kidney function chased by the accumulation of glomerular extracellular matrix, glomerular sclerosis and tubular fibrosis. Diabetic kidney disease is reported in about 15%–25% of type I diabetes patients and 30%–40% of patients with type II diabetes. Health problems associated with diabetic nephropathy have been discussed by Baig *et al.* [15], Fioretto ad Mauer [16] and Sheela *et al.* [17]. The pathophysiology of DN comprises of hyperfiltration and development of microalbumin urine which is followed by deterioration of kidney functions associated with extracellular and cellular disruption in both places that is glomerular and tubulo-interstitial regions of kidney [18]. It also includes hypertrophy/hyperplasia of glomerulus and the tubules, thickening of tubular basement membranes, thickening of glomerular, and expansion of tubulo-interstitial as well as mesangial compartments [19].

KIDNEY STONES

Aggarwal *et al.* [20] and Das *et al.* [14] have discussed in detail kidney stones and herbal treatment of kidney stones. Renal colic is the first manifestation of renal stone disease. The formation of solid phases in urinary passages is described as "Nephrolithiasis," whereas the accumulation and aggregation of salts in renal parenchyma is termed as "Nephrocalcinosis". Nephrocalcinosis is very common and can develop or cannot into nephrolithiasis. Formation of kidney stone is a complex process including chronicle events, *viz.* crystal nucleation, its growth, aggregation, and crystal retention inside the renal tubules [14, 21].

Mankind is known to be afflicted by urinary stone disease first reported in Egyptian Mummies dated 4000 BC and references are being made in early Sanskrit documents in India between 3000 and 200 BC [20]. Urolithiasis is a common multi-factorial disease that has been recognized and documented in medical literature even by Greek and Roman physicians. In the light of these historical clues, it appears that humankind has been afflicted by urinary stones since antiquity. Depending on the socio-economic conditions and subsequent changes in dietary habits, the overall probability of stone formers differs in various parts of the world. Urolithiasis is affecting 5-9% in Europe, 4-8% in the UK, 12% in Canada, 15% in the US, 20% in Gulf countries and 11% population in India with a relapse rate of 50% in 5–10 years and 75% in 20 years [22 - 24]. The stone belts of the world are located in the countries of the Middle East, North Africa, Mediterranean regions, Southern states of USA, and North-western states of India. In India, with a prevalence rate of 15%, too high incidence of stone belts has been found to occur. Marangella *et al.* [25] discussed about the drugs for the treatment of nephrolithaisis, while Butterweck *et al.* [26] gave an account of herbal medicines in the management of nephrolithiasis.

Urolithiasis encompasses all the renal, bladder and ureteric stones [27]. Kidney stones are composed of inorganic and organic crystals amalgamated with proteins. Urinary stones can be classified according to stone composition as calcium stone, uric acid stone, struvite stone and cystine stone. Some of the other types are calcium phosphate stone, xanthine stone, DHA stone, and crixivan stone. Approximately 80% of kidney stones are primarily composed of calcium oxalate

[28 - 30]. The major predisposing factors that create an imbalance between levels of promoters and inhibitors of stone formation are low urine volumes, diet, hypercalciuria, hyperoxaluria, hyperuricosuria, hypocitraturia, hypomagnesuria, low urinary pH, cystinuria, and distal renal tubular acidosis [31]. Presently, the available drug therapy for the treatment of urinary stone includes, antibiotics (for struvite stones), allopurinol (for uric acid stone), opiates and NSAID'S (for relieving pain), and diuretics (for renal stone removal) [29]. For kidney stones that do not pass on their own by pharmacological management, the most widely preferred technique is lithotripsy. In this procedure, shock waves are used to break up a large stone into smaller pieces that can then pass through the urinary system. In case of failure with all other treatments, surgical invasive techniques have also been used like percutaneous nephrolithotomy or through ureteroscopy [27, 32].

The formation of a urinary stone, known as nephrolithiasis, urolithiasis, renal calculi or kidney stone is a serious, debilitating problem throughout the world. Struvite or Ammonium Magnesium Phosphate Hexahydrate (AMPH) is one of the components of urinary stone (calculi). Struvite stones are commonly found in women. Struvites form in humans as a result of urinary tract infection with urolithic urea splitting microorganisms. These stones can grow rapidly forming "staghorn-calculi", which is a more painful urological disorder. Therefore, it is of prime importance to study the growth and inhibition of Struvite crystals.

Urolithiasis/nephrolithiasis are commonly referred to as stone formation in any part of the urinary tract, such as kidneys, ureters, urinary bladder, and urethra. Kidney stones are generally caused by bacterial infection, while kidney stones form as a result of physicochemical or genetic derangements leading to supersaturation of the urine with stone-forming salts or, less commonly, from recurrent urinary tract infection with urease producing bacteria [33]. Stone formation is a complex process that occurs due to successive physiochemical events such as supersaturation, nucleation, growth, aggregation, and retention within the renal tubules [23].

Types of Stones

Vamsi and Latha [35] have given a detailed account of urolithiasis wherein they discussed the types of stones in the urinary system.

Physiologically

Physiologically the renal calculi differentiated as tissue attached and unattached.

1. Attached stones tend to have the detectable site of attachment to papillae with the composition of calcium oxalate (CaOx) monohydrate.

2. While the unattached calculi are distinguished by having different compositions and lack of detectable site [36].

Clinically

Based on the composition of the stone forming element in the calculi, clinically, these calculi are categorized as the following types.

• Calcium stones (CaOx alone/with calcium phosphate)

• Struvite stones (Magnesium ammonium phosphate)

• Uric acid stones

• Cystine stones

• Drug induced stones

• 2,8-Dihydroxyadenine stones

Among the kidney stones, CaOx stones constitute about 75%, struvite stones of 15%, uric acid stones of about 6%, and cystine stones of about 1-2% [37].

Calcium Stones

The Idiopathic causes are absorptive hypercalciuria, renal hypercalciuria, and resorptive hypercalciuria. The metabolic causes are hypercalcemia due to primary hyperparathyroidism, hyperoxaluria, hyperuricosuria, hypocitraturia, and hypomagnesuria. In explaining the detailed cause of each event. i. Hyperoxaluria arises due to primary hyperoxaluria of genetic disorder which enhances the hepatic oxalate production and enteric hyperoxaluria, where the colon is made to diffuse more oxalate. ii. Hyperuricosuria is evident from excessive purine intake. iii. Hypocitraturia arises due to metabolic acidosis induced by inflammatory bowel disease and chronic diarrhea. iv. Hypomagnesuria due to malabsorption of magnesium from the gut because of inflammatory bowel disease and chronic diarrhea [35].

In hypercalciuria, calcium promotes the ionization and saturation of crystallization of calcium salts and also binds with stone inhibiting substances such as citrates and glycosaminoglycans there by the events of hypercalciuria induced uroliths. The renal leak from the kidney, resorption from bone and absorption from the gut tends to be key defects in implicating the hypercalciuria individually or in combination with each other. On the other hand, excessive dietary sodium intake predisposes to uroliths by hypercalciuria and hypocitraturia. Moreover, there exists a linear relationship between urinary sodium and calcium levels, which establish a strong relationship to confer the risk of hypercalciuria induced uroliths. In addition to the above all etiological factors, protein overload, and metabolic acidosis are the other possible etiological factors in the pathogenesis of hypercalciuria induced calcium nephrolithiasis. In metabolic acidosis, the high urinary pH favors the formation of calcium-containing uroliths. The excess protein intake can predispose to calcium nephrolithiasis which was evident from the animal, metabolic and epidemiological studies [35].

Hypocitraturia corresponds to about 20-60% of calcium nephrolithiasis. As it is a major inhibitory component of calcium oxalate and calcium phosphate, lowered levels of citrate favours the risk of hypercalciuria induced calcium uroliths. Furthermore, the citrate tends to complex with calcium to form a soluble complex to prevent crystal growth. Hyperoxaluria, is another etiological factor of equal importance with hypercalciuria for inducing calcium nephrolithiasis by promoting the CaOx supersaturation in the urine. It occurs as a result of the dietary intake of oxalate-rich foods of spinach, rhubarb, beetroot, almond, nuts, etc. Hyperuricosuria, as a result of high dietary intake of protein, can attribute CaOx uroliths by the heterogeneous nucleation of uric acid [35].

Struvite Stones

These are also called infectious stones, as a consequence of persistent urease producing bacterial infections. Generally, these urease infections are caused by certain species of bacteria like *E. coli, P. mirabilus, Pseudomonas* species, *Staphylococcal* species, and *Ureaplasma urealyticum.* By secreting the urease enzyme, these bacterial species hydrolyse the urea to carbon dioxide and ammonia which can raise the urinary pH to favour the struvite stones formation. Infectious stones induced by these bacterial infections are caused by urinary tract obstructions due to ureteropelvic junction stenosis, urinary catheters, neurogenic bladder dysfunctioning, vesical ureteral reflux, medullary sponge kidney and distal renal tubular acidosis [35].

Uric Acid Stones

Uric acid stones are clinically evident when there is increased hyperuricosuria, acidic urine, and reduced volume of urine. Indeed the hyperuricosuria along with the aciduria clinically manifests the uric acid stones significantly. While elevated levels of uric acid within normal pH can be tolerated. But hyperuricosuria seems to be the sole cause for uric acid uroliths in rare conditions. The common etiological factors in inducing uric acid uroliths are dietary intake of excess protein food, gout, and recurrent monoarthritis along with acidic urine. Also, high body-mass index, type 2 diabetes, and glucose intolerance are most commonly seen in patients with uric acid uroliths [35].

In particular, obesity and type 2 diabetes conditions, impaired renal ammonium excretion and increased net acid production resulting in aciduria can favor the uric acid uroliths formation when it is associated with hyperuricosuria. The other causative factors like chronic diarrhea, gastroenterostomy, exercise-induced lactic acidosis, and high consumption of animal protein can predispose to acidic urine. Reduced urinary volume occurs as a result of chronic diarrhoea, excessive perspiration and intestinal ostomies can act as contributing factors in attributing the uric acid uroliths. The congenital enzymatic deficiencies, uricosuric agents, gout, myeloproliferative disorders, hemolytic anemia, and chemotherapy-induced tumor lysis acts as the risk factors of hyperuricosuria induced uric acid stones [35].

Cystine Stones

It constitutes of about only the least amount in all types of stones which occurs in individuals having cystinuria, an autosomal recessive disease that affects proximal tubular absorption of cystine. The solubility of cystine is about 243mg/l in normal urinary pH, while the solubility greatly increases by increasing the urinary pH. Moreover, cystine being a poorly soluble amino acid forms, tends to form cystine stones more at lower urinary acidic pH. It has also occurred as an autosomal recessive disorder of ornithine, arginine, and lysine. It affects about 1 in 20,000 individuals especially at the age of 20-30 years. They are presented as staghorn stones which are multiple and radio-opaque [35].

Drug Induced Stones

These constitute the rare forms of stones which are drug induced forms that result from various drugs like indinavir, triamterene, fluoroquinolones, primidone, tetracyclines, magnesium trisilicate, and sulfonamides. In addition to this, other drugs like calcitriol, corticosteroids, furosemide, and acidifiers can predispose the individual to hypercalciuria induced calcium uroliths. In other cases like ascorbic acid and allopurinol therapy, there exist implications of hyperoxaluria and hyperxanthuria induced lithogenesis. Topiramate, a new anti-epileptic drug also implicates the calcium uroliths by its renal tubular acidosis induced by its carbonic anhydrase enzyme. HIV-positive patients are more prone to develop these drugs induced stones when they are treated with lithogenic drugs like indinavir and sulfamides (sulfamethoxazole and sulfadiazine) [35].

2, 8-Dihydroxyadenine Stones

A rare form of stones that results from a very rare form of adenine phosphoribosyl-transferase (APRT) deficiency imherits renal stone disease, progressively ending with renal failure. In APRT deficiency condition, it accumulates large amounts of adenine which then metabolized to nephrotoxic 2, 8-dihydroxyadenine by xanthine oxidase enzyme. Since it is life-threatening, early diagnosis and treatment with allopurinol are needed [38].

Urolithiasis is a consequence of an imbalance between promoters and inhibitors of crystallization in urine [34]. Stone promoters include low urine volume, low urine pH, calcium, sodium, oxalate, and urate while stone inhibitors are citrate, magnesium (inorganic inhibitors) prothrombin fragment, glycosaminoglycans and osteopontin (organic inhibitors) [39].

PREVENTION

The following measures are opted to be the best suitable preventive measures in the management of urolithiasis [35].

• Increase uptake of water up to 2L daily.

• Maximizing the urinary output.

• Limiting the use of drugs that induce uroliths.

• Minimizing the intake of animal protein.

• Low intake of sodium.

• Lowering the dietary intake of purine and oxalate rich food.

• Limitation of dietary intake of calcium.

CONCLUSION

The urinary system, in any case, is called the renal structure. Kidneys assume such fundamental parts in eliminating unwanted materials and poisons and keeping up with body- wide homeostasis that issues of the kidneys might be dangerous. The steady loss of ordinary kidney work usually happens with various problems, including nephrotoxicity, diabetic nephropathy, polycystic kidney illness (PKD), kidney failure, kidney stones, bladder diseases, urolithiasis, urinary incontinence, and high BP.

ABBREVIATIONS

ARF – Acute Renal Failure

CRF – Chronic Renal Failure

GM - Gentamicin

REFERENCES

[1]   Jayasudha A. Anti urolithiatic and antioxidant activity of fruit extract of *Cuminum cyminum* Linn. In rats. M Pharm dissertation, Rajiv Gandhi University of Health Sciences, Bangalore, Karnataka, India 2011.

[2]   Beirne GJ, Brennan JT. Glomerulonephritis associated with hydrocarbon solvents: mediated by antiglomerular basement membrane antibody. Arch Environ Health 1972; 25(5): 365-9.
[http://dx.doi.org/10.1080/00039896.1972.10666187] [PMID: 4568564]

[3]   Eugene B, Stephen L. Principles of international medicine. 15th ed. New York: McGraw- Hill Medical Publishing Division 2001; pp. 1535-626.

[4]   Adesia A. A. Protective effects of ethanolic extract of *Psidium guajava* on Adriamycin-induced nephrotoxicity and genototoxicity in rats. PhD thesis, University of Ibadan, Nigeria 2013.

[5]   Weinberg JM. The cellular basis of nephrotoxicity.Diseases of the Kidney. Boston: Little Brown 1993; pp. 1031-237.

[6]   Perazella MA. Drug-induced nephropathy: an update. Expert Opin Drug Saf 2005; 4(4): 689-706.
[http://dx.doi.org/10.1517/14740338.4.4.689] [PMID: 16011448]

[7]   Lopez-Novoa JM, Quiros Y, Vicente L, Morales AI, Lopez-Hernandez FJ. New insights into the mechanism of aminoglycoside nephrotoxicity: an integrative point of view. Kidney Int 2011; 79(1): 33-45.
[http://dx.doi.org/10.1038/ki.2010.337] [PMID: 20861826]

[8]   Quiros Y, Vicente-Vicente L, Morales AI, Lopez-Novoa JM. LopezHerna'ndez FJ. An intergrative overview on the mechanism underlying the renal tubular cytotoxicity of gentamicin. Technol Soc 2011; 119(2): 245-56.
[PMID: 20829429]

[9]   New PS, Lubash GD, Scherr L, Rubin AL. Acute renal failure associated with carbon tetrachloride intoxication. JAMA 1962; 181: 903-6.
[http://dx.doi.org/10.1001/jama.1962.03050360089019c] [PMID: 14479306]

[10]   Taher SM, Anderson RJ, McCartney R, Popovtzer MM, Schrier RW. Renal tubular acidosis associated with toluene "sniffing". N Engl J Med 1974; 290(14): 765-8.
[http://dx.doi.org/10.1056/NEJM197404042901403] [PMID: 4815223]

[11]   Gutch CF, Tomhave WG, Stevens SC. Acute renal failure due to inhalation of trichloroethylene. Ann Intern Med 1965; 63: 128-34.
[http://dx.doi.org/10.7326/0003-4819-63-1-128] [PMID: 14305960]

[12]   Das M, Garg K, Singh GB, Khanna SK. Attenuation of benzanthrone toxicity by ascorbic acid in guinea pigs. Fundam Appl Toxicol 1994; 22(3): 447-56.
[http://dx.doi.org/10.1006/faat.1994.1050] [PMID: 8050639]

[13]   Cerdá J, Bagga A, Kher V, Chakravarthi RM. The contrasting characteristics of acute kidney injury in developed and developing countries. Nat Clin Pract Nephrol 2008; 4(3): 138-53.
[http://dx.doi.org/10.1038/ncpneph0722] [PMID: 18212780]

[14]   Das S, Vasudeva N, Sharma S. Kidney disorders and management through herbs: A review. J Phytopharmcol 2019; 8(1): 21-7.
[http://dx.doi.org/10.31254/phyto.2019.8106]

[15]   Baig RM, Gillani WS, Sulaiman SA, Krishna RD, Narayanan K. Epidemiology of diabetic nephropathy in the poor patients from rural south-east India. Int J Nutr Food Sci 2011; 4(1): 53-61.

[16]   Fioretto P, Mauer M. Histopathology of diabetic nephropathy. Semin Nephrol 2007; 27(2): 195-207. [http://dx.doi.org/10.1016/j.semnephrol.2007.01.012] [PMID: 17418688]

[17]   Sheela N, Jose MA, Sathyamurthy D, Kumar BN. Effect of silymarin on streptozotocin-nicotinamid--induced type 2 diabetic nephropathy in rats. Iran J Kidney Dis 2013; 7(2): 117-23. [PMID: 23485535]

[18]   Kanwar YS, Wada J, Sun L, *et al.* Diabetic nephropathy: mechanisms of renal disease progression. Exp Biol Med (Maywood) 2008; 233(1): 4-11. [http://dx.doi.org/10.3181/0705-MR-134] [PMID: 18156300]

[19]   Mason RM, Wahab NA. Extracellular matrix metabolism in diabetic nephropathy. J Am Soc Nephrol 2003; 14(5): 1358-73. [http://dx.doi.org/10.1097/01.ASN.0000065640.77499.D7] [PMID: 12707406]

[20]   Aggarwal A, Singla SK, Tandon C. Urolithiasis: phytotherapy as an adjunct therapy. Indian J Exp Biol 2014; 52(2): 103-11. [PMID: 24597142]

[21]   Khan SR. Animal models of kidney stone formation: an analysis. World J Urol 1997; 15(4): 236-43. [http://dx.doi.org/10.1007/BF01367661] [PMID: 9280052]

[22]   Dawson PA, Russel CS, Lee S, McLeay SC, van Dongen JN, Cowley DM, *et al.* Urolithiasis and hepatotoxicity are linked to the anion transporter in mice 2010; 120-3. [http://dx.doi.org/10.1172/JCI31474]

[23]   Yadav RD, Alok S, Jain SK, Verma A, Mahor A, Bharti JP, *et al.* Herbal plants used in the treatment of urolithiasis: a review. Int J Pharaceut Sci Res 2011; 2(6): 1412-20.

[24]   Moe OW. Kidney stones: pathophysiology and medical management. Lancet 2006; 367(9507): 333-44. [http://dx.doi.org/10.1016/S0140-6736(06)68071-9] [PMID: 16443041]

[25]   Marangella M, Vitale C, Bagnis C, Petrarulo M, Tricerri A. Use of drugs for nephrolithiasis. Clin Cases Miner Bone Metab 2008; 5(2): 131-4. [PMID: 22460995]

[26]   Butterweck V, Khan SR. Herbal medicines in the management of urolithiasis: alternative or complementary? Planta Med 2009; 75(10): 1095-103. [http://dx.doi.org/10.1055/s-0029-1185719] [PMID: 19444769]

[27]   Lawrence A, Koya MP. Management of urolithiasis – a review. Samoa Med J 2009; 41-3.

[28]   Stamatiou KN, Karanasiou VI, Lacroix RE, *et al.* Prevalence of urolithiasis in rural Thebes, Greece. Rural Remote Health 2006; 6(4): 610. [PMID: 17155848]

[29]   Heilberg IP, Schor N. Renal stone disease: Causes, evaluation and medical treatment. Arq Bras Endocrinol Metabol 2006; 50(4): 823-31. [http://dx.doi.org/10.1590/S0004-27302006000400027] [PMID: 17117307]

[30]   Coe FL, Parks JH, Asplin JR. The pathogenesis and treatment of kidney stones. 1992; 327(16): 1141-52. [http://dx.doi.org/10.1056/NEJM199210153271607]

[31]   Barbas C, García A, Saavedra L, Muros M. Urinary analysis of nephrolithiasis markers. J Chromatogr B Analyt Technol Biomed Life Sci 2002; 781(1-2): 433-55. [http://dx.doi.org/10.1016/S1570-0232(02)00557-3] [PMID: 12450673]

[32]   Tiselius HG. Who forms stones and why. Eur Urol 2011; 10(5): 408-14.

[http://dx.doi.org/10.1016/j.eursup.2011.07.002]

[33] Alok S, Jain SK, Verma A, Kumar M, Sabharwal M. Pathophysiology of kidney, gall bladder and urinary stones treatment with herbal and allopathic medicine: A review. Asian Pac J Trop Dis 2013; 3(6): 496-504.
[http://dx.doi.org/10.1016/S2222-1808(13)60107-3]

[34] Tiwari A, Soni V, Londhe V, Bhandarkar A, Bandawane D, Nipate S. An overview on potent indigenous herbs for urinary tract infirmity: Urolithiasis. Asian J Pharm Clin Res 2012; 5(1): 7-12.

[35] Vamsi S, Latha P. Urolithiasis – An updated review over genetics, pathophysiology and its clinical management. Int J Pharm Pharm Sci 2014; 6(11): 23-31.

[36] Grases F, Costa-Bauzá A, Ramis M, Montesinos V, Conte A. Simple classification of renal calculi closely related to their micromorphology and etiology. Clin Chim Acta 2002; 322(1-2): 29-36.
[http://dx.doi.org/10.1016/S0009-8981(02)00063-3] [PMID: 12104078]

[37] Das I, Gupta SK, Ansari SA, Pandey VN, Rastogi RP. *In vitro* inhibition and dissolution of calcium oxalate by edible plant *Trianthema monogyna* and pulse *Macrotyloma uniflorum* extracts. J Cryst Growth 2005; 273: 546-54.
[http://dx.doi.org/10.1016/j.jcrysgro.2004.09.038]

[38] Osborne CA, Lulich JP, Swanson LL, Albasan H. Drug-induced urolithiasis. Vet Clin North Am Small Anim Pract 2009; 39(1): 55-63.
[http://dx.doi.org/10.1016/j.cvsm.2008.09.004] [PMID: 19038650]

[39] Santhoshi B, Chidrawar VR, Rao VUM. A brief review on the potential medicinal plants and screening models of urolithiasis. Int J Appl Biol Pharm Technol 2015; 6(1): 37-45.

CHAPTER 2

Screening Models of Nephroprotection, Nephrocurative and Antiurolithiatic Plants

Abstract: Renal issue stay persistent among the exceptional worldwide medical issues. It's a gradually reformist issue which may cause end-stage renal disease (ESRD). Till date, different screening models have been effectively evolved to reenact human infections, including chronic kidney disease (CKD). In this chapter, screening models for evaluating the biological activity of plant extracts in nephroprotection, nephrocuration and antiurolithiasis are given. This is a single point reference to the researchers.

Keywords: Antiurolithiasis, Assay methods, Nephrocuration, Nephrolithiasis, Nephroprotection, Screening models.

INTRODUCTION

Throughout the most recent forty years, it has become progressively clear that the kidney is antagonistically influenced by a variety of synthetics that man is presented to as prescriptions, modern and ecological synthetic substances, and an assortment of normally happening substances. The degree of openness shifts from minute amounts to exceptionally high portions. Openness might be over a significant stretch or restricted to a solitary occasion, and it very well might be because of a solitary substance or to different synthetics. The conditions of openness might be a coincidental, unplanned, or purposeful excess or remedial need. A few synthetic compounds cause an intense physical issue, while others produce chronic renal changes that may prompt end-stage renal disappointment and renal malignancies. Nephrotoxicants (as remedial medications, mechanical or ecological synthetics) may represent roughly half of all instances of intense and persistent renal disappointment. The essential proportion of kidney work is glomerular filtration rate which springs from serum and urine creatinine fixations. Decrease of glomerular filtration rate (GFR) by half, characterizes CKD in animal models. In any case, GFR can't be dependably assessed in animal models. Consequently, in animal investigations of CKD, huge changes in biomarkers of renal capacity, including blood urea nitrogen (BUN) and creatinine are not just adequate to evaluate the kidney work. What's more, urinary protein discharge, presence of common entanglements identified with CKD in people like normochromic sickliness, hyperphosphatemia, hyperparathyroidism, hyper kalemia and so forth are the highlights evaluated in animal models of CKD [1].

Different animal models are created utilizing various strategies inside the space of CKD to inexact the human illness. The accompanying subtleties have practical experience in key data on *in vivo* models of CKD created through unconstrained, obtained and hereditary strategies.

IN VIVO ANIMAL MODELS

Spontaneous Models [1]

These models could be created by different metabolic or immunological techniques.

Lupus Nephritis

Advancement of Lupus nephritis by resistant complex-interceded glomerulonephritis is one such model. Mouse models including MRL/lpr and NZB/W have the ability to foster lupus nephritis unexpectedly looking like human histological discoveries identified with CKD. Studies in mouse models of lupus nephritis have been helpful in understanding the essential pathogenesis of immune system kidney infection. Demise because of renal disappointment has been distinguished as a significant end-point of these examinations.

Aging

Since aging can cause movement of renal disability and scarring, rodents of more than two years of age could be utilized as a model of CKD. It is liked to utilize male rodents of this model because of right on time and extreme side effects of scarring than in females.

Spontaneously Hypertensive Rats

These types of rodents are another trial model that can be utilized in research purposes identified with CKD. Biochemical and histopathological highlights identified with CKD could be noticed beginning from the sixth week in immediately hypertensive rodent model.

CKD as a Result of Intense Kidney Injury

The general danger of CKD after a serious scene of ischemic intense kidney injury is valuable in creating animal models of CKD. Long haul interstitial fibrosis and reformist renal inadequacy are the trademark highlights of this model. This model is researched most usually in rodents and mice. Renal fibrosis is clear during the chronic period of the infection.

Intrinsic Insufficiency of Nephrons

Munich Wistar Frömter rodent is a hereditary model with intrinsic insufficiency in nephron number. Their nephron number is 30–50%, not exactly ordinary. These animals are inclined to foster hypertension in adulthood. Munich Wistar Frömter rodents foster proteinuria at ten weeks old enough and display critical glomerulosclerosis by nine months

Acquired Models [1]

Animal models of CKD have been created for utilizing surgical and chemical strategies causing nephrotoxicity.

Surgical Methods

5/6 Nephrectomy

Decrease in renal mass tentatively by subtotal nephrectomy causes reformist glomerulosclerosis and tubulointerstitial fibrosis, related to CKD. It is a simple technique for prompting sickness in bigger creatures like rodents and rabbits. A few strategies are accessible to foster CKD utilizing this model. One methodology is the uninephrectomy followed by ligation of polar parts of the renal supply route. It is a strategy regularly acted in rodents. Another methodology is the careful extraction of around half of the leftover kidney, fourteen days after uninephrectomy. This methodology can be utilized both in rodents and mice. A blend of the over two models, which ties at least one part of the mouse renal vein, and afterward eliminates extra renal mass to accomplish an absolute 5/6 nephrectomy.

The nephrectomy technique is exceptionally subject to careful mastery and consequently the accessibility of working facilities. Since the movement of renal disappointment is firmly connected with the amount of tissue infarcted or extracted, it's identified with moderately enormous between individual and between lab varieties.

Unilateral Ureteral Obstruction (UUO)

This is an *in vivo* model helpful in analyzing the components of tubulointerstitial fibrosis related to human renal illness. It is feasible to incite this model both in rodents and mice without explicit strain reliance. Decrease in the renal blood stream and glomerular filtration rate is commented inside 24 hrs following kidney deterrent. Interstitial irritation tops at 2–3 days and rounded widening, cylindrical decay and fibrosis start from multi week after UUO. The test model would arrive at the end stage by around fourteen days following the technique.

ANIMAL MODELS OF CHRONIC NEPHROTOXICITY [1]

Thinking about the limitations in surgical models, the usage of non-surgical choices that utilize nephrotoxic specialists appear to be gainful. Following are not many models for the animal models created utilizing nephrotoxicants.

Adenine Induced CKD

The advancement of an animal model for CKD dependent on the admission of adenine, was first proposed by Yokowaza in 1982 [2]. Oral intake of adenine blended in with the food at 0.75% w/w was performed for the advancement of the trial model. Adenine and its metabolite, 2, 8-dihydroxyadenine, accelerate in the renal tubules and structure precious stones causing degenerative changes in renal tubules and the interstitium. The utilization of oral adenine causes impediment of renal tubules, which hinders the discharge of nitrogenous substances. This prompts morphological, biochemical and histopathological changes in kidneys looking like CKD in people. Grown-up creatures create hyperphosphatemia, auxiliary hyperparathyroidism, bone infection, and vascular calcification following oral administration of adenine.

High dreariness and mortality were seen in the above cases because of starvation and unhealthiness as opposed to renal disappointment in animals. As an answer, Adenine is blended in a casein-based chow, in which the casein successfully eliminates the natural smell and taste of adenine.

Another new model is for the enlistment of CKD by means of intraperitoneal adenine to defeat the high bleakness and mortality. It is by all accounts a better model than oral adenine administration for the acceptance of CKD since it is more common-sense, advantageous and exact because of the direct passage of the medication to the fundamental course. Adenine model is a superior option for the careful models of CKD because of a few reasons. It is a helpful strategy which can be utilized to initiate renal disappointment, with almost no between singular varieties throughout a brief timeframe. The level of decrease in renal capacity is additionally generally homogeneous.

Adriamycin Induced CKD

Adriamycin (doxorubicin) is an anthracycline drug utilized in malignant growth chemotherapy. It is a cytotoxic anti-infection secluded from societies of *Streptomyces peucetius* var. *caesius*. It is a notable inducer of renal injury in rodents, which mirrors the highlights in human CKD. Adriamycin isn't fundamentally used and is collected mostly in the kidney causing nephrotoxicity. The ideal portion of Adriamycin which may demonstrate nephrotoxicity relies upon species, strain, sexual orientation, age, source and bunch of the exploratory creatures. The ideal course of administration in a large portion of the examinations is intravenous utilizing the tail vein. Not withstanding, skin putrefaction in case of tissue extravazation is a fundamental entanglement related to tail vein infusion. Substernal intracardiac approach, intrarenal course, direct infusion of the renal vein and intraperitoneal organization are different courses of organization. Despite the fact that intraperitoneal organization is a simple technique to manage the medication, because of variable assimilation through the peritoneal layer and irregularity in acceptance of renal injury contrasted and the intravenous course makes this strategy less ideal. Male rodents are more helpless than female rodents to Adriamycin prompted nephropathy. Adriamycin actuated nephropathy model is an exceptionally reproducible model of renal injury with adequate mortality and dismalness.

Diabetic Nephropathy

Diabetic nephropathy is a significant reason for human CKD. A few mouse models have been created to summarise the pathogenesis of diabetic nephropathy. The pancreatic β-cell poison streptozotocin (STZ) is regularly used to display Type 1 diabetes to foster nephropathy in trial models. Primary similitude among glucose and STZ brings about transportation of STZ into pancreatic β-cells, with ensuing obliteration prompting hyperglycaemia. Mice are infused with a higher portion of STZ on sequential days because of their protection from STZ than in rodents. Further, Akita mice are utilized to foster type 1 diabetes mellitus. An unconstrained point change in the Akita mice prompts misfolding of insulin, coming about in pancreatic β-cell disappointment. This may bring about supported hyperglycaemia with significant degrees of albuminuria and nephropathy related renal histopathological changes.

Other Models of Chronic Nephrotoxicity

Poisons, heavy metals and natural medications are accounted for as possible reasons for CKD in people. Backing for the above discoveries came as few animals considered were incited by nephrotoxic renal illness. Folic corrosive and aristolochic corrosive nephropathy are two such models which cause intense kidney injury which will arrive at interstitial fibrosis. Intraperitoneal administration of nutrient folic corrosive during a high measurement (250ug/g BW) might be a typical strategy for prompting inconsistent interstitial fibrosis inside the persistent stage (28–42 days). Intraperitoneal infusion of aristolochic corrosive week after week has prompted reformist fibrosis and renal disappointment seriously in male mice inside the investigations, including this model. The outcomes were practically similar to the discoveries in adenine initiated models. Future utilization of cyclosporine A can prompt renal fibrosis in humans. On the side of this hypothesis, a rodent model has been created by controlling cyclosporin A (7.5 mg/kg/day and 15 mg/kg/day s.c.) for multi day time frame inside the examinations including CKD.

Cisplatin (cDDP; cisdiamminedichloroplatinum II) is another powerful antitumor specialist utilized in the treatment of strong tumors. Nephritic impedance is the principal genuine antagonistic outcome revealed in patients treated with cisplatin. These discoveries have intersection rectifier to the occasion of cisplatin inspired harmful models for the trials on CKD. The salt eating routine evoked model is another solid decision. Dislike in oral purine organization, salt is immediately ingested by mice. Further, the proportion of urinary salt discharge is useful in exact watching of dietary admission. A brief period of time (one to three weeks) for the enlistment of cutting edge CKD might be an additional benefit of this model.

Radiation Nephropathy

Animal models with nephropathy could be produced by therapeutic irradiation. Nonetheless, the chance of instigating illness is less (20%) contrasted with different techniques for acceptance. Intense endothelial wounds, persistent reformist optional sclerosis with corresponding tubulointerstitial fibrosis are the trademark highlights of radiation nephropathy.

MODEL FOR ASSESSING THE NEPHROPROTECTIVE ACTIVITY

Adesia [3] has given details of methods for assessing the nephrotoxicity, which are given below.

Biochemical Parameters

The nephroprotective action can be evaluated utilizing different biochemical parameters like ALT, AST, ALP, total protein, serum bilirubin, and serum antioxidant enzymes alongside histopathological investigations of kidney tissue which are given underneath.

Experimental Animals

Male or female Wistar rats, weighing somewhere in the range of 150 and 200 g are to be utilized for the nephroprotective action. The rats are housed in polypropylene confines and kept up at 24 ± 2 °C under 12 h light/dull cycle and took care of not indispensable with standard pellet diet and ought to have free admittance to water. They are at first accustomed for the investigation convention and study convention is to be supported by the Institutional Ethical Committee according to the necessities of the Committee for the Purpose of Control and Supervision of Experiments on Animals (CPCSEA), India or according to the Organisation for Economic Co-operation and Development (OECD/OCDE) or NIH guidelines. Prior to directing the trial, ethical clearance must be gotten from the Institutional Animal Ethical Committee of the Institution where the work is being completed.

Acute Oral Toxicity Studies

Wistar male albino rats 150–200 g are kept up under standard husbandry conditions, and are utilized for all arrangements of trials. The acute oral toxicity study is to be completed according to the OECD rules, got draft rules 423, got from CPCSEA, Ministry of Social Justice and Empowerment, Government of India. Animals are permitted to take standard research center feed and faucet water.

Evaluation of Nephroprotective Activity by Animal Model

In the Paracetamol-initiated kidney injury model, Paracetamol (2 g/kg) suspension utilized 0.1% Tween 80, is regulated to all animals with the exception of cotrol group. Cystone (100 mg/kg p.o.) is utilized as a norm. The animals are isolated into six gatherings of six each. Group 1, which filled in as should be expected control getting 1.5% Tween 80. Gathering/group 2 got paracetamol (2 g/kg, p.o.) single portion on sixth day. Gathering 3 got synthetic (2 g/kg, p.o.) single portion and cystone (100 mg/kg, p.o.) all the while for 7 days. Gathering 4, 5, and 6 got substance (2 g/kg, p.o.) various dosages and plant separate (100, 200, 300mg/kg, p.o.) all the while for 7 days. On the seventh day of the beginning of separate treatment, the rodents are anesthetized by light ether sedation and the blood is removed from retro orbital plexus. It is permitted to coagulate for 30 min and serum is isolated by centrifugation at 2500 rpm. The serum is utilized to appraise serum glutamate pyruvate transaminase, serum glutamate oxaloacetate transaminase, and ALP.

Assortment of Blood Tests and Planning of Post-Mitochondrial and Microsomal Parts of Kidney Samples

Prior to the end of the investigations, rodent feed is removed to quick the rodents and their sheets changed. Be that as it may, drinking water is given not indispensable. Rodents are forfeited by cervical disengagement. Blood tests are gathered via cardiovascular cut into heparinized cylinders and kidneys promptly eliminated, washed in super cold 1.15% KCl, smudged, and gauged. The kidneys are then minced with scissors in 3 volumes of super cold 100 mM potassium phosphate cradle, pH 7.4 and homogenized in a Teflon homogenizer. The homogenates are later centrifuged at 12,500 g for 15 minutes at 4°C and the supernatants termed the postmitochondrial fractions (PMF) is taken and recentrifuged at 100,000g for 1hr using the L5-50B ultracentrifuge Beckman to get the microsomal pellets which are resuspended in 0.25M sucrose solution. Aliquots of this suspension are stored at -20°C and thawed before use.

RENAL FUNCTION TESTS

Plasma Creatinine Estimation

Creatinine responds with basic picric acid to the structure a red tautomer of creatinine picrate. Absorbance is corresponding to concentration of creatinine [4]. 3.5 mL of picric acid in a test tube is added 0.5 mL of plasma test. The blend is centrifuged for 5 minutes. To 3 mL of the supernatant is added 0.2 mL of 4N NaOH. This response blend is hatched for 10 minutes and the absorbance is then perused at 520 nm and the creatinine concentration decided.

Blood Urea Nitrogen Estimation

Measurement of plasma urea is by the technique for Weatherburn [5] utilizing diagnostic Randox Kit. The standard of this response depends on the condensation of diacetyl with urea to frame the chromogen, diazine. Since diacetyl is unsteady, it is normally produced in the response framework from diacetyl monoxime. The response of diacetyl and urea gives diazine which absorbs firmly at 540 nm. Thiosemicarbazide and Fe (III) are added to the framework to upgrade and settle the shading. Test in copy, (0.1 mL) is added into a widespread container containing 19.9 ml of distilled water and the combination is shaken quite well. Aliquot of the combination is moved into a test tube and to it is added 1 mL of shading reagent followed by 1 mL of acid reagent. The blend is warmed in bubbling water shower for 20 minutes. It is then cooled and the absorbance read at 520 nm against blank. The concentration of urea in mg/100 mL is then calculated from a calibration curve.

Determination of Catalase Activity

Catalase activity is measured by the technique for Sinha [6]. This strategy depends on the way that dichromate in acetic acid is reduced to chromic acetic acid derivation when warmed within the sight of H_2O_2, with the development of perchromic acid as an unsteady transitional. The chromic acetic acid derivation at that point created is estimated colorimetrically at 570-610 nm. The catalase arrangement is permitted to part H_2O_2 for various periods. The response is halted at a specific time by the expansion of dichromate/acidic corrosive blend and the leftover H_2O_2 is controlled by estimating chromic acetic acid derivation colorimetrically subsequent to warming the response combination.

Colorimetric determination of H_2O_2*:* Various volumes of H_2O_2, going from 10 to 100 mmoles are taken in little test tubes and 2 mL of dichromate/acetic acid is added to each. The expansion of the reagent momentarily delivered a flimsy blue accelerates of perchromic acid. Resulting warming for 10 minutes in a bubbling water shower changed the shade of the answer for stable green because of the development of chromic acetic acid derivation. Subsequent to cooling at room temperature, the volume of the response blend is made to 3 mL and the optical density estimated with a spectrophotometer at 570 nm. The concentrations of the standard Vs absorbance were plotted.

Determination of catalase activity of samples: 1 mL of the test sample is mixed with 49 mL of distilled H_2O_2 to produce 1 in 50 dilutions of the sample. The test combination contained 4 mL of H_2O_2 (800 µmoles) and 5 mL of phosphate buffer in a 10 mL flat bottom flask. Mix rapidly, diluted enzyme preparation (1 mL) with the reaction mixture by a twirling movement. The response is had at room temperature. A 1 mL segment of the response combination is removed into 2 mL dichromate/acetic acid reagent at 60 seconds spans. The hydrogen peroxide substance of the removed sample is measured by the technique depicted previously.

Determination of Superoxide Dismutase (SOD) Activity

Superoxide dismutase activity is determined by the method of Misra and Fridovich [7]. This technique is based on the inhibition by superoxide dismutase, of the spontaneous autoxidation of adrenaline to adrenochrome at pH of 10.2 [8]. The reaction is performed at 30°C in 1 mL of 50 nM sodium carbonate buffer, pH of 10.2 having 0.3 mm adrenaline and 0.1 mm EDTA. The amount of enzyme required to block the change in absorbance at 480nm by 50%. 1 mL of sample diluted in 9 mL of distilled water to produce a 1 in 10 dilution is known as one unit of activity. 0.2 mL of the diluted sample is mixed with a 2.5 mL of 0.05M carbonate buffer at a pH of 10.2 to equilibrate in the spectrophotometer and the reaction initiated by the adding a freshly prepared 0.3 mL adrenaline to the mixture which is quickly mixed by inversion. Blank having 0.3 mL of adrenaline substrate, and 0.2 mL of distilled water. The increment in absorbance at 480 nm is checked at regular intervals for 150 seconds.

Determination of Reduced Glutathione Level

The technique for Beutler *et al.* [9] can be adopted in determining the degree of diminished glutathione (GSH). The diminished type of glutathione involves in many occasions the heft of cell non-protein sulfhydryl groups. This technique is hence founded on the advancement of a generally steady (yellow) shading when 5', 5'-dithiobis - (2-nitrobenzoic corrosive) (Ellman's reagent) is added to sulfhydryl compounds. The chromophoric item coming about because of the response of Ellman's reagent with the diminished glutathione, 2 – nitro---thiobenzoic corrosive has a molar assimilation at 412 nm. 0.2 mL of test is added to 1.8 mL of distilled water and 3 mL of the precipitating solution is blended in with test. The combination is then permitted to represent around 5 minutes and afterward separated. Toward the finish of the fifth moment, 1 ml of filtrate is added to 4 mL of 0.1M phosphate support. At long last 0.5 mL of the Ellman's reagent is added. A clear is set up with 4 mL of the 0.1M phosphate support, 1 mL of diluted precipitating solution (3 sections to 2 pieces of refined water) and 0.5 mL of the Ellman's reagent. The optical density is estimated at 412 nm. GSH fixation is relative to the absorbance at that frequency and the gauge is acquired from the GSH standard.

Estimation of Glutathione-S-Transferase Activity

The estimation can be done by the method proposed by Habig *et al.* [10]. The rule depends on the way that all known glutathione-S-transferase exhibit a generally high action with 1-chloro-2, 4,- dinitrobenzene as the subsequent substrate, thusly, the customary measure for glutathione-S-transferase activity uses 1-chloro-2, 4,-dinitrobenzene as a substrate. At the point when this substance is formed with diminished glutathione, its ingestion greatest movements to a more extended frequency. The ingestion increments at the new frequency of 340nm give an immediate estimation of the enzymatic response. The mechanism for the assessment is arranged and the response is permitted to run for 1 moment each time before the absorbance is perused against the blank at 340 nm. The absorbance is estimated utilizing UNICAM Spectrophotometer.

Determination of Lipid Peroxidation

As per the method of Varshney and Kale [11], lipid peroxidation is dictated by estimating the arrangement of thiobarbituric acid reactive substances (TBARS). Under acidic condition, malondialdehyde (MDA) created from the peroxidation of unsaturated fat films and food items respond with the chromogenic reagent, 2-thiobarbituric corrosive to yield a pink shaded complex with most extreme absorbance at 532 nm. The pink chromophore is promptly extractable into natural solvents like butanol. 0.4 mL of the kidney PMF is blended in with 1.6 mL of Tris-KCl buffer to which 0.5 mL of 30% TCA is added. At that point 0.5 mL of 0.75% TBA is added and put in a water bath for 45 minutes at 80°C. This is then cooled in ice and centrifuged at 3000. The clear supernatant is gathered and absorbance estimated against a reference at 532 nm. The MDA level is determined by the strategy for Adam-Vizi and Seregi [12]. Lipid peroxidation in units/mg protein or gram tissue is processed with a molar extinction coefficient of 1.56×105 M^{-1}cm^{-1}.

Determination of Renal Glucose-6-Phosphatase Activity

This is completed by the strategy for Swanson [13]. Glucose-6-phosphatase, a multifunctional enzyme goes about as a phosphohydrolase and phosphotransferase. The response includes the development of covalently bound compound inorganic phosphate (Pi) moderate, which responds with an assortment of Pi acceptors like water (Phosphohydrolase capacity) and glucose (Phosphotransferase work). The inorganic phosphate freed is complexed with ammonium molybdate, which is reduced by iron sulfate to give a blue shaded item. The inorganic phosphate delivered is estimated colorimetrically at 700 nm. The mixture which comprised of 0.15 mL, 0.04 M glucose-6-phosphate, 0.2 mL of 1.0 M sodium acetate at a pH of 5.8, 0.15 mL of test and 0.5 mL of distilled water (last volume 1.0 mL) is incubated for 30 minutes at 37°C. The response is ended by adding 0.5 mL of TCA. Protein accelerate is eliminated by centrifugation. 0.5 mL of supernatant is added to 5.0 mL of ammonium molybdate, at that point 0.2 mL of sodium acetic acid derivation and 0.8 mL of ferrous sulfate arrangement. The optical density is estimated at 700 nm in the wake of shaking. Substrate is added to the blank after stopping the reaction and product to the standard after stopping the reaction.

IN VITRO NEPHROPROTECTIVE ACTIVITY

Epiflourescence Staining

Dual-staining procedure is used with epifluorescence microscopy which allows the detection of live cells and dead cells. In this method, 10 mL of phosphate buffered saline (PBS) suspended with normal kidney cells (vero cells) and 50 µL of the selected plant extracts were incubated with 200 µL of the suspension at the concentration of 500 mg/mL. Another 200 µL of the suspension is incubated with gentamicin followed by the addition of vitamin E, which is used as a positive control. To the above suspensions 50 µL of ethidium bromide and 50 µL of acridine orange are added and is incubated for 1 hr. After the incubation the cells are viewed under epiflourescence microscope, in which the live cells emit green color and dead cells emit red color [14].

Cytoprotective Assay

Cytoprotective test is the test utilized to asses cell feasibility utilizing 3-(4,--dimethythiazol-2-yl)- 2,5-diphenyl tetrazolium bromide (MTT), which colorimetrically estimates the decrease of yellow MTT by mitochondrial succinate dehydrogenase. The MTT enters the cells and passes into the mitochondria where it is diminished to an insoluble, shaded (dull purple) formazan item. The harmfulness to the cells is brought about by hatching of cells with gentamicin. The cells are then solubilized with a natural dissolvable (for example isopropanol), and the delivered, solubilized formazan reagent is estimated spectrophotometrically. Plate vero cells of 0.1×10^6 of every 100 µL PBS are put in 96 wells (level base). The cells are then hatched with 50 µL of MTT arrangement in the grouping of 1 mg/mL for 48 hr at 37°C. 150 µL of dimethyl sulfoxide (DMSO) is added to the formazon item created by the viable cells. The absorbance at 630 nm is estimated utilizing microplate spectrophotometer (Bio-Tek Instruments, USA) [14].

Docking Studies

The *in vitro* nephroprotective screening docking analysis against nephrotoxic proteins are carried out using the molecules identified from test sample using liquid chromatography mass spectrometry/mass spectrometry analysis. The marker compounds of sample are used in molecular docking studies. These inhibitors are employed in docking studies and for subsequent docking simulations. This is to understand the mechanism behind [14].

SCREENING MODELS OF MEDICINAL PLANTS FOR TREATING UROLITHIASIS

Urolithiasis is normally alluded as stone deposition in any place of the urinary tract like kidneys, ureters, urinary bladder and urethra. Diverse *in vitro* and *in vivo* models are utilized for deciding different system profiles of testing concentrate or mixtures against various pathophysiological conditions and furthermore for urolithiasis. Santhoshi *et al.* [15] have given a detailed account on screening models of medicinal plants for treating urolithiasis.

Preclinical Animal Models of Urolithiasis

Ethylene Glycol Induced Urolithiasis in Rats

Ethylene glycol ($C_2H_6O_2$) chemically ethan-di-ol accepted as a solvent and antifreeze agent in automobile [16]. $C_2H_6O_2$ is rapidly absorbed and metabolized in liver to glycolic acid via alcohol dehydrogenase and aldehyde dehydrogenase. This is oxidized to glyoxylic acid and then to oxalic oxalate by glycolate oxidase, in this way causing hyperoxaluria and it is the significant danger factor for urolithiasis. In rats, urolithiasis can be induced at a dose of 0.75% v/v po for 28 days through drinking water.

Healthy male wistar rats weighing in the range of 120-200g are suitable for the study. Animals are divided into four groups each containing six animals. Group-I is a control and vehicle is given for 28 days, whereas Group II-IV as positive control, standard and test groups and are given ethylene glycol as per the dose mentioned in the above for 28 days. Group –III & IV are given cystone at a dose of 750 mg/kg, p.o acts as a standard and test drug respectively for the same 28 days. On the last day i.e., on 28th, urine and serum of the all groups are collected evaluated and compared [17].

Diet Induced Model

In this model, an adjusted lithogenic diet comprises of 30% lactose having 3.68% sucrose, 30% lactose, 10% fat, 23.4% protein, 5.3% fiber, 6.9% minerals like Ca, and P; Mg, vit D 4.5 IU/g vit A 22 IU/g, vit. E 49 IU/g. and 1% ethylene glycol is used for induction of urolithiasis.

Healthy male wistar rats weighing in the range of 120-200g are suitable for the study. Animal are divided into four groups each containing six animals. Gathering I filled in as control and taken care of with ordinary lab diet. Gathering II, III, IV filled in as unhealthy control, standard and test separately and they are given adjusted lithogenic diet for 28 days. Simultaneously group III and IV are given standard drug and test drug respectively from day 1 to day 28 as preventive regimen. Various biological samples are gathered, estimated and analysed [18].

By Sodium Oxalate

This is an acute model used to study the urolithiasis activity causing hyper-oxaluria at a dose of 70 mg/kg bw given i.p. for a period of 1 week.

Healthy male Wistar rats weighing in the range of 120-200g are suitable for the study. Animals are divided into four groups each containing six animals. Group I as control, Group II-IV serves as positive control, standard and test groups respectively and given with sodium oxalate for 7 days, Group III, IV group are given cystone 750 mg/kg, p.o as standard drug and test drug respectively. Blood samples are withdrawn from all the groups and compared to obtain results [19].

By Zinc Disc Implantation

Male Wistar rats weighing in the range of 200-250 g are used to study the zinc disc implantation induced urinary bladder calculi model. Sodium pentobarbitone at a dose of 40 mg/ kg bw, i.p is used for producing anaesthesia in rats.

A suprapubic cut is made and urinary bladder is uncovered. A little cut is made at the highest point of the bladder and a formerly weighed sterile zinc circle of 2 to 48 mg/kg is embedded into the bladder and the cut is shut with a solitary stitch utilizing absorbable catgut. The midsection is shut in layers and this is performed for each rodent and every one of the rodents is recuperated for multi week. Toward the finish of 28 days treatment every one of the rats are estimated for its various parameters and then compared [20].

Xenoplantation Model

Stone particles from male patient with renal stones are extricated by percutaneous lithotomy. The chose stone is cut with a heavy-handed contrivance into areas with a width of 2-3 mm, gauged and kept up in a sterile climate, before use.

Multi week old male rats weighing around 250-300 g are chosen and randomized into 3 gatherings like control, standard and test. Sodium pentobarbital at a dose of 50 mg/kg bw is used for induction of anaesthesia in rats and the bladder is uncovered by a suprapubic entry point. Following this, a 4-5 mm entry point is made at the highest point of bladder and one arranged stone molecule is embedded in each rodent and afterward the bladder and the suprapubic cut is shut individually. Ethylene glycol is provided in drinking water at a last grouping of 1% from the subsequent (day 1) postoperatively for about a month. Following a month, kidney and urinary bladder are analyzed and the kidneys are got dried out in an evaluated ethanol arrangement and installed in paraffin. Renal stones arrangement was surveyed by von Kossa histochemical staining. Bladder stones are collected, gauged and kept up in 75% ethanol for 24 hrs, preceding the stones being implanted in auto-polymerizing pitch and separated dynamically with diamond wire found to choose the best area sheet. Separated squares are then fixed on a glass slide with thermoplastic paste and cleaned progressively utilizing a 1, 200 coarseness sandpaper and a blend of alumina cleaning compounds (3, 1 and 0.3 μm) with a little volume of water, until it was feasible to notice the center obviously under a transmitted light microscope [21].

Chemical (TPA/DMT) Induced Urolithiasis in Weaned Rats

Calculi is instigated in the urinary lot of weanling Fischer rodents (post pregnancy day 28) in under about fourteen days by openness to terephthalic acids (TPA) at 3-5% in the eating regimen or dimethylterephthalate (DMT) at 1-3% of diet. Indicated rodents of 24 are haphazardly partitioned into 4 groups gatherings, each gathering containing 6 rodents each. Gathering – I, II, III, and IV goes about as control got vehicle, disease control (positive control) got TP)/DMT for about fourteen days, standard got TPA/DMT and cystone at 750 mg/kg bw p.o and the last gathering i.e IV fills in as test got TPA/DMT in addition to test drug. After the treatment time frame different blood examples are gathered and the parameters are estimated and looked at [22].

Urinary Calculi by Sulfamonomethoxine in Pigs

Five 45-60 kg Yorkshine-Durox cross-reproduced pigs within a farrow-to-finish herd with commercial crossbred are used in the study. The pigs were fed on a regimen of sulfamonomethoxine at 50 mg/kg bw po twice a day. The affected pig's clinical history included streptococcal disease and toxoplasmosis, which are analyzed in the third week, diagnosed with toxoplasmosis and then infused with sulfamonomethoxine at 50 mg/kg bw [23].

Mild Tubular Damage in Hyperoxaluric Rodents Initiates Renal Lithogenesis

It is a two stage or two hit model of lithogenesis used to evaluate the anti-urolithiatic activity. In the initial step it is utilized to initiate crystalluria which is essential advance however not adequate to actuate urolithiasis. In the second step it causes tubular damage that incites lithiasis [24].

IN-VITRO MODELS

In Vitro Crystallization

It is the time course estimation of turbidity changes because of the crystallization in artificial urine on expansion of 0.01M sodium oxalate. The precipitation of calcium oxalate at 37°C and pH 6.8 has been concentrated by the estimation of turbidity at 620 nm utilizing UV/Visible spectrophotometer. Artificial urine: sodium chloride 105.5 mmol/l, potassium chloride 63.7 mmol/1, sodium phosphate 32.3 mmol/1, ammonium hydroxide 17.9 mmol/1, sodium sulfate 16.95 mmol/1, calcium chloride 4.5 mmol/1, magnesium sulfate 3.85 mmol/1, sodium citrate 3.21 mmol/l, sodium oxalate 0.32 mmol/1, and ammonium chloride 0.0028mmol/1. The artificial urine was arranged fresh each time and pH was set at 6.0.

Method: Four test tubes are taken and moved artificial urine of 1 ml into each test tube and marked as control (1), negative control (2), standard (3) and test (4).Test tube 1 and 2 are added with 0.5 ml of distilled water, aside from test tube (1) all the test tubes are added with 0.5 ml of 0.05 M sodium oxalate and 3 and 4 test tubes are added with standard and test drug separately. Test tubes are left to represent 10 minutes. Following 10 minutes, the absorbance was estimated in UV-Spectrophotometer at 620 nm and thought about. Microscopy of urine should likewise be possible utilizing a light microscope instrument with an objective of 40 X and an eye piece of 10 X [25].

Nucleation Assay

At pH 6.5, 3 mmol/l calcium chloride solution and 0.5 mol/l sodium oxalate solution are prepared in a buffer having Tris 0.05 mol/l and NaCl 0.15 mol/l. The two solutions are separated through a 0.22 μm channel; 33 ml of calcium chloride solution is blended in with 3.3 ml of the test at various concentrations. Crystallization is begun by adding 33 ml of sodium oxalate. The final mixture is blended at 800 rpm utilizing a PTFE-covered mixing bar. The temperature is kept up at 37°C. The absorbance is observed at 620 nm after each 1 min. The rate hindrance created by test is determined as [1-(Tsi/TSC)]x100, Where Tsc is the turbidity incline within the sight of the inhibitor [26].

Growth Assay

Inhibitory movement against CaOx stone development is estimated utilizing the seeded, solution depletion assay a test arrangement of 10 mM Tris-HCl having 90 mM NaCl is acclimated to pH 7.2 with 4N HCl in 1.5 mg/ml. At pH 5.7, stone slurry is set up in 50 mM sodium acetate buffer. CaOx monohydrate gem seed is added to an answer containing 1 mM $CaCl_2$ and 1 mM $Na_2C_2O_4$. The response of $CaCl_2$ and $Na_2C_2O_4$ with stone seed prompted the statement of CaOx (CaC_2O_4) on the gem surfaces, consequently diminishing free oxalate that is noticeable by Spectrophotometer at λ214 nm. At the point when test is added into this solution, consumption of free oxalate particles will diminish if the test represses CaOx gem development. Pace of decrease of free oxalate is determined utilizing the standard worth and the worth following 30-second brooding with or without test. The overall inhibitory action is determined as follows: % Relative inhibitory action =[(C-S)/C]x100, where C is the rate of reduction of free oxalate with no test and S is the rate of reduction of free oxalate with a test [26].

Calcium Phosphate Assay

Assay of Calcium phosphate (CaP) is studied on *in vitro* homogeneous mixture of beginning mineral stage development for CaP, its resulting development and demineralization by utilizing 5.0 ml sample which is set up by adding 0.5 ml of 50 mM $KH_2 PO_4$, 0.5 of 50 mM $CaCl_2$, 2.5 ml of Tris support prepared by mixing 210 mM NaCl and 0.1 mM tris HCl and expanding volume of test going from 0.2 ml to 1.5 ml by in this way diminishing the volume of water going from 1.5 ml to 0.0 ml. This mixture is centrifuged at 4500 rpm and precipitate so acquired are disintegrated in 5 ml of 0.1 N HCl. This 5 ml sample for mineralization. For the development, in the beginning, 5 ml samples are arranged utilizing standard conventions; of course 5 ml are re-developed on similar cylinders with the augmentations of expanding volumes of the test. Calcium and phosphate are then assessed on the accelerates acquired and broke down in 0.1 N HCl. In the event of control, no test is added. Test (T) checks the demineralization, again 5 ml framework is arranged having no test added to that and precipitate are acquired. To these precipitates, 2.5 ml of Tris and expanded volumes of test going from 0.2

ml to 1.5 ml with in this way diminished volume of water is added and afterward centrifuged at 4500 rpm for 15 min. Calcium and phosphate are then assessed in supernatant got after centrifugation. The Ca^{2+} and HPO_4^{2-} particles are assessed by the strategies separately. Rate hindrance of mineral stage within the sight of test is determined as % inhibition= $((C-T)/C)x100$, where T is the convergence of Ca^{2+} or HPO_4^{2-} particle of the hastens framed in test having test going from 0.2 ml to 1.5 ml in the test frameworks and C is the grouping of Ca^{2+} or HPO_4^{2-} particle of the precipitate shaped in charge frameworks which had refined water (Millipore) and no test [26].

Calcium Oxalate Crystal Assay

Inhibitory movement of test is likewise kept an eye on calcium oxalate stone development. A 4 ml sample is set up to check the impact of the test in repressing development of calcium oxalate stones. In this framework, 1 ml of 4 mM calcium chloride and 4 mM sodium oxalate are added to a 1.5 ml solution containing 90 Mm NaCl buffered with 10 mM Tris HCl at pH of 7.2. To this 30 μl of calcium oxalate monohydrate stone slurry is added. Utilization of oxalate starts following calcium oxalate monohydrate slurry option and is checked for 600 sec by vanishing of absorbance at 214 nm. At the point when test is added into this arrangement, consumption of free oxalate particles will diminish if test hinders calcium oxalate gem development. Rate of reduction of free oxalate is determined utilizing the gauge esteem and the worth after 30 sec hatching with or without the test. The overall inhibitory action is determined $=((CS)/C)x100$, where C is the rate of decrease of free oxalate with no test and S is the pace of decrease of free oxalate with a test [26].

Lactate Dehydrogenase Leakage Assay

The 6.6 mM Nicotinamide adenine dinucleotide NADH and 30 mM sodium pyruvate are set up in 0.2M Tris at pH of 7.3 and response is started with the expansion of 50 μl of the test and the vanishing of NADH is checked at 340 nm, for 5 min at a time frame min. The % Lactate dehydrogenase LDH discharge is determined by isolating the action of LDH in the supernatant by the LDH movement estimated after complete cell lysis accomplished by sonication [26].

CONCLUSION

The renal framework pathologies have a wide scope of clinical introductions. The consideration of researchers has been attracted to the utilization of medicinal plants for the treatment or the board of different renal framework issues, including kidney stones. Various screening techniques for *in vivo* animal models, *in vitro* research facility tests, are accessible to assess the nephroprotection. Renal function tests like Plasma creatinine assessment, BUN assessment, determination of catalase activity, SOD activity, reduced glutathione level, glutathione--transferase activity, lipid peroxidation, renal glucose-6-phosphatase activity beneficial for estimation of elements of the renal framework.

REFERENCES

[1]   Amarasiri SS, Attanayake AP, Jayatilaka KA, Mudduwa LK. Animal models of chronic kidney disease: Screening tool to investigate nephroprotective effects of natural products. Intern J Pharmaceut Chem & Analysis 2018; 5(2): 52-8.

[2]   Claramunt D, Gil-Peña H, Fuente R, *et al.* Chronic kidney disease induced by adenine: a suitable model of growth retardation in uremia. Am J Physiol Renal Physiol 2015; 309(1): F57-62.
        [http://dx.doi.org/10.1152/ajprenal.00051.2015] [PMID: 25972508]

[3]   Adesia A. Protective effects of ethanolic extract of *Psidium guajava* on Adriamycin-induced nephrotoxicity and genototoxicity in rats. PhD thesis, University of Ibadan, Nigeria 2013.

[4]   Henry RJ. Clinical chemistry: Principles and tecniques. 2nd ed., Harper and Row 1974.

[5]   Weatherburn MW. Urease-Berthelot method colorimetric manual. Anal Chem 1967; 39: 971.
        [http://dx.doi.org/10.1021/ac60252a045]

[6]   Sinha AK. Colorimetric assay of catalase. Anal Biochem 1972; 47(2): 389-94.
        [http://dx.doi.org/10.1016/0003-2697(72)90132-7] [PMID: 4556490]

[7]   Misra HP, Fridovich I. The univalent reduction of oxygen by reduced flavins and quinones. J Biol Chem 1972; 247(1): 188-92.
        [http://dx.doi.org/10.1016/S0021-9258(19)45773-6] [PMID: 4401581]

[8]   Valerino DM, McCormack JJ. Xanthine oxidase-mediated oxidation of epinephrine. Biochem Pharmacol 1971; 20(1): 47-55.
        [http://dx.doi.org/10.1016/0006-2952(71)90470-9] [PMID: 5570640]

[9]   Beutler E, Duron O, Kelly BM. Improved method for the determination of blood glutathione. J Lab Clin Med 1963; 61: 882-8.
        [PMID: 13967893]

[10]   Habig WH, Pabst MJ, Jakoby WB. Glutathione S-transferases. The first enzymatic step in mercapturic acid formation. J Biol Chem 1974; 249(22): 7130-9.
        [http://dx.doi.org/10.1016/S0021-9258(19)42083-8] [PMID: 4436300]

[11]   Varshney R, Kale RK. Effects of calmodulin antagonists on radiation-induced lipid peroxidation in microsomes. Int J Radiat Biol 1990; 58(5): 733-43.
        [http://dx.doi.org/10.1080/09553009014552121] [PMID: 1977818]

[12]   Adám-Vizi V, Seregi A. Receptor independent stimulatory effect of noradrenaline on Na,K-ATPase in rat brain homogenate. Role of lipid peroxidation. Biochem Pharmacol 1982; 31(13): 2231-6.
        [http://dx.doi.org/10.1016/0006-2952(82)90106-X] [PMID: 6127081]

[13]   Swanson MA. Phosphatases of liver. I. Glucose-6-phosphatase. J Biol Chem 1950; 184(2): 647-59.
        [http://dx.doi.org/10.1016/S0021-9258(19)50999-1] [PMID: 15428449]

[14]   Kiruba, Arun KP, Brindha P. *In vitro* studies on nephroprotective efficacy of *Cynodon dactylon* and *Gmelina asiatica.* Asian J Pharm Clin Res 2014; 7(4): 111-20.

[15]   Santhoshi B, Chidrawar VR, Uma Maheshwara Rao V. A brief review on the potential medicinal plants and screening models of urolithiasis. Int J Appl Biol Pharm Technol 2015; 6(1): 37-45.

[16] Saha S. R.J. Verma RJ. Efficacy of *Dolichos biflorus* in the management of nephrotoxicity. Asian Pac J Trop Biomed 2012; 2(3): S1471-6.
[http://dx.doi.org/10.1016/S2221-1691(12)60440-7]

[17] Shah BN, Raiyani KD, Modi DC. Antiurolithiatic activity studies of *Momordica charantia* Linn. fruits. Int J Pharm Res Tech 2011; 1(1): 6-11.

[18] Vidhya G, Sumithra G, Anandhan R, Anand G. Antiurolithiatic activity of *Nardostachys jatamansi* DC on modified lithogenic diet induced urolithiasis in rats. Int J Adv Pharma Gen Res 2013; 1(2): 52-63.

[19] Ramesh C, Kumar D, Einstein J. Saleem, Girish. Antiurolithiatic activity of woodbark of *Cassia fistula* in rats. J Pharm Biomed Sci 2010; 2: 12.

[20] Ahmad A, Garg R, Sharma S. Evaluation on antiurolithiatic activity of *Bryophyllum pinnatum* of rats. Int J Pharm Sci Health Care 2013; 6(3): 1-33.

[21] Wang S, Xu Q, Huang X, Lin J, Wang J, Wang X. Use of a calcium tracer to detect stone increments in a rat calcium oxalate xenoplantation model. Exp Ther Med 2013; 6(4): 957-60.
[http://dx.doi.org/10.3892/etm.2013.1233] [PMID: 24137297]

[22] Wolkowski-Tyl R, Chin TY, Popp JA, Heck HD. Chemically induced urolithiasis in weanling rats. Am J Pathol 1982; 107(3): 419-21.
[PMID: 7081391]

[23] Wei-Dong S, Zhang KC, Wang JY, Wang X. Sulfamonomethoxine- induced urinary calculi in pigs. World Acad Sci Eng Technol 2009; 3: 9-29.

[24] Gambaro G, Valente ML, Zanetti E, *et al.* Mild tubular damage induces calcium oxalate crystalluria in a model of subtle hyperoxaluria: Evidence that a second hit is necessary for renal lithogenesis. J Am Soc Nephrol 2006; 17(8): 2213-9.
[http://dx.doi.org/10.1681/ASN.2005121282] [PMID: 16790510]

[25] Kumar GP, Arun M, Rishi K. Evaluation of *Tinosopora cordiofolia* for antiurolithiatic potential. J Pharm Biomed Sci 2011; 9: 14.

[26] Rathod N, Chitme HR, Chandra R. *in vivo* and *in vitro* models for evaluating anti-urolithiasis activity of herbal drugs. Intern J Pharmaceut Res Bio-Sci 2014; 3(5): 309-29.

CHAPTER 3

Medicinal Plants with Nephroprotective, Nephrocuratve and Antiurolithiatic Activitites

Abstract: Medicinal plants are important sources of drugs for the treatment of several ailments, including kidney disorders. In this chapter, published work on nephroprotective, nephrocurative and antiurolithiatic plants has been reviewed. Plants are listed species wise and species are arranged in alphabetical sequence. Under each species, the plant part, extract, solvent, method of assay, nephrotoxin and the results of the studies have been given.

Keywords: Antiurolithiatic, Kidney disorders, Kidney stones, Nephrocurative, Nephroprotective.

INTRODUCTION

Medicinal plants are important sources of drugs for the treatment of several ailments, including kidney disorders. Several reviews have been published on Nephroprotective activity of medicinal plants; these include Javaid *et al.* [1] Lakshmi *et al.* [2], Dhole *et al.* [3], Peesa [4], Ahmad *et al.* [5], Sundararajan *et al.* [6], Janakiram and Jayaprakash [7], Sabiu *et al.* [8], Rad *et al.* [9], Vaya *et al.* [10], Al-Snafi and Talab [11] and Das *et al.* [12]. Published work on medicinal plants with anti-urolithiactic effects has been reviewed by Prasad *et al.* [13], Butterweck and Khan [14], Pareta *et al.* [15], Yadav *et al.* [16], Joy *et al.* [17], Nagal and Singla [18], Aggarwal *et al.* [19], Rathod *et al.* [20], Al-Snafi [21, 22] and Kasote *et al.* [23]. Phytotherapy in the management of kidney disorders in Nigeria and South Africa was reviewed by Sabiu *et al.* [8]. Bioactive compounds from Unani medicinal plants and their application in urolithiasism were reviewed by Makbul *et al.* [24]. Zeng *et al.* [25] reviewed the protective roles of flavonoids and flavonoid-rich plant extracts against urolithiasis.

In the following pages, publications on medicinal plants with nephroprotective, nephrocurative and antiurolithiatic activities are reviewed. Plants are arranged species wise and species are arranged in alphabetical sequence. The reviews on each species are in chronological order.

Abelmoschus Moschatus Medik. Family: Malvaceae

Christina and Muthumani [26] evaluated the protective effect of the hydro-alcoholic extract of *Abelmoschus moschatus* against urolithiasis in male Wistar albino rats. Simultaneous administration of the extract of *A. moschatus* orally for 28 days along with ethylene glycol (0. 75%) increased urinary magnesium level and decreased the urinary calcium, oxalate, phosphate levels. It also increased the urinary volume thereby reducing the tendency for crystallization.

Some experienced people in Manado, Indonesia, reported that *A. moschatus* plants can be used to treat kidney stones. Djamhuri and Khildah [27] determined the activity and the effective dose of *A. moschatus* leaf extract as an inhibitor of kidney stone formation. Ethanol extract of *A. moschatus* leaves had an inhibitory activity of kidney stones formation in all dose variation and the most effective one was at a dose of 150 mg/kg BW.

Abutilon indicum (L.) Sweet Family: Malvaceae

Lakshmi *et al*. [28] evaluated the protective effect of ethanol extract of *Abutilon indicum* (EEAI) against cisplatin-induced nephrotoxicity in albino Wistar rats. There were significant differences in serum BUN and creatinine levels between the control group and cisplatin treated groups. The result suggested that EEAI at 200 and 400mg/kg administered 7 days before cisplatin treatment significantly prevented the increase of serum creatinine, BUN, uric acid, total proteins, total cholesterol, alkaline phosphatase, and albumin concentrations and markedly decreased cisplatin-induced renal damage as confirmed by biochemical assays and histopathological studies.

The effects of ethanolic extract of *A. indicum* (EEAI) on acetaminophen induced nephrotoxicity were investigated by Reddy *et al*. [29]. The EEAI was given orally concurrent with oral administration of acetaminophen treatment with EEAI prevented the acetaminophen - induced nephrotoxicity and oxidative impairments of the kidney, as evidenced by a significantly reduced level of serum creatinine, BUN, serum alkaline phosphatase, serum uric acid, serum total proteins and total cholesterol. The nephroprotective effects of EEAI were confirmed by a reduced intensity of renal cellular damage, as evidenced by histological findings. EEAI administered at 400 mg/kg was found to show greater protective effects than that at 200 mg/kg.

Shanmugapriya *et al*. [30] evaluated the anti nephrotoxic activities of the whole plants of *Abutilon indicum* and *Boerhavia diffusa*, their formulation and individual extracts in *in vivo* models against nephrotoxicity in rats, induced with GM. The effect of ethanolic extract of *Abutilon indicum* and *Boerhavia diffusa* formulation and individual extract at a dose level of 200 mg/kg was compared in GM-induced nephrotoxicity. Administration of ethanolic extract of formulation prevented severe alterations of biochemical parameters like urea, uric acid, creatinine, sodium, and potassium.

Jesurun and Lavakumar [31] investigated the protective effect of *A. indicum* root in GM induced nephrotoxicity in Wistar albino rats. Animals treated with extract showed significant improvement in biochemical parameters and histopathological changes compared to animals treated with GM. The protective effect was highly significant at the dose of 300 mg/kg of extract.

Gum Arabic - *Acaica* species – Family: Fabaceae

Arabic gum (AG), a complex polysaccharide, is mainly obtained from *Acacia senegal* and *Acacia seyal* trees. Al-Majed *et al.* [32] tested the nephroprotective effect of Arabic gum against GM-induced nephrotoxicity using a rat model. Treatment with AG protected the rats from GM-induced nephrotoxicity, as evident by the normalisation of biochemical parameters like urine volume, serum creatinine and urea. AG totally prevented the GM-induced rise in kidney tissue contents of MDA. Kidney histology of the tissue from GM-treated rats showed necrosis and desquamation of tubular epithelial cells in the renal cortex as well as interstitial nephritis, whereas it was very much comparable to control when AG was co-administered with GM.

Mahmoud *et al.* [33] evaluated the effects of *Zingiber officinale* Roscoe (Ginger), Arabic gum (AG), and *Boswellia* on both acute and chronic renal failure (CRF) and the mechanisms underlying their effects. Ginger and AG showed renoprotective effects in both models of renal failure. These protective effects may be attributed at least in part to their anti-inflammatory properties as evident by attenuating serum C-reactive protein levels and antioxidant effects as evident by attenuating lipid peroxidation marker, MDA levels, and increasing renal SOD activity.

Acalypha indica L. Family: Euphorbiaceae

Sathya and Kokilavani [34] evaluated the antilithiatic activity of *Acalypha indica* supplementation on ethylene glycol induced nephrolithiasis in male Wistar albino rats. Supplementation with ethanolic extract of *A. indica* (200mg/kg b.wt.dose-1 day-1oral-1) restored the levels of enzymatic and non-enzymatic antioxidants such as GST, glucose-6-phosphate dehydrogenase (G-6-PD), GR, SOD, CAT, GPx, GSH, vitamin C and vitamin E in liver and kidney and it brought back the values to near normal range in liver and kidney.

Achyranthus aspera L. Family: Amaranthaceae

The ethanolic extract of leaves of *Achyranthus aspera* was screened by Awari *et al*. [35] for antilithiatic activity in male albino Wistar rats. Supplementation with ethanolic extract of leaves of *A. aspera* significantly reduced the elevated urinary calcium and oxalate ion concentration in the urine, *i.e.*, calcium, oxalate, phosphate, confirming the stone inhibitory effect. Also, it elevated the urinary concentration of magnesium, which is considered as one of the inhibitors of crystallisation. The high urine creatinine level observed in ethylene glycol treated rats was also reduced following treatment with the extract. The histopathological findings also showed signs of improvement after treatment with the ethanolic extract.

Farook *et al*. [36] investigated the inhibition of mineralization of urinary stone-forming minerals by leaves, fruits and seeds of *A. aspera*. The study suggests that the fruit juice and seed extract is moderate to a good inhibitor of CaOx, calcium carbonate and calcium phosphate mineralization while leaves extracts are poor inhibitors.

Aggarwal *et al*. [37] investigated the inhibitory potency of *A. aspera* on nucleation and the growth of the CaOx crystals as well as on oxalate-induced cell injury of renal tubular epithelial (NRK 52E) cells *in vitro*. *A. aspera* extract exhibited concentration-dependent inhibition of the growth of CaOx crystals but a similar pattern of inhibition was not observed with an increase in the plant extract concentration for the nucleation assay. When NRK 52E cells were injured by exposure to oxalate, *A. aspera* extract prevented the injury in a dose-dependent manner. On treatment with the different concentrations of the plant, the cell viability increased and the LDH release decreased in a concentration-dependent manner.

Aggarwal *et al*. [38] evaluated the efficacy of *A. aspera* in preventing and reducing the growth of CaOx stones in ethylene glycol induced nephrolithiatic model. Upon administration of aqueous extract of *A. aspera* (500 and 1000 mg/kg body wt.), levels of renal injury markers (LDH and alkaline phosphatase) were normalized with a decrease in serum urea and serum creatinine. Concurrent treatment reduced changes in the architecture of renal tissue and also decreased the size of crystals, thereby helping in quick expulsion of the crystals.

Christi and Senthamarai [39] evaluated the antiurolithiatic activity of aqueous and alcoholic extract of leaves *A. aspera* using ethylene glycol induced hyperoxaluria model in rats. Extract exerted its antilithogenic property by decreasing the calcium and oxalate ion concentration or increasing magnesium and citrate excretion. The extract at a dose of 200mg/kg produced a significant reduction in

MDA and increased GSH and antioxidant enzymes likes SOD and CAT. Methanolic extract showed better results than aqueous extract.

Achyranthes indica L. Family: Amaranthaceaee

Pareta *et al.* [40] investigated the inhibitor effect of hydroalcoholic extract of *Achyranthes indica* on the crystallization of CaOx in synthetic urine. The addition of inhibitor with various concentrations (10%, 20%, and 40%) enabled authors to give information on the percentage of inhibition. By comparing the photomicrographs of with and without inhibitor, authors concluded that hydroalcoholic extract of the extract of *A. indica* remarkably inhibits crystal formation in CaOx urinary lithiasis.

Acorus calamus L. Family: Araceae

Prasad *et al.* [41] reported the effect of *Acorus calamus* on nickel chloride ($NiCl_2$)-induced renal oxidative stress, toxicity, and cell proliferation response in male Wistar rats. Prophylactic treatment of rats with *A. calamus* (100 and 200 mg/kg body weight po) daily for 1 wk resulted in the diminution of $NiCl_2$-mediated damage, as evident from the downregulation of GSH content, GST, GR, LPO, H_2O_2 generation, BUN, serum creatinine, DNA synthesis, and ODC activity with concomitant restoration of GPx activity.

Palani *et al.* [42] investigated the nephroprotective and antioxidant activities of ethanol extract of *A. calamus* (AC) at two dose levels of 250 and 500 mg/kg B/W on acetaminophen (APAP) induced toxicity in male albino rats. AC inhibited the hematological effects of APAP. AC significantly increased activities of renal SOD, CAT, GSH, and GPx and decreased MDA content of APAP-treated rats. Histopathological changes also showed the protective nature of the AC extract against APAP induced necrotic damage of renal tissues.

The extracts of *A. calamus* protected the renal tissue effectively from cisplatin-induced toxicity. Treatment of cisplatin-administered animals with the plant extract could prevent the drug-induced oxidative damage in the renal tissue, as evidenced by the decreased levels of lipid peroxidation and enhanced activities of the antioxidants in the renal tissue. Cisplatin treatment increased serum urea level to 41.3 +/- 2.86 mg/dL and administration of the extract *A. calamus* brought down the level to 30.12 +/- 0.95 mg/dL. Serum creatinine levels were increased to 1.1 +/- 0.02 mg/dL following cisplatin administration, and treatment with extract *A. calamus* brought this down to 0.61 +/- 0.06 mg/dL. The histopathological observations indicated that treatment with the *A. calamus* extract restored the cisplatin-induced structural alterations in the renal tissue [43].

Ghelani *et al.* [44] investigated the diuretic and antiurolithiatic activities of an ethanolic extract of *A. calamus* rhizome (EEAC). EEAC (750 mg/kg, p.o.) produced significant increase in urine volume and urinary excretion of Na^+ and K^+ electrolytes in a pattern comparable to that of furosemide. In ethylene glycol induced urolithiatic model, EEAC significantly decreased excretion and deposition of various urolithiatic promoters as compared to urolithiatic control in a pattern comparable to that of Cystone. The EEAC supplementation also prevents the impairment of renal functions.

Adiantum capillus-veneris L. Family: Adiantaceae

Ahmed *et al.* [45] evaluated the effect of the hydro alcoholic extract of *Adiantum capillus-veneris* on CaOx crystallisation by *in vitro* study. Extract of *A. capillus-veneris* inhibited the crystallization in solution; less and smaller particles were observed in the presence of extract. The rate of nucleation was not inhibited but number of crystals was found to be decreased. The extract also inhibited crystal aggregation.

Ahmed *et al.* [46] investigated the antiurolithiasic effect of the hydroalcoholic extract of *A. capillus-veneris* in male Sprague Dawley rats. Urine microscopy showed a significant reduction in the number of crystals in test groups. Serum levels of calcium, phosphorous, and blood urea were found to be decreased significantly in all the groups. In both the test groups, serum creatinine level was found to be similar as in plain control. The animals treated with extract of *A. capillus-veneris* showed much improvement in body weight. In treated groups, histopathology showed almost normal kidney architecture.

Adonis aestivalis L. Family: Ranunculaceae

Lithiasis was induced by feeding the rats with 0.75% ethylene glycolated water for 28 days. Ethylene glycol treatment raised the urinary calcium, phosphate, oxalate and protein levels significantly in the lithiatic group, where magnesium level showed a significant decrease. However, treatment with *Adonis aestivalis* (divided doses of extract of 60 mg/kg of body weight daily by gavages) attenuated the elevated parameters and inhibited stone formation [47].

Aegle marmelos (L.) Correa Family: Rutaceae

Kore *et al.* [48] evaluated the nephroprotective activity of an aqueous extract of leaves of *Aegle marmelos* (AEAM) in Wistar rats. AEAM significantly reduced the elevated MDA levels and increased GSH and CAT concentration. AEAM reduced serum creatinine, urea and BUN level in GM toxicity indicating a nephroprotective effect.

The protective activity of hydro-alcoholic (HAEAM) and ethyl acetate (EAEAM) extracts of *A. marmelos* leaves was evaluated by Dwivedi *et al.* [49] against nephrotoxicity induced by cisplatin (CP). EAEAM (400 mg/kg) decreased the creatinine levels and BUN and restored the activities of renal antioxidant enzymes, decreased the lipid peroxidasde (LPO) levels, and increased SOD levels, GSH and CAT.

Aerva javanica (Burm.f.) Juss. ex Schult. Family: Amaranthaceae

Movaliya *et al.* [50] investigated the protective activity of aqueous extract of *Aerva javanica* roots in cisplatin induced renal toxicity in rats. The aqueous extract at the dose level of 400 mg/kg body weight was found to normalize the elevated biochemical markers (blood urea, serum creatinine, total protein and serum albumin, urine volume, urine PH) and bring about a marked recovery in kidneys as evidenced microscopically.

Padala and Ragini [51] investigated the potential activity of *A. javanica* in the treatment of renal calculi. Treatment with aqueous, methanol and ethyleacetate extract of *A. javanica* roots significantly reduced the elevated urinary oxalate, showing a regulatory action on endogenous oxalate synthesis. The increased deposition of stone forming constituents in the serum and urine of calculogenic rats was also significantly lowered.

Aerva lanata (L.) Juss. Family: Amaranthaceae

The efficacy of *Aerva lanata* as antilithic agent using a urolithic rat model was tested by Selvam *et al.* [52]. Increased urinary excretion of calcium, oxalate, uric acid, phosphorus and protein in hyperoxaluric rats was brought down significantly by the administration of *A. lanata*. Decreased magnesium excretion in hyperoxaluric rats was normalized by drug treatment. The drug increased the urine volume, thereby reducing the solubility product with respect to CaOx and other crystallizing salts such as uric acid, which may induce epitaxial deposition of CaOx.

The ethanol extract of *A. lanata* was studied by Shirwaikar *et al.* [53] for its nephroprotective activity in cisplatin- and GM-induced acute nephrotoxicity in albino rats. In the curative regimen, the extract at dose levels of 75, 150 and 300 mg/kg showed dose-dependent reduction in the elevated blood urea and serum creatinine and normalized the histopathological changes in the curative regimen. In the GM model, the rats in the preventive regimen also showed good response to the ethanol extract at 300 mg/kg.

Soundararajan *et al*. [54] evaluated the protective effect of *A. lanata* on CaOx urolithiasis in rats. Administration of *A. lanata* aqueous suspension (2g/kg body wt/dose/day for 28 days) to CaOx urolithic rats had reduced the oxalate synthesizing enzymes, diminished the markers of crystal deposition in the kidney.

Farook *et al*. [36] investigated inhibition of mineralization of urinary stone forming minerals by *A. lanata*. Inhibition efficiencies of leaves, seeds and fruits of *A. lanata* have been investigated in different models. Study suggests that the fruit juice and seed extract is moderate to good inhibitor of CaOx, calcium carbonate and calcium phosphate mineralization. Relatively poor inhibition of mineralization by leaves extracts was reported.

The effect of ethanolic extract of *A. lanata* was studied by Soumya *et al*. [55] on mercuric chloride induced renal damage in rats. Oral administration of ethanolic extract of *A. lanata* (200mg/kg and 400 mg/kg) effectively inhibited the levels of marker enzymes, antioxidant enzymes, lipid profile, protein and lipid peroxidation as compared to the normal groups. Fatty infiltration, fatty degeneration and necrosis observed in mercuric chloride treated groups were completely absent in histology of the liver and kidney sections of the animals treated with the ethanolic extract. It is stipulated that the extract treated groups were partially protected from hepatocellular damage caused by mercuric chloride.

Nirmaladevi *et al*. [56] evaluated the antilithiatic potential of aqueous dried flowers of *Aerva lanata* against ethylene glycol induced renal calculi in albino wistar rats. Ethylene glcol administration elevated urinary calcium with high urinary oxalate which might lead to CaOx stone formation. Administration of *A. lanata* extracts significantly lowered urinary calcium and oxalate.

Aesculus hippocastanum L. Family: Sapindaceae

Elmas *et al*. [57] investigated the preventive effects on oxidative stress and TGF-β-related diabetic nephropathy in streptozotocin (STZ)-induced diabetic nephropathy in rats by *Aesculus hippocastanum* (AH). Glomerular area, the severity of sclerosis, fibronectin immunoexpression, and levels of MDA, TGF-β, BUN, creatinine, and proteinuria were decreased in the diabetes +AH group. AH extract ameliorated diabetic nephropathy without decrease in blood glucose levels. AH seeds showed beneficial effects on the functional properties of the kidney and microscopic improvements in diabetic nephropathy.

Ageratum conyzoides (L.) L. Family: Asteraceae

Aqueous leaf extract of *Ageratum conyzoides* was studied by Sumalatha *et al*. [58] for its antiurolithiatic activity. CaOx urolithiasis was induced by administration of

GM and calculi producing diet. Aqueous leaf extract of *A. conyzoides* exhibited significant effect in preventing CaOx stone formation and also in dissolving the preformed CaOx stones in the kidney along with significant effect on *in vitro* antioxidant parameters.

Bhuvaneswari *et al.* [59] evalauated the anti-urolithiatic activity of aqueous, ethyl acetate and ethanolic extracts of whole plant of *A. conyzoides*. The results of the study proved that all the plant extracts at a dose level of 500 mg/kg significantly reduced calcium and oxalate concentration in the excreted urine and the deposition of the same in the kidney, while the highest reduction in the calcium and oxalate in the urine and kidney was noted with the ethanol extract.

Agrimonia eupatoria L. Family: Rosaceae

Significant uricosuric activity has been documented for *Agrimonia eupatoria* infusions and decoctions (15% w/v), following their oral administration to male rats at a dose of 20 ml/kg body weight (equivalent to 3 g dry plant powder) [60].

Ajuga iva (L.) Schreb. Family: Lamiaceae

Inhibition of CaOx monohydrate crystal growth using aqueous extract of aerial part of *Ajuga iva* was investigated by Beghalia *et al.* [61]. Activity was tested in bioassays. In the presence of plants extract, the length and the width of the crystals were reduced. The average length of the crystals grown in the presence of the inhibitors was less than that of the control sample. The extract inhibited potently the nucleation, growth and aggregation phases. Inhibition was 89.97% at 25% concentration, 95.22% at 50% concentration, 97.01% at 75% concentration and 96.06 at 100% concentration.

Alcea rosea L. [Syn.: *Althaea rosea* (L.) Cav.] Family: Malvaceae

Hydroalcoholic extract of *Alcea rosea* roots significantly reduced the kidney CaOx deposits compared to ethylene glycol group. Administration of *A. rosea* extract also reduced the elevated urinary oxalate due to ethylene glycol [62].

Alisma orientale (Sam.) Juzep Family: Alismataceae

Suzuki *et al.* [63] examined the effect of *Alismatis rhizoma*, on the formation, growth and aggregation of CaOx crystals. Takusha had a strong inhibitory effect on the aggregation and growth when the concentration was above 10 mg/ml. In measuring the metastable limit by the microplate method, Takusha had a mild inhibitory effect on the formation of crystals above the concentration of 1000 mg/ml. In the undiluted urine system, the formation and growth of CaOx crystals precipitated in response to a load of sodium oxalate were measured. Takusha had a strong inhibitory effect at concentrations of 100 to 1000 mg/ml. In the continuous flow crystallizer system, nucleation rate, growth rate and crystal mass were decreased in proportion to the increase of added Takusha.

Allanblackia gabonensis (Pellegr.) Bamps. Family: Clusiaceae

The aqueous suspension of the stem bark of *Allanblackia gabonensis* showed significant protective activity against acetaminophen-induced nephrotoxicity in rats. Pre-treatment with 100 and 200 mg/kg significantly reduced the serum level of MDA, increase in enzymatic antioxidant activities (SOD and CAT) and non enzymatic antioxidant (GSH) levels [64].

Allium cepa L. Famiy: Liliaceae

Ige *et al.* [65] evaluated the protective effect of *Allium cepa* extract, on cadmium-induced renal toxicity. Renal clearance and 24 h urine volume were significantly reduced in rats treated with cadmium. Renal clearance was also reduced in rats treated with cadmium and *A.cepa* extract, though this decrease was only significant when compared with the control group. Pre-treatment and post treatment with *A.cepa* extract in cadmium-treated rats produced mild protective potentials. However, co-treatment with *A. cepa* extract during cadmium administration showed significant antioxidative potentials in preventing cadmium-induced nephrotoxicity.

Allium sativum L. Family: Liliaceae

Kaur *et al.* [66] investigated the effect of garlic oil and propylene glycol, which is a constituent of many drug preparations containing aspirin, steroids and antibiotics, on young and aged mice. Male albino mice were given garlic oil with propylene glycol as a vehicle, to study the effects on certain parameters of the kidney. Garlic oil decreased the activities of transaminases and phosphatases, and lipid peroxide levels, while propylene glycol counteracted the effects of garlic oil. These results suggest that garlic oil may check or reverse the harmful effects of propylene glycol and might thereby protect the system against its toxic effects.

Maldonado *et al.* [67] investigated if aged garlic extract (AGE), an antioxidant, has a protective role in nephrotoxicity. In nephrotoxicity model there was an increase in BUN and plasma creatinine, the decrease in plasma GPx activity and the urinary increase in N-acetyl-beta-D-glucosaminidase activity and total protein, and necrosis of proximal tubular cells. These alterations were prevented or ameliorated by AGE treatment. Furthermore, AGE prevented the GM-induced increase in the renal levels of oxidative stress markers: nitrotyrosine and protein carbonyl groups and the decrease in Mn-SOD, GPx, and GR activities.

The effect of garlic on GM nephrotoxicity was investigated by Pedraza-Chaverri *et al*. [68]. GM nephrotoxicity was made evident by tubular histological damage, enhanced BUN and urinary excretion of N-acetyl-beta-D-glucosaminidase, and decreased creatinine clearance. These alterations were prevented or ameliorated in GM + GA group. The rise in lipoperoxidation and the decrease in Mn-SOD and GPx activities observed in the GM group, were prevented in the GM + GA group. Cu, Zn-SOD activity and Mn-SOD and Cu, Zn-SOD content did not change. CAT activity and content decreased in the GM, GA, and GM + GA groups. CAT mRNA levels decreased in the GM group. The protective effect of garlic is associated with the prevention of the decrease of Mn-SOD and GPx activities and with the rise of lipoperoxidation in renal cortex.

Effect of *Allium sativum* against mercuric chloride induced toxicity in albino rats was studied by Abirami and Jagadeeswari [69]. Simultaneous administration of garlic along with mercuric chloride, produced a pronounced neproprotective effect against mercuric chloride induced toxicity in rats by restoring the normal levels of biochemical parameters.

Al-Qattan *et al*. [70] investigated the hypoglycaemic effects of garlic on the kidney structure of streptozotocin-induced diabetic rats. Compared to normal levels, non-treated diabetic serum glucose and protein clearance were 330% and 185%, respectively. Compared to non-treated diabetic rats, garlic-treated diabetic rats serum glucose and protein clearance levels decreased by 45% and 50%, respectively. In garlic -treated rats, these renal structural changes changes (*e.g.* capsular space shrinkage, glomerular hypertrophy and diffusion, glomerular and microvascular eosinophilic precipitation, and cytoplasm fragmentation and retraction) although evident were less prominent.

Gulnaz *et al*. [71] examined the preventive effects of garlic oil on acetaminophen induced nephrotoxicity in male albino rats. Garlic oil pretreatment significantly reduced acetaminophen induced nephrotoxicity as evidenced by amelioration of histological changes in size of glomerulus. Garlic oil also reduced deleterious effects of acetaminophen on tubules of kidney as evidenced by absence of vacuolation and granularity of epithelial cells of proximal and distal convoluted tubules and, protein casts in thick ascending limb of loop of Henle in rats. Value of serum urea and that of serum creatinine was restored.

Savas *et al*. [72] examined the effect of oral application of garlic oil (GO) on rats after renal ischemia-reperfusion (I/R) injury. The serum urea, creatinine, and cystatin C levels were significantly higher in I/R group compared to I/R+GO group. The serum and tissue antioxidant markers (TAC, CAT) were significantly lower in I/R group than I/R+GO group. The serum oxidant markers (TOS, MPO,

NO, and PC) were significantly higher in I/R group than I/R+GO group. Also oral application of GO was effective in decreasing of tubular necrosis score.

Abdelaziz and Kandeel [73] evaluated the effect of garlic extract in ameliorating amikacin-induced nephrotoxicity. Garlic extract significantly decreased the levels of NO, MDA and total antioxidant capacity. Furthermore, they increased the level of reduced GSH. These results were coinciding with the lower levels of urea, uric acid and creatinine. Semi-quantitative analysis of cellular infiltration, necrosis of tubular cells and tubular cellular damage indicated the protective effect of the used plant materials in reducing renal damage induced by amikacin.

Bagheri *et al.* [74] examined the preventive effect of garlic juice on renal reperfusion injury in rats. Garlic juice significantly decreased serum urea levels in the reperfusion + garlic group compared with the reperfusion group. Preteatment with garlic juice also resulted in significant increase in urine potassium compared to reperfusion. Fractional excretions of sodium and creatinine clearance were also improved. On histological examination, rats pretreated with garlic juice had nearly normal morphology.

Anusuya *et al.* [75] investigated the *in vivo* protective potential of ethanolic extract of garlic against cisplatin induced nephrotoxicity in Wistar male rats. Treatment with ethanolic extract of garlic rendered a protective effect by boosting up the antioxidant levels and reverting back the markers like urea, creatinine, uric acid and BUN to near normalcy. The garlic extract at higher dose also had no significant biochemical alterations in normal rats.

Nasri *et al.* [76] investigated the ameliorative effects *A. sativum* on GM-induced nephrotoxicity. However, the levels of Serum creatinine and BUN in animals treated with GM and garlic were significantly lower than those in GM treated animals. These parameters were also lower in animals treated with GM and garlic, when compared with animals treated with GM and saline. Postadministration of garlic after GM treatment or co-administration of garlic and GM significantly attenuated the damage score.

Rafieian-Kopaei *et al.* [77] evaluated the preventive and curative effects of garlic, metformin (MF) and their combination on GM-induced tubular toxicity in Wistar rats. GM injection significantly increased the serum BUN and Cr. Administration of MF, garlic or their combination with or after injection of GM (high doses) could atenuate BUN and Cr.

Aloe vera (L.) Burm.f. (Syn.: *A. barbadensis* Mill.) Family: Asparagaceae

Chatterjee *et al.* [78] evaluated the protective effects of the aqueous leaf extract of

Aloe vera (*AEAV*) on GM and Cisplatin–induced nephrotoxic Wistar rats. In the GM nephrotoxic rats, 100-200 mg/kg bodyweight per day of the extract significantly attenuated elevations in the serum creatinine, total protein and BUN levels in dose related fashion and no treatment related effect on uric acid and ions, and attenuated the GM-induced tubulonephrosis. Similar effects were also recorded in the Cisplatin model of acute renal injury.

Alpinia galanga (L.) Willd. Family: Zingiberaceae

The protective effect of the alcoholic extract of the rhizomes of *Alpinia galanga* was evaluated by Kaushik *et al.* [79] for the treatment of diabetes-induced nephropathy in rats. After 40 days of treatment, *A. galanga* significantly decreased glycaemia, BUN, urine albumin and increased body weight in diabetes-nephropathic rats. The extract (200 mg/kg) decreased MDA significantly GSH, increased SOD and CAT in the rats, compared with nephropathic control. The extract (100 and 200 mg/kg, respectively) lowered total cholesterolemia, blood triglycerides, blood LDL cholesterol, but increased blood HDL cholesterol. Overall, atherogenic index was decreased significantly.

Althaea officinalis L. Family: Malvaceae

Talebi *et al.* [80] investigated the effect of *Althaea officinalis* flower extract (AOFE) against nephrotoxicity induced by GM in male rats. GM significantly increased serum levels of BUN and creatinine as well as the pathological damage score. Low dose of AOFE did not decrease the nephrotoxicity induced by GM while the high dose of AOFE aggravated renal toxicity. Although AOFE acts as an antioxidant, at the doses used in this study did not ameliorate nephrotoxicity induced by GM.

Amaranthus spinosus L. Family: Amaranthaceae

Amuthan *et al.* [81] evaluated the diuretic potential of *A. spinosus* aqueous extract (ASAE) in rats. ASAE produced increase in Na(+), K(+), Cl(-) excretion, caused alkalinization of urine, showed strong saluretic activity and carbonic anhydrase inhibition activity. These effects were observed predominantly at 500mg/kg dose and there was no dose-response relationship.

Ethanol extract of *A. spinosus* root was investigated by Kengar *et al.* [82] for protective activity in CCl_4 induced nephrotoxicity in male albino rats. The results revealed the deleterious histopathological alterations in kidney associated with glomerular and tubular degenerations in CCl_4 intoxicated rat. Treatment of *A. spinosus* roots especially at 450 mg dose protects the kidney by improving disrupted metabolisms and antioxidant defence against CCl_4 induced oxidative damage in 15 days' protective experimental schedule.

Ammannia baccifera L. Family: Lythraceae

Prasad *et al.* [83] investigated the antiurolithic activity of *Ammannia baccifera* in male albino rats. The ethanolic extract of *A. baccifera* (2g/kg/day, p.o.) was effective in reducing the formation of stone and also in dissolving the pre-formed one. Four weeks after implantation of zinc discs there was a significant increase in the urinary excretion of calcium, magnesium and oxalate. Treatment with *A. baccifera* has significantly reduced calcium and magnesium levels in the prophylactic group while it has reversed the levels of these ions to normal values in the curative group.

Ammi majus L. Family: Apiaceae

Ahsan *et al.* [84] evaluated the effect of *Ammi majus* fruit on experimentally-induced urolithiasis. The effects obtained by *A. majus* were not significant.

A. majus with confirmed antioxidant effect could be used in diabetic nephropathy and myocardial injury [85].

Ammi visnaga (L.) Lam. Family: Apiaceae

The effect of *Ammi visnaga* seeds on kidney stones is mainly because of highly potent diuretic activity and amelioration of uraemia and hyperbilirubinemia by seeds of *A. visnaga* [87].

The oral administration of an aqueous extract prepared from the fruits of *A. visnaga* as well as two major constituents khellin and visnagin prevent crystal deposition in stone-forming rats [87, 88]. The histopathological examination of the kidneys revealed that Khella extract (KE) significantly reduced the incidence of CaOx crystal deposition. In addition, KE significantly increased urinary excretion of citrate along with a decrease of oxalate excretion. Comparable to the extract, khellin and visnagin significantly reduced the incidence of CaOx deposition in the kidneys. However, both compounds did not affect urinary citrate or oxalate excretion indicating a mechanism of action that differs from that of the extract. For KE, a reasonably good correlation was observed between the incidence of crystal deposition, the increase in citrate excretion and urine pH suggesting a mechanism that may interfere with citrate reabsorption.

The prophylactic effects of *A.visnaga* may be attributed to its diuretic activity to maintain the oxalate, below the supersaturation to precipitate as CaOx.

Ammodaucus leucotrichus Coss Family: Apiaceae

Inhibition of CaOx monohydrate crystal growth using aqueous extract of fruits of *Ammodaucus leutotrichus* was investigated by Beghalia *et al*. [61]. Activity was tested in bioassays. In the presence of plants extract, the length and the width of the crystals were reduced. Extracts plants inhibited potently the nucleation, growth and aggregation phases. Inhibition was 94.98% at 25% concentration, 96.87% at 50% concentration, 97.25% at 75% concentration and 97.85 at 100% concentration.

Andrographis paniculata (Burm. f.) Nees Family: Acanthaceae

Muangman *et al*. [89] investigated the effect of the usage of *Andrographis paniculata* following extracorporeal shock wave lithotripsy (ESWL). The results showed that post ESWL pyuria and hematuria in patients receiving *A. paniculata* were reduced to 0.69 and 0.55 time of pre ESWL value.

Rao *et al*. [90] reported that the root extract of *A. paniculata* is useful in preventing the incidence of long-term complications of diabetic nephropathy. Singh *et al*. [91] reported that the aqueous extract (whole plant) of *A. paniculata* exhibited a significant renoprotective effect in GM-induced nephrotoxicity in male Wistar albino rats. Aqueous extract of *A. paniculata* attenuated the GM-induced increase in serum creatinine, serum urea, and BUN levels by 176.92%, 106.27%, and 202.90%, respectively.

Nephroprotective activities of root extracts of *A. paniculata* (AP), in GM-induced renal failure in Wistar rats, was investigated by Singh *et al*. [92]. Oral administration of Pt. ether, $CHCl_3$ and MeOH extracts of AP patently prevented GM induced elevated levels of SCr, SU and UP. The results were also supported by measuring the urine volume voided by each rat separately, of all the groups with time. The extent of protection offered by various extracts increased with the increasing time of treatment and polarity of the solvents. The signs of GM nephrotoxicity in rats were significantly mitigated by Pt. ether and $CHCl_3$ extracts whereas the maximal alleviation of ARF was caused by MeOH root extract.

Pratibhakumari and Prasad [93] investigated the protective effect of the methanol extract of *A. paniculata* (MEAP) in experimentally induced nephrolithiatic rats. All the elevated biochemical parameters in EG received group were declined in the MEAP treated groups at dosage of 200 and 400mg/kg. Urinary protein, phosphorus and calcium also declined in both MEAP treatment groups than the lithiatic groups. Serum creatinine declined significantly in high dose received group than its low dose in both post and co treatment groups. A dose dependent effect was observed in all the serum parameters except BUN. Kidney phosphorus and calcium of preventive regime which received MEAP at a high dose of 400mg/kg showed a clear dose dependent effect than the curative regimes.

Annona squamosa L. Family: Annonaceae

Deshmukh and Patel [94] assessed the protective activity of the aqueous extract of *Annona squamosa* in 5/6 nephrectomized animals. Nephrectomized rats (5/6) showed a significant rise in plasma urea and creatinine levels with a stable fall in urine creatinine. Treatment with *A. squamosa* extract (300 mg/kg bw) lead to a significant fall in the plasma urea and creatinine values with partial restoration to normal values along with a significant rise in the activity of SOD.

Apium graveolens L. Family: Apiaceae

The effect of *Apium graveolens* in reducing calcium deposits from renal parenchyma was studied by Al-Jawad *et al.* [95] in rabbit models with induced nephrocalcinosis by a large dose of oxalic acid. *A. graveolens* significantly reduced BUN, serum creatinine and serum Na+ levels in addition to non-significant reduction in serum K+. It caused a significant reduction in calcium deposition in renal parenchyma after 10 days treatment. This effect was attributed to its diuretic effect.

Arctium lappa L. Family: Asteraceae

Grases *et al.* [96] studied the effects of *Arctium lappa* to prevent and treat stone kidney formation in female Wistar rats. The infusion does not affect calciuria and citraturia values, they do not diminish calcinuria or increase the crystallization inhibitory capacity of the urine. Authors are of the opinion that the beneficial effect caused by this herb infusion on urolithiasis can be attributed to some disinfectant action, and tentatively to the presence of saponins. Gurocak and Kupeli [97] also reported antiurolithiactity property of *A. lappa*.

Arctostaphylos uva-ursi (L.) Spreng. Family: Ericaceae

Grases *et al.* [96] studied the effects of *Arctostaphylos uva-ursi* to prevent and treat stone kidney formation in female Wistar rats. The infusion does not affect calciuria and citraturia values, they do not diminish calcinuria or increase the crystallization inhibitory capacity of the urine. The beneficial effect caused by this herb infusion on urolithiasis can be attributed to some disinfectant action, and tentatively to the presence of saponins.

Aristolochia albida Duch. Family: Aristolochiaceae

Guinnin *et al.* [98] evaluated the effects of *Aristolochia albida* used in virus hepatitis treatment, on the liver and kidneys. The hepatic and renal parameters investigated are transaminases (AST, ALT), alkaline phosphatase (ALP), bilirubin (free and conjugated), urea, total protein, creatinine. Several doses (250 mg/kg, 500 mg/kg, 750 mg/kg) of the ethanolic extract of *A. albida* were used to evaluate effective dose for liver and kidneys. Biochemical analysis showed a significant decrease in transaminases (AST, ALT), alkaline phosphatase (ALP), bilirubin (free and conjugated) at 750 mg/kg. Concerning renal parameters, authors noticed that *A. albida* don't reduce significantly urea level.

Aristolochia indica L. Family: Aristolochiaceae

Arivazhagan and Vimaastalin [99] evaluated the protective activity of *Aristolochia indica* in GM induced nephrotoxicity in Wistar rats. Treatment with *A. indica* leaves (500mg/kg) significantly restored the levels of serum creatine, urea, sodium, protein and potassium. Significantly increase the antioxidant defence enzye levels of SID, GPx and CAT on treatment with *A.indica*.

Artocarpus heterophyllus Lam. Family: Moraceae

Bhattacharjee and Dutta [100] examined the possible nephroprotective role methanolic and aqueous extracts of *Artocarpus heterophyllus* bark against GM-induced nephrotoxicity. The plant extracts showed a remarkable nephroprotective activity against GM-induced nephrotoxicity. In GM-induced nephrotoxicity there was a significant elevation of uric acid, urea and creatinine level. Treatment with both the extracts (100mg/kg and 200mg/kg) significantly reduced the biochemical level in a dose dependant manner which proved its nephroprotective activity. There was also significant increase in RBC count and haemoglobin level by both the extracts. Histopathological study of kidney further confirmed the activity.

Asparagus racemosus Willd. Family: Asparagaceae

Christina *et al.* [101] evaluated the antilithiatic potential of the ethanolic extract of *Asparagus racemosus* in albino Wistar rats. Ethylene glycol elevated the urinary concentration of calcium, oxalate, and phosphate, thereby contributing to renal stone formation. The ethanolic extract, however, significantly reduced the elevated level of these ions in urine. Also, it elevated the urinary concentration of magnesium, which is considered as one of the inhibitors of crystallization. Following treatment with the extract the high serum creatinine level observed in ethylene glycol-treated rats was also reduced. Histopathological findings also showed signs of improvement after treatment with the extract.

Aqueous extract of *A. racemosus* roots was evaluated by Kumar *et al.* [102] for its antiurolithiatic potential in albino Wistar rats. Two doses of extract for prophylactic and curative groups were used. Administration of the drug has resulted in reduction in the weight of stones compared to the control group, but was not significantly reduced.

Jagannath *et al.* [103] investigated the effect of ethanolic extract of *A. racemosus* on urolithiasis in rats. The rats treated with ethanolic extract of *A. racemosus* at doses 800 and 1600 mg/kg significantly reduced the serum concentrations of calcium, phosphorus, urea, and creatinine. Histopathology of the kidneys revealed less tissue damage and were almost similar to control rats.

Astragalus membranaceus (Sisch.) Bunge Family: Fabaceae

Li *et al.* [104] aimed to systematically review the randomized and semi-randomized control trials to ascertain its role in the treatment of DN. PUBMED, MEDLINE, Chinese journal full-test database (CJFD), Chinese biological and medical database were searched by computer and manual searching. Astragalus injection had more therapeutic effect in DN patients including renal protective effect (BUN, SCr, CCr and urine protein) and systemic state improvement (serum albumin level) compared with the control group.

Atriplex halimus L. Family: Amaranthaceae

Inhibition of CaOx monohydrate crystal growth using aqueous extract of leaves of *Atriplex halimus* was investigated by Beghalia *et al.* [61]. Activity was tested in bioassays. The average length of the crystals grown in the presence of the inhibitors was less than that of the control sample. The extract inhibited potently the growth and aggregation phases. Inhibition was 63.12% at 25% concentration, 67.18% at 50% concentration, 91.64% at 75% concentration and 89.26 at 100% concentration.

Azadirachta indica A. Juss. Family: Meliaceae

Ezz-Din *et al.* [105] investigated the protective effect of *Azadirachta indica* (neem) leaves against cisplatin-induced nephrotoxicity. Neem leaves showed significant protection as evidenced by the decrease of elevated serum ALT, AST, gamma glutamyl transpeptidase, alkaline phosphatase, total bilirubin, creatinine, uric acid and urea. This improvement of physiological function was associated with high protection against histopathological injury induced by cisplatin on kidney.

Hwisa *et al.* [106] investigated the antiurolithiatic activity of aqueous plant extract of *A. indica* (wrongly spelt in the paper as *Melia Azadirachta*) in male Wistar albino rats. A significant increase in urinary excretion of calcium, oxalate, magnesium and phosphate was observed after four weeks of implantation of zinc discs. Treatment with aqueous extract of *A.indica* caused a significant reduction in stone weight and urinary excretion of electrolytes in both the preventive and curative group of animals as compared to those of control groups. The aqueous extract of *A. indica* prevents urolithiasis by 59% and dissolve the pre-formed magnesium ammonium phosphate type of stones by 46%.

Azima tetracantha Lam. Family: Salvadoraceae

Konda *et al.* [107] evaluated the effect of root extract of *Azima tetracantha* (ATR) in Wistar albino rats. Rats treated with ATR showed significant improvement in biochemical parameters and histopathological changes compared to glycerol treated group. The protective effect was highly significant at 500 mg/kg. Both *in vitro* and *in vivo* assays showed significant antioxidant activity. The *in vitro* activity was comparable to vitamin-C.

Bacopa monnieri (L.) Wettst. Family: Plantaginaceaae

Bacopa monniera methanol extract (mBME) was evaluated by Shahid and Subhan [108] against CCl_4 induced renal damage in rats. Pretreatment with mBME (40 mg/kg) for 14 days decreased the serum ALT, AST and creatinine levels and protected kidneys from the toxicological influence of CCl_4. The EC_{50} for the DPPH free radical scavenging assay of revealed that mBME had an efficient antioxidant potential.

Balanites aegyptica (L.) Delile Family: Zygophyllaceae

Water extract of *Balanites aegyptica* was tested by Patel *et al.* [109] for its *in vitro* antilithiatic/anticalcification activity by the homogenous precipitation method. Extract of *Balanites aegyptica* showed less activity than peptone.

Barleria prionitis L. Family: Acanthaceae

Atif *et al.* [110] investigated the antiurolithiatic activity of hydro-alcoholic and aqueous leaf extract of *B. prionitis* in albino rats. Preventive regimen (PR) and Curative regimen (CR) of *B. prionitis* hydro-alcoholic extract (Alc.E) 400 mg/kg and aqueous extract (Aq. E) 400 mg/kg significantly lowered the increased urinary and serum parameters whereas preventive regimen and curative regimen of *B. prionitis* Alc. E 200 mg/kg and Aq. E 200 mg/kg were less significant. The histopathological evaluations of kidney samples were in support of the obtained result.

Barringtonia acutangula (L.) Gaertn. Family: Lecythidaceae

Nephroprotective activity of extracts of *Barringtonia acutangula* leaves was investigated by Mishra *et al.* [111] against GM-induced acute nephrotoxicity in Wistar rats. The extracts of root significantly attenuated the nephrotoxicity by elevation of body weight, CAT, GPx and SOD or lowering urine LDH and creatinine, serum urea; serum creatinine and LPO respectively.

Bauhinia purpurea L. Family: Fabaceae

Lakshmi *et al.* [112] evaluated the ethanol extract of leaves and unripe pods of *Bauhinia purpurea* for its protective effects on GM-induced nephrotoxicity in rats. Effect of concurrent administration of ethanol extract of leaves of *B. purpurea* and unripe pods of *B. purpurea* at a dose of 300 mg/kg/d was determined. GM-induced glomerular congestion, blood vessel congestion, epithelial desquamation, accumulation of inflammatory cells and necrosis of the kidney cells were found to be reduced in the groups receiving the leaf and unripe pods extract of *B. purpurea* along with GM. The extracts also normalized the GM-induced increase in serum creatinine, serum uric acid and BUN levels. This is also evidenced by the histopathological studies.

Sivanagi Reddy *et al.* [113] evaluated the protective activity of ethanolic extract of stem bark of *B. purpurea* against paracetamol induced nephrotoxicity in rats. Biochemical parameters like increase in the levels of serum GOT, GPT, ALP, total bilirubin, triglycerides, BUN, creatinine and urea and reduction in the levels of total protein in paracetamol induced groups are retrieved significantly in a dose dependant manner by treatment with ethanolic extracts of *B purpurea* stem bark at three different doses (100, 200 and 400 mg/kg).

Rana *et al.* [114] evaluated the nephroprotective activity and antioxidant potential of *B. purpurea* unripe pods (BPE) and bark (BBE) against cisplatin-induced nephrotoxicity. Administration of BBE and BPE at doses of 200 and 400 mg/kg caused a dose-dependant reduction in the rise of blood urea, serum creatinine and urine glucose, and there was a dose-dependant increase in creatinine clearance compared with negative control. There was increased CAT and GSH and decreased MDA levels in cisplatin-induced Group, while BBE 400 and BPE 400 treatments significantly reversed the changes toward normal values. Histological examination of the kidney revealed protection in treated animals compared with untreated Group.

Bauhinia variegata L. Family: Fabaceae

The protective activity of the ethanolic extract of *Bauhinia variegata* whole stem against cisplatin-induced nephropathy was investigated by Pani *et al*. [115] by an *in vivo* method in rats. Administration of ethanol extract at dose levels of 400 and 200 mg/kg (b.w.) to cisplatin-intoxicated rats attenuated nephrotoxicity in a dose-dependent manner. Ethanol extract at 400 mg/kg decreased the serum level of creatinine and urea associated with a significant increase in body weight and urine volume output as compared to the toxic control group. Nephroprotective potential of the ethanol extract at 400 mg/kg (b.w.) was comparable to that of the standard drug cystone.

Sharma [116] and Sharma *et al*. [117] evaluated the antioxidant and nephroprotective effect of ethanolic and aqueous extracts of root of *B. variegata* in GM induced nephrotoxicity in rats. Both the extracts produced significant nephroprotective activity in GM-induced nephrotoxicity model as evident by decrease in elevated serum creatinine, serum urea, urine creatinine and BUN levels, which was further confirmed by histopathological study. GM-induced glomerular congestion, blood vessel congestion, and epithelial desquamation, accumulation of inflammatory cells and necrosis of the kidney cells were found to be reduced in the groups receiving the root extract of *B. variegata* along with GM.

Prusty *et al*. [118] carried out the protective activity of methanolic extract of leaves of *B. variegata* by GM-induced nephrotoxicity. Extract has reduced the increased creatinine levels when compared to the control group. Normal serum creatinine levels are 0.7 ± 0.02, that of the GM-treated group was 1.25 ± 0.05, that of plant treated group was 0.86 ± 0.02, Levels of BUN were 24.4 ± 0.97, 76.11 ± 0.92, 28.03 ± 0.2 respectively. The levels in urinary parameters of all the groups were also altered by the leaf extract. Urinary parameters, creatinine of normal, control and methanolic leaf extract group were 69 ± 0.86, 194.5 ± 1.77, 137.67 ± 2.08 and urea were 17.73 ± 0.1, 32.67 ± 0.73, 19.12 ± 0.18 respectively. Decrease in the body weight of rats was also observed and that was significantly less when methanolic group was compared with the control group.

Benincasa hispida Thunb. Family: Cucurbitaceae

Patel *et al*. [119] investigated protective effect of ethanolic extract of *Benincasa hispida* seeds (BHE) in hyperoxaluria and renal cell injury. Supplementation with BHE significantly reduced the elevated urinary oxalate, showing a regulatory action on endogenous oxalate synthesis. BHE significantly lowered the urinary excretion and kidney retention levels of oxalate, protein and calcium. Moreover, elevated serum levels of sodium, creatinine and calcium, phosphorus were significantly reduced by the extracts.

The protective effect of hydro-alcoholic extract of *B. hispida* whole fruit extract was investigated in paracetamol-induced nephrotoxicity in rats. Treatment with *B. hispida* whole fruit extract at doses of 200 and 400 mg/kg bw prevented the paracetamol induced nephrotoxicity and oxidative impairments of the kidney, as evidenced by a significantly reduced in kidney weight, blood urea, blood creatinine, urinary glucose, urinary potassium level and also increased body weight, urine volume, urinary creatinine and blood total protein level. *B. hispida* whole fruit extract significantly increased the tissue GSH levels and reduced lipid peroxidation levels. Furthermore, it was confirmed by the histopathological observation that the degenerative changes caused by paracetamol were also restored by treatment with hydro-alcoholic extract of *B. hispida* whole fruit extract [120]. It also showed nephroprotective activity against mercury poisoning in rats [121].

Berberis aristata Sims Family: Berberidaceae

Sreedevi *et al.* [122] evaluated the protective effect of decoction of root bark of *Berberis aristata* against cisplatin-induced renal toxicity in rats. The effect of decoction of root bark of *B. aristata* was examined in terms of BUN, serum creatinine, urinary protein, urine to serum creatinine ratio, lipid peroxidation and histological aspects of kidney. The decoction of root bark significantly reversed the all the effects induced by cisplatin in dose dependent manner. The plant decoction also effectively protected from cisplatin-induced effects in prophylactic regimen. The above results are substantiated by histological studies.

Berberis baluchistanica Ahrendt Family: Berberidaceae

Pervez *et al.* [123] explored the protective effect of *Berberis baluchistanica* against GM-induced nephrotoxicity in rabbits. The crude hydro-methanolic extract at various doses (100, 200 and 300 mg/kg body weight) elicited strong nephroprotective effects by restoring various biomarkers which were deranged by GM such as creatinine, urea, serum uric acid levels in plasma and urine output creatinine clearance, urinary protein and γ-glutamyl transferase level in urine in a dose dependent manner. The mediators involved in oxidative stress such as MDA, reduced GSH, GPx, and CAT levels were significantly modulated in kidney tissue homogenate. Correspondingly, there was a significant recovery in kidney weight and % loss in body weight compared to GM group.

Berberis integerrima Bunge Family: Berberidaceae

Protective effect of aqueous extract of *Berberis integerrima* root (AEBIR) was evaluated by Ashraf *et al*. [124] for renal function in diabetic rats induced by STZ. Streptozotocin induced a significant rise in fasting blood glucose, serum creatinine, BUN, urine glucose, urine protein, urine albumin, and water intake and a significant decrease in body weight, serum protein, urine urea, and urine creatinine. There was a significant restoration of these parameters to near normal after administration of the AEBIR and also by the standard drug, glibenclamide. The activity of the extract at dose of 500 mg/kg in all parameters except blood glucose and urine glucose was more than that of the standard drug, glibenclamide. Histopathological changes of kidney samples were comparable with respective control.

Berberis lycium Royle Family: Berberidaceae

Anwar *et al*. [125] investigated the sub-acute protective effect of *Berberis lycium* root bark extracts against cisplatin-induced nephrotoxicity. Aqueous and methanol extracts (200 and 400 mg/kg) significantly reduced the serum creatinine, urea and uric acid levels. Moreover, GST, CAT activity and tGSH content were significantly increased and MDA level was decreased. Histopathological examination showed that both extracts efficiently reversed the morphological changes and damage induced by cisplatin.

Berberis vulgaris L. Family: Berberidaceae

Bashir *et al*. [126] evaluated antiurolithic potential of the crude aqueous-methanol extract of *Berberis vulgaris* root bark (Bv.Cr) in male Wistar rats. Bv.Cr (50 mg/kg) inhibited CaOx crystal deposition in renal tubules and protected against associated changes including polyuria, weight loss, impaired renal function and the development of oxidative stress in kidneys.

Jyothilakshimi *et al*. [127] evaluated the anti-urolithiasis potential of ultra-diluted homeopathic potency of *B. vulgaris* root bark. Administration of ethylene glycol to rats increased the levels of the stone-forming constituent's calcium, phosphorus and uric acid, in urine. Levels were normalized by *B. vulgaris* treatment. The decrease in the urolithiasis inhibitor magnesium in urine was prevented by treatment with *B. vulgaris*. Serum creatinine levels were largely normalized by *B. vulgaris* treatment. Hyperoxaluria induced renal damage was evident from the decreased activities of tissue marker enzymes and an apparent escalation in their activity in the urine in control animals; this was prevented by *B. vulgaris* treatment.

Bergenia ciliata (Haw.) Sternb. Family: Saxifragaceae

Alcohol, butanol, ethyl acetate extracts and isolated phenolic compounds from *Bergenia ciliata* leaves were evaluated for their potential to dissolve experimentally prepared kidney stones- CaOx and calcium phosphate, by an *in-vitro* model [128]. At 10 mg concentration phenolic compound P(1) isolated from the ethyl acetate fraction of the leaves, demonstrated highest dissolution of both stones when compared to test extracts. However, it was more effective in dissolving calcium phosphate stones (67.74%) than oxalate (36.95%).

Saha and Verma [129] evaluated the effect of *B. ciliata* extract on kidney of ethylene glycol induced urolithiasis in adult female Wistar rats. Administration of *B. ciliata* extract along with ethylene glycol showed significant protective effect in body weight and organ weight with few stray areas of calcifications in glomeruli. Moreover, *B. ciliata* extract showed higher renoprotective index than standard drug cystone at the same dose level.

Saha and Verma [130] evaluated the effectiveness of an extract obtained from the rhizomes of *B. ciliata* on the inhibition of CaOx crystallisation *in vitro*. The extract of *B. ciliata* was significantly more effective in inhibiting the nucleation and aggregation of COM crystals in a dose-dependent manner than was Cystone. Moreover, the extract induced more CaOx dihydrate crystals, with a significant reduction in the number and size of COM crystals.

Bergenia ligulata Engl. Family: Saxifragaceae

Joshi *et al.* [131] reported that herbal extracts of *B. ligulata* inhibit growth of CaOx monohydrate crystals *in vitro*. Bashir and Gilani [132] investigated the antiurolithic effect of *B. ligulata* rhizome (BLR) using *in vitro* and *in vivo* methods. BLR inhibited CaOx (CaC_2O_4) crystal aggregation as well as crystal formation in the metastable solutions. BLR caused diuresis in rats accompanied by a saluretic effect. In an animal model of urolithiasis, developed in male Wistar rats by adding 0.75% ethylene glycol (EG) in drinking water, BLR (5-10 mg/kg) prevented CaC_2O_4 crystal deposition in the renal tubules. The lithogenic treatment caused polyuria, weight loss, impairment of renal function and oxidative stress, manifested as increased MDA and protein carbonyl contents, depleted reduced GSH and decreased antioxidant enzyme activities of the kidneys, which were prevented by BLR.

The effect of CaOx urolithiasis urinary risk factor of ethanolic extract of *Bergenia ligulata*, *Nigella sativa* and their combination have been studied by Harsoliya *et al.* [133] in albino rats. From this study it was deduced that the possible effect of the ethanolic extract of *Bergenia ligulata, Nigella sativa* and their combination can be assigned to be positive effect on the main urolithiasis risk factors.

Beta vulgaris L. Family: Amaranthaceae

The inhibitory potential of *Beta vulgaris* leaf and root aqueous extracts against CaOx crystallization under *in vitro* condition was investigated by Saranya and Geetha [134]. Leaf and root aqueous extracts of *B. vulgaris* inhibit the crystal nucleation, aggregation and growth. When compared with leaf aqueous extract, root aqueous extract of beet root showed better inhibitory activity. Extracts inhibited the crystallization in solution; less and smaller particles were observed in the presence of extracts. The extracts prevented the aggregation and growth of formed CaOx particles and it kept the crystals as dispersed.

Betula utilis D. Don Family: Betulaceae

Shah *et al.* [135] evaluated the antiurolithiatic activity of alcoholic extract of *Betula utilis* in male Wistar rats. The administration of alcoholic extract of *Betula utilis* to rats with ethylene glycol-induced lithiasis significantly reduced all the elevated biochemical parameters (calcium, phosphate, oxalate, creatinine, BUN and uric acid), restored the urine pH to normal and increased the urine volume significantly when compared to the model control.

Biophytum sensitivum (L.) DC. Family: Oxalidaceae

Pawar and Vyawahare [136] investigated the anti-urolithiatic activity of standardized methanolic extract of whole plant of *B. sensitivum* (MBS) in rats. A significant decrease in urinary output was observed in the disc-implanted animals, which was prevented by the MBS treatment. Supplementation with MBS caused significant improvement in glomerular filtration rate and protein excretion. The elevated levels of serum creatinine, uric acid, and BUN were also prevented by the MBS treatment. The MBS treatment showed reduced formation of deposition around the implanted zinc disc. The higher dose of MBS (400 mg/kg) found more effective.

Chandavarkar *et al.* [137] evaluated the nephroprotective activity of different extracts of whole plant of *Biophytum sensitivum* in Wistar albino rats. Methanol and aqueous extracts of *B. sensitivum* possesses nephroprotective activity. The elevations of serum urea and creatinine produced by GM were considerably reduced and showed histopathological changes in the kidneys to normal.

Boerhavia diffusa L. Family: Nyctaginaceae

Raut *et al.* [138] investigated the effect of *Boerhavia diffusa* on anticrystal activity. The effect was assayed on microcrystals in 24-well microplates *in vitro*. The aqueous extract of *B. diffusa* has not shown crystal dissolving activity against MSUM.

In vitro study had been carried out by Chauhan *et al.* [139] on growth and inhibition of struvite crystals in the presence of herbal extract of *B. diffusa* by using single diffusion gel growth technique. After the gelation, equal amount of supernatant solution of 1.0 M magnesium acetate prepared with 0.5 and 1% concentrations of the herbal extract of *B. diffusa* were gently poured on the set gels in the respective test tubes in the aseptic medium. As the concentration of *B. diffusa* increased, the inhibition of crystals also increased in the gel media as well as the dissolution of crystals at the gel-liquid interface increases. The defragmentation of some grown crystals was also noticed.

The protective effect of *B. diffusa* leaf extract against mercury chloride toxicity was studied by Indhumathi *et al.* [140] in rats. Group 2 rats were administered intraperitonially with mercuric chloride (200mg/kg/b.w) is a nephrotoxicant for 5 days. Group 3 animals were administered with mercuric chloride followed by aqueous extract of *B. diffusa* leaves 200mg/kg/bw orally for 10 days. The elevated serum levels of Alkaline phosphatase, Acid phosphatase, AST, ALT, Lactate DHase, Urea, LPO, and Creatine were seen in mercuric chloride treated rats. Antioxidant enzymes such as GPx, reduced GSH, Vitamin C and CAT were elevated in animals treated with *B. diffusa* aqueous extract.

Pareta *et al.* [141] investigated the protective effect of aqueous extract of *B. diffusa* roots (BDE) in hyperoxaluric oxidative stress and renal cell injury. Oxalate excretion significantly increased in hyperoxaluric animals as compared to control which was protected in BDE-treated animals. BDE treatment significantly reduced level of MDA and improved the activity of antioxidant enzymes followed by reduction in BUN and serum creatinine. BDE reduced the number of CaOx monohydrate crystals in the urine. Histological analysis depicted that BDE treatment inhibited deposition of CaOx crystal and renal cell damage.

Effect of plant extract of *B. diffusa* was determined by Yasir and Waqar [142] on the formation of CaOx crystals. Effect on the number, size and type of CaOx crystals was observed. Results showed significant activity of the extract against CaOx crystallization at different concentrations. Size of the crystals gradually reduced with the increasing concentration of the extract. The number of CaOx monohydrate crystals which are injurious to epithelial cells gradually reduced and the highest concentration of extracts (100 mg/ml), completely disappeared.

Control of crystal size and formation of COD rather than COM crystals, in combination with the diuretic action of extracts is an important way to control urolithiasis.

The alcoholic extract of roots of *B. diffusa* (ABED) was evaluated by Chitra *et al.* [143] for its antilithiatic activity in Adult male albino Wistar rats. The AEBD reduced the elevated levels of crucial ions, *viz.* calcium, phosphate, uric acid and oxalate ions in urine. Also, it elevated the concentration of urinary magnesium, which is considered as one of the inhibitor of crystallization. The histopathological studies confirmed the induction as degenerated glomeruli, necrotic tubule and inflammatory cells was observed in the section of kidney from animals treated with ethylene glycol. This was reduced, however after treatment with AEBD.

Kulkarni *et al.* [144] evaluated the nephroprotective and anti-nephrotoxic properties of roots of *B. diffusa* by using GM induced nephrotoxic model in Wistar strain albino rats. The drug has shown both nephroprotective and anti-nephrotoxic action. Nephrotoxicity can be reversed as evidenced from the biochemical parameters as well as histopathology. Srinivas and Arun Kumar [145] assessed the effects of *B. diffusa* roots on urolithiatic rats. From the study, it was found that the alcoholic extract of plant parts was effective in *in-vivo* anti-urolithiatic activity on induced CaOx crystals in rats and found noteworthy in treatment of renal calculosis.

Karwasra *et al.* [146] evaluated the nephroprotective role of *B. diffusa* in cisplatin-induced acute kidney injury. *B. diffusa* at a dose of 200 mg/kg body weight significantly ameliorated increased serum creatinine, BUN, oxidative stress and inflammatory markers. In parallel to this, it also exhibited antiapoptotic activity through the reduction of active caspase-3 expression in kidneys.

Boldoa purpurascens Cav. Family: Nyctaginaceae

Boldoa purprasacens is used in traditional medicine in Cuba as antiurolithiatic. Mosquera *et al.* [147] evaluated the *in vitro* and *in vivo* antiurolothiatic activity of an aqueous extract from the leaves of *B. purpurascens*. The aqueous extract of *B. purpurascens* inhibited the slope of nucleation and aggregation of CaOx crystallization, and decreased the crystal density. It also inhibited the growth and caused the dissolution of CaOx crystals. At a dose of 400 mg/kg the extract reduced the concentration of uric acid in urine, as well as the serum concentration of uric acid and creatinine. Histopathologic analysis of the kidneys of the same treatment group revealed reduced tissue damage; the results were almost similar to the untreated healthy control group.

Bombax ceiba L. Family: Malvaceae

Gadge and Jalalpure [148] investigated the efficacy of *Bombax ceiba* fruit extracts as curative agents in experimentally induced CaOx urolithiatic rats. Supplementation with aqueous and ethanol extracts of *B. ceiba* fruit significantly reduced the elevated urinary oxalate, showing a regulatory action on endogenous oxalate synthesis. The increased deposition of stone forming constituents in kidneys of calculogenic rats was also significantly lowered with curative treatment of aqueous and ethanol extract.

Brassica nigra (L.) K.Koch Family: Brassicaceae

The protective effect of the methanol extract of *Brassica nigra* leaves was investigated by Rajamurugan *et al.* [149] against D-galactosamine (D-GalN)-induced nephrotoxicity in Wistar rats. The *B. nigra* pretreated groups (200 and 400 mg/kg bw) showed significant reduction in the DGalN-induced toxicity as obvious from biochemical parameters. Histopathological observations confirm the protective effect of *B. nigra* leaf extract by reduction in renal tissue damage. Results are comparable with that of the standard.

Brassica oleracea var. *gongylodes* Family: Brassicaceae and *Desmostachya bipinnata* Family: Poaceae

Naga Kishore *et al.* [150] evaluated the effects of *Brassica oleracea* var. *gongylodes* and *Desmostachya bipinnata* in combination and alone on experimentally-induced urolithiasis. Daily oral treatment with almost all extracts not only significantly decreased the quantity of CaOx deposited in the kidneys but also reverted all the biochemical changes induced by CaOx urolithiasis. Aqueous extract of both plants in combination and in alone was found to be significant when compared with standard and control group.

Brassica rapa L. Family: Brassicaceae

A study was conducted by Kim *et al.* [151] to evaluate the protective effect of the ethanol extract of the roots of *Brassica rapa* (EBR) in cisplatin-induced nephrotoxicity. Pretreatment of cells with EBR prevented cisplatin-induced decreases in cell viability and cellular GSH content. The effect of EBR was then investigated in rats given EBR for 14 d before cisplatin administration. Rats given EBR showed lower blood levels of BUN and creatinine, and of urinary LDH. EBR prevented the rise of MDA production and the induction of AO and XO activities. This extract also recovered the reduced activities of GPx, SOD and CAT.

Bridelia retusa (L.) A. Juss. Family: Phyllanthaceae

Cordeiro and Kaliwal [152] investigated nephroprotective activity of ethanolic and aqueous extracts of the stem bark of *Bridelia retusa* in CCl_4 treated female mice. The protective activity of the extracts was justified by the significant decrease in the weights of adrenal glands when compared to CCl_4 treated group and the weights of ovary was increased to that of the normal control group. The enzyme activity of ALT and LDH in the liver while that of ALT, AST, LDH and AKP (Alkaline phosphotase) in the kidney were significantly lowered in all the groups treated with extracts when compared to CCl_4 treated group and were found to be brought almost to normal control. The enzyme activity of ACP in the kidney was significantly increased in all the groups treated with extracts when compared to CCl_4 treated group and were found to be brought almost to normal control. The ATPase enzyme activity of kidney was significantly increased with respect to that of CCl_4 treated group.

Bryophyllum pinnatum (Lam.) Oken (Syn.: *Kalanchoe pinnata* Pers.) Family: Crassulaceae

Harlalka *et al.* [153] evaluated the protective effects of aqueous extract of *Bryophyllum pinnatumm* (Syn.: *Kalanchoe pinnata*) on GM-induced nephrotoxicity in rats. GM-induced glomerular congestion, peritubular and blood vessel congestion, epithelial desquamation, accumulation of inflammatory cells and necrosis of the kidney cells were found to be reduced in the group receiving the leaf extract of *B. pinnatum* along with GM. This extract also normalized the GM-induced increases in urine and plasma creatinine, blood urea and BUN levels.

Hydroalcoholic extract of *B. pinnatum* was found to exert significant diuresis and antiurolithitic activity when given by oral and ip routes to rats [154].

Effect of *B. pinnatum* extract was determined by Yasir and Waqar [142] on the CaOx crystals formatiom. Results showed significant activity of the extract against CaOx crystallization at different concentrations. Size of the crystals gradually reduced with the increasing concentration of the extract. The number of CaOx monohydrate crystals which are injurious to epithelial cells gradually reduced and at the highest concentration of extracts (100 mg/ml) completely disappeared. Control of crystal size and formation of COD rather than COM crystals, in combination with the diuretic action of extracts is an important way to control urolithiasis.

Clinical efficacy and safety profile of *B. pinnatum* juice for treatment of lithiasis by performing a non comparative open clinical study was carried out by Gahlaut *et al.* [155]. Patients having <10mm stones were treated with fresh juice of *B.*

pinnatum leaves in a single dose of 10 ml/day × 30 days. Among the 23 patients who underwent the treatment, 64% patients had medium renal stones (<10mm in diameter) and 36% had small sized (<5mm in diameter) stones at different locations. A clinical effective improvement was observed in 87% patients while 13% patients showed moderate improvement. Out of five patients of colilithiasis three patients showed effective improvement and two patients showed moderate improvement. Biochemical assays showed that oxalate excretion and super-saturation of CaOx was decreased in treated patients.

Evaluation of anti-urolithiatic effect of aqueous extract of *B. pinnatum* leaves in male Wistar rats was carried out by Shukla *et al.* [156]. Aqueous extract of leaves of *B. pinnatum* reduced urine oxalate level significantly, as compared with ethylene glycol control. Serum creatinine and blood urea level were improved significantly in all aqueous extract of leaves of *B. pinnatum*-treated groups. Relative kidney weight and CaOx depositions were found significantly reduced in animals received ABP as compared with untreatedGroup.

Phatak *et al.* [157] explored anti-urolithiatic activities of *B. pinnatum* leaves extract by utilizing different *in-vitro* models. In dissolution models, the extract of *B. pinnatum* has greater capability to dissolve CaOx. The extract of *B. pinnatum* exhibited inhibitory action in both of nucleation and aggregation assays to significant level.

Effects on experimentally induced *in vivo* lithiatic model was investigated by Yadav *et al.* [158], who found that treatment with leaf extract of *B. pinnatum* effectively reversed oxidative and histological damages in kidneys as well as attenuated the evaluation in urinary parameters and serum biochemical parameters of animals exposed to EG.

Butea monosperma (Lam.) Taub. Family: Fabaceae

Protective effect of *Butea monosperma* flowers (BMF) against GM-induced nephrotoxicity in male Wistar rats was evaluated by Maheshwari *et al.* [159]. Methanol extract of *B. monosperma* (BMF) at a dose rate of 100 mg/kg p.o. and 200 mg/kg p.o. showed a significant reduction in serum creatinine, BUN and serum urea levels. These effects were predominant with 200 mg/kg.

Sonkar *et al.* [160] evaluated the nephroprotective potential of *B. monosperma*. Nephrotoxicity was induced by GM. Urine creatinine, serum urea, and BUN were found to be significantly increased in rats treated with only GM; whereas, treatment with the ethanolic extract of leaf of *B. monosperma* reversed the effect of GM.

Brijesh *et al.* [161] investigated the possible benefits of n-butanolic fraction (NBF) of *B. monosperma* flowers in doxorubicin (DOX) induced nephritic syndrome in rats. NBF significantly reduced proteinuria, hypoalbuminemia, dyslipidemia and restored renal antioxidant enzymes activities like SOD, CAT and GSH. Histopathological studies have supported biochemical findings with no evidence of vacuolization and reduction of glomerular sclerosis in NBF treated rats.

The effect of aqueous extracts of dried seeds powder of *B. monosperma* against Ethylene glycol induced renal calculi in albino Wistar rats has been studied Sikandari *et al.* [162]. Oral administration of *B. monosperma* aqueous suspension to ethylene glycol induced urolithic rats (2g/kg body wt/day) had reduced the concentration of calcium, oxalate, BUN, creatinine, phosphorous, and diminished the crystals deposition in the kidneys.

Caesalpinia bonduc (L.) Roxb. [Syn.: *C. bonducella* (L.) Fleming] Family: Fabaceae

Noorani *et al.* [163] evaluated the protective effect of methanolic leaf extract of *Caesalpinia bonduc* on GM-induced nephrotoxicity in rats. Administration of methanolic extract of *C.bonduc* before gentamicin exposure prevented severe alterations of biochemical parameters and disruptions of liver structure. This was supported by histopathological study.

Calendula officinalis L. Family: Asteraceae

Protective role of the flower extract of *Calendula officinalis* against and cisplatin-induced nephrotoxicity has been shown [164]. Possible mechanism of action of the flower extract may be due to its antioxidant activity and reduction of oxygen radicals [165].

Calotropis procera (Aiton) Dryand Family: Apocynaceae

The possible nephroprotective activities of the ethanolic extract of *Calotropis procera* root in female rats were investigated by Dahiru *et al.* [166]. Administration of 150 and 300 mg/kg bw of the ethanolic extract of *C. procera* root did not protect the liver and kidney from CCl_4 - induced toxicity. Pretreatment with the extract rather potentiated the toxicity induced by CCl_4.

Protective role of aqueous extract of *C. procera* flowers on GM-induced nephrotoxicity in rabbit model was evaluated by Javed *et al.* [167]. Co-administration of plant extract with GM reduced the GM induced toxic effects by restoring the renal function markers *i.e.* BUN, serum urea, serum creatinine and electrolytes indicating the protective potential of plant extract. Disturbance in hematological parameters induced by GM was attenuated by the administration of plant extract. In addition, *C. procera* extract increased the antioxidant enzyme CAT and decreased the serum total oxidant status along with protective effects evidenced by histopathological evaluation.

Canarium schweinfurthii Engl. Family: Burseraceae

Okwuosa *et al.* [168] evaluated the protective effects of aqueous and methanol extracts of stem bark of *Canarium schweinfurthii* on acetaminophen-induced nephrotoxicity in rats. Blood urea and serum creatinine levels were significantly higher in acetaminophen and negative control groups compared to baseline control group and the AE and ME groups. Histopathological examination showed that the extracts presereved the renal histoarchitecture while the acetaminophen and negative control groups showed varying degrees of inflammatory cells infiltration, necrosis, tubular casts, tubular erosion and increased urinary pole.

Capparis spinosa L. Family: Capparaceae

Kalantar *et al.* [169] investigated the protective effect of *Capparis spinosa* extract on cyclophosphamide-induced nephrotoxicity in mice. A significant increase in the levels of MDA, Cr, and BUN and a reduction of GSH by CP administration. Pre-treatment with CSE decreased the levels of MDA, Cr, and BUN. GSH increased in all doses, but the most significant alteration was observed in the doses of 200 and 400 mg/kg. The nephroprotective effect of the CSE was confirmed by the histological examination of the kidneys.

Tlilia *et al.* [170] explored the nephroprotective effect of methanolic extract of *C. spinosa* leaves (MECS).

Carica papaya L. Family: Cucurbitaceae

Olagunju *et al.* [171] evaluated nephroprotective activity of seed extract of *Carica papaya* in CCl_4-induced renal toxicity in rats. Elevations in the measured biochemical parameters were significantly attenuated in rats pre-treated with the graded oral doses of the extract, in dose related fashion. Maximum nephroprotection was offered by the extract at 400 mg/kg/day CPE which lasted up to 3 hours post-CCl_4 exposure and these biochemical evidences were corroborated by improvements in the renal histological lesions induced by CCl_4 intoxication.

The fruit of *C. papaya* used in indigenous medicine for the treatment of urinary stones. Nayeem *et al.* [172] evaluated the antiurolithatic effects of the aqueous and alcoholic extracts of the fruit of *C. papaya* on ethylene glycol (EG) induced urolithiatic rats. Treatment with aqueous and alcoholic extracts of *C. papaya* fruit significantly reduced the elevated urinary oxalate, showing a regulatory action on endogenous oxalate synthesis. The increased deposition of stone forming constituents in the kidneys of calculogenic rats was also significantly lowered by curative and preventive treatment using aqueous and alcoholic extracts of the fruits of *C. papaya*.

Debnath *et al*. [173] investigated the protective evaluation of ethanolic extract of the papaya seed against Cisplatin-inducede nephrotoxicity. The ethanolic extract exhibited protection against cisplatin-induced nephrotoxicity, which were proved by the gross behavioural studies, histopathological, renal function and biochemical studies. Antioxidant studies and Histopathological investigations also supported the nephroprotective activity of these seeds.

Carthamus tinctorius L. Family: Asteraceae

The aqueous and alcoholic seed extracts of *Carthamus tinctorius* were tested by Patil *et al*. [174] on rats to assess nephroprotective activity using body weight, serum urea, serum creatinine and diuretic activity by using urine volume, urine concentration of Na+, K+ and Cl-. The extracts contained flavonoids, steroids and alkaloids and showed significant nephroprotective and diuretic activities.

The effects of Flos carthami (FC) (600 and 1200 mg/day, by gastric gavages), was evaluated on CaOx formation in ethylene glycol (EG)-fed rats. Kidney tissue was histopathologically examined using a polarized light microscope, and crystal deposits were evaluated by a semi-quantitative scoring method; these scores were significantly lower in the FC groups (600 and 1200 mg/day) than in the placebo group [175].

Carum carvi L. Family: Apiaceae

Sadiq *et al*. [176] assessed the effect of aqueous extract of *Carum carvi* seeds in experimentally induced diabetic nephropathy (DN) in rats. 60 mg/kg body weight of *C. carvi* dose significantly decreased the levels of the biochemical parameters like serum levels of glucose, urea, creatinine, total urinary protein and microalbuminuric levels.

The protective effect of aqueous extract of *C. carvi* seeds was evaluated in experimentally induced diabetic nephropathy (DN) in rats. 30 and 60 mg/kg body weight of *C. carvi* significantly decreased the levels of the biochemical parameters. High dose of *C. carvi* aqueous seeds extract (60 mg/kg) showed renoprotection against STZ induced diabetic nephropathy in rats. The renoprotective effect of *C. carvi* essential oil (10 mg/kg of body weights orally) was also studied in diabetic rats. Diabetic rats showed an increase in the serum level of glucose, and decrease in GPx. 10 mg/kg body weight of *C. carvi* oil significantly corrected these parameters. The kidney of *C. carvi* essential oil treated rats showed marked improvement with minor pathological changes [177].

Carum copticum (L.) Benth. & Hook.f. Family: Apiaceae

Swamiranga Reddy *et al.* [178] evaluated the antiurolithiatic activity of *Carum copticum* seeds on ethylene glycol induced urolithiasis in male albino rats. Parameters like urea, uric acid, creatinine, calcium, potassium in serum analysis and ultrasound scanning were used assess the activity. Three different doses *i.e.*, 100, 200 and 300 mg/kg body weight of *C. copticum* were used. The results indicated that the dose 300 mg/kg body weight of *C. copticum* is efficient dose when compared with standard drug of Cystone.

Cassia auriculata L. Family: Fabaceae

The ethanol extract of the roots of *Cassia auriculata* was studied by Shirwaikar *et al.* [179] for its protective activity in cisplatin- and GM-induced nephrotoxicity in male albino rats. In the cisplatin model, the extract at doses of 300 and 600 mg/kg body wt. reduced elevated blood urea and serum creatinine and normalized the histopathological changes in the curative regimen. In the GM model, the ethanol extract at a dose of 600 mg/kg body wt. reduced blood urea and serum creatinine effectively in both the curative and the preventive regimen.

Cassia fistula L. Family: Fabaceae

Sodium oxalate induced urolithiasis in rats model was used to evaluate anti-urolithiatic activity of the wood bark extracts of *Cassia fistula* in wistar rats [180]. Methanolic and aqueous extracts showed significant increase in the elimination of normal urine parameters and there by reduced their concentration in the serum when compared to control group. In the urine microscopy and histology of the kidney samples, control group showed maximum crystal deposition, kidney samples of the animals pretreated with methanolic extract and aqueous extract showed moderate to mild crystal deposition. In evaluation of diuretic activity, methanolic and aqueous extracts of *Cassia fistula* were significantly increased urine output and elimination of sodium and chlorides when compared to normal group.

Cassia occidentalis L. Family: Fabaceae

The protective activity of the 70% hydroalcoholic extract of *Cassia occidentalis*

(HACO) was assessed by Gowrisri *et al.* [181] against GM-induced nephrotoxicity in rats. The treatment with HACO (200 and 400 mg/kg body weight) markedly reduced GM-induced elevation of urinary sodium, potassium electrolytes, urinary glucose, blood urea and creatinine levels. It also increased the body weight and urinary creatinine. The comparative histopathological study of kidney exhibited almost normal architecture as compared to control group.

Ntchapda *et al.* [182] assessed the putative diurtic properties of *C. occidentalis* leaves' aqueous extract. Administration of *C.occidentalis* increased the urinary excretion of 107.58% at the higher dose tested, compared to negative control.. Acutely, the extract induced Na^+ and Cl^- elimination, whereas subchronically an increase in K^+ elimination was also observed. The extract also improved the kidney function indexes and oxidative stress markers. These effects were dose-dependent and comparable with positive control observations.

Casuarina equisetifolia L. Family: Casuarinaceae

El-Tantawy *et al.* [183] carried out the protective activity of methanolic extract of *Casuarina equisetifolia* leaves in GM-induced nephrotoxicity in Wistar rats. Administration of plant extract at a dose of 300 mg/kg once daily for 4 weeks restored normal renal functions and attenuated oxidative stress.

Cedrus deodara (Roxb.) G. Don Family: Pinaceae

The petroleum ether extract of the heart wood of *Cedrus deodara* (PECD) was assessed by Ramesh *et al.* [184] for its diuretic and anti-urolithiatic activity. PECD (100 and 200 mg/kg) was orally gavaged daily 1 h before sodium oxalate (NaOx) administration for 10 days. Concomitant administration of PECD for 10 days along with NaOx prevented elevated serum biochemical levels due to the elimination of these in urine. Histology of the kidneys also indicated that PECD treatment had protected against NaOx induced nephroliathiasis.

Ceiba pentandra (L.) Gaertn. Family: Malvaceae

The effect of oral administration of aqueous and alcohol extracts of bark of *Ceiba pentandra* on CaOx urolithiasis has been studied in male albino wistar rats by Choubey *et al.* [185]. Supplementation with aqueous and alcohol extracts of bark of *Ceiba pentandra* significantly reduced the elevated urinary oxalate showing a regulatory action on endogenous oxalate synthesis. The increased deposition of stone forming constituents in the kidneys of calculogenic rats was significantly lowered by preventive treatment using aqueous and alcohol extracts.

Celosia argentea L. Family: Amaranthaceae

Traditionally *Celosia argentea* seeds were used as diuretic. Joshi *et al.* [186] evaluated antiurolithiatic activity of ethanolic extract of *C. argentea* seeds in ethylene glycol induced urolithiasis in rats. Treated groups showed significant antiurolithiatic activity which was comparable with the standard drug.

Kachchhi *et al.* [187] evaluated the antiurolithiatic activity of methanolic extract of *C. argentea* roots (CaME) in male albino wistar rats. Treatment groups significantly prevented improvement in urinary pH, diuresis and body weight. All the treatments significantly prevented the rise in promoters like calcium, oxalate, uric acid, and inorganic phosphate and increased the levels of magnesium and citrate like inhibitors in various biological samples. Renal function impairment and oxidative stress was also prevented by the treatment as observed by BUN and creatinine analysis and analysis of MDA, proteins, CAT and histopathology respectively.

Centratherum anthelminticum (L.) Kuntze Family: Asteraceae

Ashok *et al.* [188] investigated the potential of *Centratherum anthelminticum* in the treatment of renal calculi against ethylene glycol induced nephrolithiasis in rats. Petroleum ether, chloroform and alcoholic extracts of *C. anthelminticum* seeds were evaluated for antiurolithiatic activity. Supplementation with alcoholic extract of *C. anthelminticum* seeds significantly reduced the elevated levels of oxalae, calcium and phosphate in urinary excretion. Curative and preventive treatment using alcohol extract significantly lowered the increased deposition of stone forming constituents in the kidneys of calculogenic rats.

Galani and Panchal [189] evaluated the protect effect of treatment of methanolic extract of *C. anthelminticum* seeds (CAE) (200 mg/kg and 400 mg/kg, p.o.) against ethylene glycol induced nephrolithiasis in rats. Simultaneous treatment with CAE significantly reduced stone forming promoters (calcium, oxalate, phosphate, creatinine, urea, uric acid), enhanced stone forming inhibitors (magnesium) with significant antioxidant activity in a dose dependent manner. Antiurolithiatic effect of CAE was also confirmed by histopathological changes in kidney tissue. The protective action of CAE was comparable to Cystone.

Ceratonia siliqua L. Family: Fabaceae

The protective effect of *Ceratonia siliqua* pods and leaves was investigated by Ahmed [190] using cisplatin-induced renal damage in mice. The concentration of serum creatinine and urea in the *C. siliqua* pods (200 mg/kg body weight) treated group were reduced to 57.5% and 51.5%, respectively, with respect to the control group. Cisplatin induced decline of renal antioxidant enzymes such as SOD, CAT, GPx activities, but the treatment of carob pods and leaves significantly attenuated the cisplatin-induced nephrotoxicity. Both pods and leaves of carob at 100 and 200 mg/kg increased the concentration of reduced GSH and protected against the increase of cisplatin-induced lipid peroxidation. The treatment of carob pods and leaves (100 and 200 mg/kg, p.o.) improved the activity of lysosomal enzymes nearly to the normal group.

Ceropegia bulbosa Family: Apocynaceae

Hydroalcoholic extract from leaves of *C.bulbosa* possess significant antiurolithiatic activity in rats [191].

Cestrum nocturnum Family: Solanaceae

Saleem *et al.* [192] evaluated the protective and curative effects of methanolic extract of *Cestrum nocturnum* leaves in rabbits against GM-induced nephrotoxicity. A significant decrease was found in total oxidant status, BUN, serum creatinine and uric acid levels whereas albumin level increased significantly. Histopathological studies also revealed nephroprotective and nephrocurative effects.

Chamaerops humilis L. Family: Arecaceae

Beghalia *et al.* [193] studied the effect of herbal extract of *Chamaerops humilis* on the CaOx crystals *in vitro*. Extract of *C. humilis* was studied as inhibitor. The crystallisation of CaOx monohydrate occurred in the absence of inhibitor and was calculated at 5, 10, 15, 20, 25 and 30 minutes, by polarised light microscopy. The same procedure was followed for the study of CaOx monohydrate crystallisation in the presence of *C. humilis* extract. A series of concentrations of 25, 50, 75, and 100% of these extracts were studied. With the addition of *C. humilis* the best inhibitory concentrations 94.86% and 93.07% were encountered at the concentration of 25% and 50% respectively after 30 minutes.

Inhibition of CaOx monohydrate crystal growth using aqueous extract of sheath of *C. humilis* was investigated by Beghalia *et al.* [193]. Activity was tested in bioassays. In the presence of plants extract, the length and the width of the crystals were reduced. It was found that extracts of plants used in this study inhibited potently the growth phase. Inhibition was 94.86% at 25% concentration, 93.07% at 50% concentration, 88.54% at 75% concentration and 88.66 at 100% concentration.

Chenopodium album L. Family: Amaranthaceae

Sikarwar *et al.* [194] evaluated the effect of methanolic (CAME) and aqueous extracts (CAAE) of leaves of *Chenopodium album* on experimentally-induced urolithiasis in rats. The treatment with CAME or CAAE for 28 days significantly attenuated the EG-induced elevations in the urine and plasma levels of calcium, phosphorus, urea, uric acid and creatinine along with decrease in urine volume, pH and oxalates. The treatments also decreased renal tissue oxalate and deposition of oxalate crystals in kidney due to EG treatment. The effects of CAME and CAAE were comparable to standard antilithiatic agent, cystone.

Cicer arietinum L. Famiy: Fabaceae

The diuretic and anti-nephrolithiasis activities of *Cicer arietinum* ethanolic seed extract were evaluated in albino rats. The extract decreased urinary stones in the kidney with good diuretic property [195].

Biglarkhani *et al.* [196] assessed the efficacy and safety of *C. arietinum* in patients with renal stone. In the *C. arietinum* group, complete stone dissolution occurred in 9 (23.7%) patients and reduced stone size was observed in 17 (44.7%) patients while no response to treatment was observed in placebo group. The mean stone size was reduced from 7.15 ± 1.34 mm to 4.28 ± 3.09 mm in the *C. arietinum* group and was increased from 7.08 ± 1.09 mm to 7.15 ± 1.09 mm in the placebo group. The changes of the urinary volume and magnesium level were significantly higher in the treatment group. .

Cichorium intybus L. Family: Asteraceae

Noori and Mahboob [197] evaluated the protective effect of *Cichorium intybus* on Cisplatin – induced toxicity in male Albino Wistar rats. At a dose of 500 mg/kg b.w. of *C. intybus* pretreatment showed partial counter action on the electrolytes imbalances and Na+ -K+ -ATPase activity.

Cinnamomum tamala (Buch.-Ham.) Nees & Eberm. Family: Lauraceae

Ullah *et al.* [198] investigated the nephroprotective effect of *Cinnamomum tamala* against GM-induced nephrotoxicity in rabbits. Animals treated with GM and *C. tamala* significantly protected rabbit kidney from structural and functional changes associated with GM.

Cinnamomum zeylanicum Blume Family: Lauraceae

Mishra *et al.* [199] evaluated the ameliorative effect of the cinnamon oil upon early stage diabetic nephropathy owing to its antioxidant and antidiabetic effect.

Histological studies of the kidney proved the protective effect of cinnamon oil by reducing the glomerular expansion, eradicating hyaline casts, and decreasing the tubular dilatations. Their results indicate that the volatile oil from cinnamon contains more than 98% cinnamaldehyde and that it confers dose-dependent, significant protection against alloxan-induced renal damage, the maximum decrease in fasting blood glucose having been achieved at the dose of 20 mg/kg.

Ullah *et al*. [200] explored the nephroprotective effects of the plant. *C. zeylanicum* significantly attenuated renal functional and histological changes associated with GM as assessed by urea, creatinine, uric acid, electrolytes, urinary protein, and histopathological examination. The plant extract successfully proved to have strong nephroprotective properties, especially against aminoglycosides induced nephrotoxicities.

Cissampelos pareira L. Family: Menispermaceae

Reddy *et al*. [201] examined the protective activity of the whole plant extract of *Cissampelos pareira* in paracetamol induced nephrotoxic rats. The treatment with 70% hydroalcoholic extract of *C. pareira* whole plant (HACP) (200 and 400 mg/kg body weight, p.o) markedly reduced paracetamol induced elevation of urinary sodium, potassium electrolytes, urinary glucose, blood urea and creatinine levels. It also increased the body weights and urinary creatinine. In addition treatment with HACP significantly restored the tissue SOD, CAT, GSH and reduced the LP.

Reddy *et al*. [202] evaluated the potential nephroprotective and antioxidant activity of hydroalcoholic *C. pareira* whole plant extract using GM-induced rats. For acute toxicity testing rats administered with the extract at a dose 2 g/kg, the result showed no toxicity. Hydroalcoholic *C. pareira* whole plant extract (200 and 400 mg/kg p.o) significantly decreased the elevated urinary glucose levels in the urine, decrease the elevated urea and creatinine levels in blood and increase the urinary creatinine levels in GM-induced nephrotoxic rats. There were a dose dependent decreasing and increasing of lipid peroxidation, GSH levels in hydoalcoholic extract treated groups respectively.

Sayana *et al*. [203] evaluated the antiurolithic activity of aqueous extract of roots of *C. pareira* (AQERCP) in 2% ammonium chloride and 0.75% ethylene glycol-induced urolithiasis in albino rats. Rats treated with 3 doses of AQERCP significantly reduced urinary calcium, uric acid and increased urinary magnesium levels, reduced serum calcium, creatinine and increased serum magnesium. Histopathology of kidneys in groups treated with AQERCP at 200 mg/kg and 400 mg/kg doses revealed less tissue damage and the cytology of nephrotic tissue was almost similar to the control rats.

Citrullus colocynthis (L.) Schrad. Family: Cucurbitaceae

The nephroprotective effect of *Citrullus colocynthis* fruits extract was investigated in streptozotocin induced diabetes in rats. *C. colocynthis* fruits extract caused significant decrease in blood glucose, urea, creatinine, microalbuminuria and uric acid, while, GSH, GPx and SOD were significantly increased in comparison with diabetic untreated group. The histopathological findings coincided with biochemical findings in both diabetic and treated groups [204].

Komolafe *et al*. [205] investigated the effect of four herbal extracts and their efficacy on the histomorphometry of the kidney in STZ induced diabetic rats. The histology and morphometric analysis revealed that the kidney in the group treated with *C. colocynthis* showed significant increase in density compared to control.

Ullah *et al*. [206] explored the protective potentials of *C. colocynthis* against GM induced nephrotoxicity due to its strong antioxidant properties. Authors reported that co-theapy of *C. colocynthis* with GM for twenty one days, failed to protect renal injury associated with GM in spite of its strong antioxidant properties.

Citrus aurantium L. Family: Rutaceae

Ullah *et al*. [207] evaluated the protective role of *C. aurantium* against GM induced renal damage. Animals treated with co-administration of *C. aurantium* and GM protected renal damage expected with GM, assessed by known functional and morphological parameters, significantly different from animals treated with GM.

Citrus limon (L.) Osbeck Family: Rutaceae

Influence of inhibition of citric acid and lemon juice to the growth of calcium hydrogen phosphate dihydrate urinary crystals was investigated by Joshi and Joshi [208]. The growth velocity measurements indicated maximum inhibition in case or calcium chloride + lemon juice + natural urine containing solution.

Analysis by Touhami *et al*. [209] showed that the rats treated with ethylene glycol (EG)/ammonium chloride (AC) alone had higher amounts of calciumin the kidneys compared to negative control rats. This EG/AC-induced increase in kidney calcium levels was inhibited by the administration of lemon juice. Histology showed that rats treated with sEG/AC alone had large deposits of CaOx crystals in all parts of the kidney, and that such deposits were not present in rats also treated with either 100% or 75% lemon juice.

Kulaksizoglu *et al*. [210] studied the effects of *Citrus limon* and *Citrus sinensis* juices on CaOx crystallization *in vitro*. The effects on CaOx crystal growth of trisodium citrate, lemon and orange juices were examined. The effects of lemon and orange juices were evaluated by the addition of 50 ml of juices. Lemon juice was also found to inhibit the rate of crystal nucleation and aggregation. But orange juice did not have any effect on the CaOx crystallization.

Citrus medica L. Family: Rutaceae

Chauhan and Joshi [211] carried out study on growth and inhibition of struvite crystals in the presence of the juice of *Citrus medica* by using single diffusion gel growth technique. From the study of growth-inhibition behavior of struvite crystals, it was found that *C. medica* inhibits the growth of the crystals.

Shah *et al*. [212] evaluated the effect of *C. medica* in urolithiasis induced by ethylene glycol model. Both cystone and extract of *C. medica* showed significant increase in physical parameters and stone forming inhibitors and significant decrease in stone forming promoters. Degree of oxidative stress reduced with cystone and in treatment group.

Al-Yahya *et al*. [213] evaluated the protective activity of the ethanolic extract of *C. medica* 'Otroj' (EEOT) against GM-induced renal toxicity in rats. Administration of EEOT significantly protected kidney tissues against nephrotoxic effect of GM as evident from amelioration of the marker enzymes and lipid peroxidation and elevated NP-SH and TP levels, besides some indices of histopathological alterations. The MTT-test showed a 48% protection at a concentration of 1 mg/ml.

Citrus paradisii Macfad. Family: Rutaceae

Goldfarb and Asplin [214] studied the effect of grapefruit juice consumption on urinary chemistry and measures of lithogenicity. Urine volume and creatinine excretion were the same during the control and experimental periods. The results do not demonstrate an effect of grapefruit juice for increasing lithogenicity. The basis of the observations of epidemiological studies remain unexplained.

Trinchieri *et al*. [215] investigated changes in urinary stone risk factors after administration of a soft drink containing grapefruit juice. Seven healthy subjects, with no history of kidney stones, were submitted to an acute oral load (20 ml/kg body weight over 60 min) of a soft drink containing grapefruit juice diluted (10%) in mineral water. Urinary flow was significantly increased after both grapefruit juice (46+/-26 *vs* 186+/-109 ml/h) and mineral water (42+/-16 *vs* 230+/-72 ml/h) compared to baseline. Compared to mineral water, grapefruit juice significantly increased urinary excretion of citrate (25.8+/-9.3 *vs* 18.7+/-6.2 mg/h), calcium (6.7+/-4.3 *vs* 3.3+/-2.3 mg/h) and magnesium (2.9+/-1.5 *vs* 1.0+/-0.7 mg/h).

Citrus fruit juices could represent a natural alternative to potassium citrate in the management of nephrolithiasis.

Citrus sinensis (L.) Osbeck Family: Rutaceae

The risk of forming CaOx stones significantly diminshed when women drank 1/2 liter of orange juice daily, their urinary pH value and citric acid excretion increased [216].

Cleistocalyx nervosum A. Cunn. ex DC. var. *paniala* (Roxb.) J.A.N. Parnell Family: Myrtaceae

Poontawee *et al.* [217] studied the effect of *Cleistocalyx nervosum* var. *paniala* fruit extract (CNFE) on cadmium-induced nephrotoxicity. Cadmium-induced nephrotoxicity was diminished in rats supplemented with CNFE, particularly at the doses of 1 and 2 g/kg..

Clerodendrum inerme (L.) Gaertn. Family: Lamiaceae

The diuretic activity of chloroform and ethanolic extract of leaves of *Clerodendrum inerme* was investigated in rats. 200 and 400 mg/kg of both extracts showed good diuretic activity after 24 hr [218].

Clerodendron trichotomum Thunb. Family: Verbenaceae

Lu *et al.* [219] assessed the action of the herb *Clerodendron trichotomum* on renal function, the extract was administered to rats and dogs. Intravenous administration of the extract elicited renal vasodilation and increased urine flow and urinary sodium excretion.

Clitoria ternatea L. Family: Fabaceae

Clitoria ternatea roots or their extract in 95% alcohol showed no significant diuretic or natriuretic effect in dogs when administered orally in non-toxic dose. Intravenous doses of the extract led to a moderate increase in the excretion of sodium and potassium in the urine, but at the same time, it showed signs of kidney damage [220].

Sarumathy *et al.* [221] evaluated the protective activity of the ethanol extract of *C. ternatea* on acetaminophen induced toxicity in rats. Increase in the levels of serum urea and creatinine along with an increase in the body weight and reduction in the levels of uric acid in acetaminophen induced groups are retrieved significantly by treatment with *C. ternatea* extracts at two different doses. The antioxidant studies reveal that the levels of renal SOD, CAT, GSH and GPx in the APAP treated animals are increased significantly along with a reduced MDA content in ethanol extract of *C. ternatea* treated groups. Apart from these, histopathological changes also reveal the protective nature of the *C. ternatea* extract against acetaminophen induced necrotic damage of renal tissues.

Coix lacryma-jobi L. Family: Poaceae

Antiurolithic property of *Coix lacryma-jobi* was assessed by Devi *et al.* [222] by subjecting different extracts of this plant for its decrystallizing property. The aqueous extract can decrystallize renal calculi.

Cola nitida (Vent.) Schott. & Endl. Family: Malvaceae

Evaluation of nephroprotective properties of aqueous and ethanolic extracts of *Cola nitida* against GM induced renal dysfunction in the albino rats was carried out by Abou *et al.* [223]. The results showed that intra-peritoneal injection of GM causes a significant decrease of total serum rate of protein and a significant raise in serum rate of creatinine and urea. The results also showed a significant increase in total protein and albumin in the urine of animals. However, changes in biochemical parameters measured were significantly attenuated in co-treated rats with the extracts of *C. nitida*. Treatment with the extracts significantly attenuated levels of serum creatinine, serum urea, serum protein, proteinuria and albuminuria.

Coleus aromaticus Benth. Family: Lamiaceae

Auqueous extract of the leaves of *Coleus aromaticus* was evaluated by Ghosh *et al.* [224] for the antiurolithiatic activity against CaOx stones in male albino rats. The water extract of *C. aromaticus* (0.5 g/kg and 1.0 g/kg, once, orally for 30 days) was found to be effective in reducing deposition of CaOx.

Combretum micranthum G. Don Family: Combretaceae

The protective effects of a hydroalcoholic extract of *Combretum micranthum* (CM) against cisplatin (CP)-induced renal damage was evaluated by Kpemissi *et al.* [225, 226] using *in vitro* human embryonic kidney (HEK)-293 cells and *in vivo* experiments. Co-treatment of HEK-293 cells with CP and CM extract at varying concentrations resulted in significant enhancement of cell growth compared to CP treatment indicating the cytoprotective activity of CM with an EC_{50} 8.136 µg/mL. Pre-treatment with CM normalized the renal function by ameliorating the CP-induced renal damage markers, oxidative stress and histopathological variations.

Commiphora wightii (Arn.) Bhandari Family: Burseraceae

Chauhan *et al.* [227] carried out study on growth and inhibition of struvite crystals in the presence of extract of *Commiphora wightii* by using single diffusion gel growth technique. From the study of growth and inhibition behavior of struvite crystals, it was found that *C. wightii* inhibits the growth of the struvite.

Raut *et al.* [138] screened anticrystal activity of *C. wightii* against basic calcium phosphate (BCP), calcium pyrophosphate (CPPD) and monosodium urate monohydrate (MSUM). The aqueous extracts of *C. wightii* have shown crystal dissolving activity against MSUM.

Convolvulus arvensis L. Family: Convolvulaceae

The diuretic effect of the *Convolvulus arvensis* root extracts were assessed by Sharma and Verma [228] in rats. The aqueous and ethanol extracts (50 and 100 mg/kg) of the root extract of *C. arvensis* produced time dependent increase in urine output. Electrolyte excretion was also significantly affected by the extracts. The aqueous extract increased the urine excretion of $Na+$, $K+$ and HCO_3-. In contrast, the ethanol extract increased the excretion of HCO_3-, decreased the loss of $K+$ and had little effect on renal removal of $Na+$. The high-ceiling diuretic, furosemide increased the renal excretion of $Na+$ and $Cl-$; but had no effect on $K+$ and HCO_3- loss.

Rajeshwari *et al.* [229] evaluated the *in vitro* anti-urolithiasis activity of leaves and flower infusions of *Convolvulus arvensis*. Crystal formation in synthetic urine was studied at different time intervals using leaf and flower infusions at different concentrations 10, 25, 50, 75,100 mg/ml each respectively. Among the two extracts when compared to control group, the inhibitory potency of leaf extract was found to be more significant, than the flower extract.

Copaifera langsdorffii Desf. Family: Fabaceae

Brancalion *et al.* [230] reported that the extract of leaves of *Copaifera langsdorffii* rich in flavonoids might prevent rats from urolithiasis by dispersing the particles of CaOx in urine to facilitate elimination, diminishing the number of calculi formed and reducing the pressure required to break the calculi.

Coriandrum sativum L. Family: Apiaceae

The acute diuretic activity of aqueous extract of the seed of *Coriandrum sativum* was evaluated in rats. The crude aqueous extract of coriander seeds increased diuresis, excretion of electrolytes, and glomerular filtration rate in a dose-dependent manner [231].

Costus afer Ker-Gawl. Family: Zingiberaceae

Ezejiofor *et al*. [232] evaluated the protective effect of the water extract of *Costus afer* leaves in male albino Wistar rats with GM-induced nephrotoxicity. The water extract of *C. afer* increased the feed intake and fluid intake in a dose dependent manner when compared with the GM-treated group. Low and medium doses of the extract reversed the deleterious effect of GM on the kidney. The extract also significantly decreased the absolute kidney weight and relative kidney weight when compared with the corresponding weights in the GM-treated group. *C. afer* significantly decreased serum sodium, blood urea, and serum creatinine levels and significantly increased serum potassium level in GM-induced nephrotoxic rats.

Costus arabicus L. Family: Zingiberaceae

de Cogain *et al*. [233] assessed the inhibitory activity of *Costus arabicus* on CaOx crystallization and the interaction of CaOx crystals with the renal epithelium. Aqueous extracts of *C. arabicus* decreased crystal growth in a concentration-dependent fashion. Precoating crystals with *C. arabicus* extract prevented their adhesion to MDCK cells, while pretreating cells did not show any effect. The extract was non-cytotoxic in concentrations of at least 1 mg/ml, which is likely above concentrations achievable in the urine following oral ingestion and excretion. No inhibitory activity was found in hexane, methyl chloride, *n*-butanol and ethyl acetate fractions of an ethanol extract of the herb. An aqueous extract *of C. arabicus* may disrupt calculogenesis by interacting with CaOx crystal surfaces.

Costus igneus N.E.Br. Family: Zingiberaceae

The effects of aqueous and ethanolic extracts of *Costus igneus* (stem) and isolated compounds lupeol and stigmasterol on CaOx urolithiasis have been studied by Manjula *et al*. [234] in male albino Wistar rats. The increased deposition of stone-forming constituents in the urine, serum, and kidney homogenate of urolithic rats was significantly lowered by treatment with aqueous and ethanolic extracts of *C. igneus* (stem), and isolated compounds lupeol and stigmasterol. After administration of aqueous and ethanolic extract of *C. igneus*, the deposition of calcium and oxalate was significantly lowered. Treatment with lupeol and stigmasterol significantly reduced the deposition of calcium and oxalate in the kidney, and also in the blood serum; the lipid profile serum total cholesterol (TC), triglycerides (TG), low-density lipoprotein (LDL) and high-density lipoprotein (HDL) levels at 50 and 100 mg/kg were significantly lowered in urolithiatic rats.

Mukundam [235] evaluated the *in vitro* antiurolithiatic activity of *Costus igneus* seeds. Both alcoholic and aqueous extracts of *C. igneus* showed their maximum efficiencies in the dissolution of CaOx crystals. Alcoholic extract was more efficient than aqueous extracts in dissolution of CaOx crystals.

Costus pictus D.Don Family: Zingiberaceae

Rajasekaran [236] evaluated the protective effect of *Costus pictus* against doxorubicin-induced nephrotoxicity. Significant changes of the serum kidney markers, albumin, urea, uric acid and creatinine, and GPx, GST, CAT, SOD, reduced GSH and lipid peroxides in the kidney of doxorubicin-treated rat were observed. Histological features were also severely affected. However, biochemical and histological changes in the extract-treated rat were non-significant, showing that the herb is nephroprotective.

Costus spiralis Roscoe Family: Zingiberaceae

The antiurolithiatic activity of the aqueous extract of *C. spiralis* was evaluated by Viel *et al.* [237] in rats. Oral treatment with the extract of *C. spiralis* (0.25 and 0.5 g/kg per day) after 4 weeks surgery reduced the growth of calculi, but it did not prevent hypertrophy of the organ smooth musculature. The contractile responses of isolated urinary bladder preparations to the muscarinic agonist bethanecol, in the presence and absence of the extract (0.3-3 mg/ml) or atropine (0.3-3 nM) did not differ among the experimental groups. The results indicate that the extract of *C. spiralis* is endowed with antiurolithiatic activity.

Crataeva adansonii DC. Family: Capparaceae

Anti-urolithiatic effect of petroleum ether extract stem bark of *Crataeva adansonii* in rats was studied by Gupta *et al.* [238]. Administration of petroleum ether extract (50 and 100 mg/kg, p.o.) of *C. adansonii* along with sodium oxalate (prophylactically) and after 7 days of sodium oxalate injection (therapeutically) significantly decreased CaOx content in urine and kidney and lipid peroxide level in liver and kidney compared with vehicle-treated group. Animals treated with petroleum ether extract of *C. adansonii* showed improved creatinine clearance as compared with vehicle group. Histological estimation of kidney treated with petroleum ether extract along with sodium oxalate strongly inhibited the growth of calculi and reduced the number of stones in kidney compared with group receiving vehicle.

Crataeva magna Lour. Family: Capparaceae

Crataeva magna bark, commonly known as Baruna, has been investigated by Mekap *et al.* [239] for its antiurolithiatic activity in rats. The ethanol extract (400 mg/kg bw) reduced the elevated levels of serum calcium (3.25 ± 0.30) and urine calcium (2.33 ± 0.18) significantly, employing lactose (30%) + ethylene glycol

(1%) induced urolithiasis model. The ethanol extract (400 mg/kg bw) reduced the urine uric acid level significantly employing both models, *viz.* lactose (30%) + ethylene glycol (1%) (0.82 ± 0.07) and ammonium chloride (2%) + ethylene glycol (0.75%) (0.85 ± 0.12) when compared to toxic group. The ethanol extract employing both models resulted in reduced serum creatinine and calcium, urine oxalate and kidney weight significantly with a marked increase in final body weight and urine volume output when compared to toxic group.

Crataeva nurvala Buch.-Ham. Family: Capparaceae

Clinical studies conducted at Banaras Hindu University, India, provide evidence that *Crataeva nurvala* can be effectively used in the management of urolithiasis, prostatic hypertrophy, neurogenic bladder and chronic urinary infections. Decoction of the bark when administered in urolithiatic cases, reduced the urinary excretion of calcium. As excretory rates increased, of sodium and magnesium it was inferred that the drug alters the relatve proportions of urinary calcium, magnesium and sodium which are involved in the formation of urinary stones. Crystallurea was also cured signifrcantly. The clinical findings were supported by data accrued from experimental urolihiasis in rats, wherein the treated animals had lighter stones, less oedema of bladder mucosa, ulceration and cellular infiltration [240].

The ability of *C. nurvala* bark to induce spontaneous passage of stones has also been demonstrated. Twenty six patients from a group of fortysix suffering from stones in the kidney, ureter and bladders were able to pass the stones within four months of treatment with the decoction [240]. This is substantiated by reports of increased tone of smooth muscle achieved by aqueous extract of the plant material [241].

The effect of oral administration of *C. nurvala* bark decoction on CaOx lithiasis has been studied in rats by Varalakshmi *et al.* [242]. The elevation of the oxalate-synthesizing liver enzyme, glycolate oxidase, produced by feeding glycollic acid was remarkably reduced with the decoction, showing a regulatory action on endogenous oxalate synthesis. Protein-bound carbohydrates were increased in the renal tissues during calculosis but these changes were not reversed with the herbal treatment. The increased deposition of stone-forming constituents in the kidneys of calculogenic rats was lowered with decoction administration. The increased urinary excretion of the crystalline constituents along with lowered magnesium excretion found in stone-forming rats was partially reversed by decoction treatment.

Effect of *C. nurvala* on the biochemistry of the small intestinal tract of normal and stone-forming rats was investigated by Varalakshmi *et al*. [243]. Treatment with *C. nurvala* bark decoction lowered levels of small intestinal (Na+,K+)-ATPases.

The action of the decoction on the small intestinal tract seems to be mediated through (Na+,K+)-ATPases, which in turn may affect the transport of metabolites.

Effect of simultaneous sodium oxalate and methionine feeding with and without Varuna (*C. nurvala*) therapy on urolithogenesis in guinea pigs was studied in 18 adult male guinea pigs by Singh *et al*. [244]. Administration of Varuna to oxalate and methionine-supplemented animals prevented either totally or partially most of the urolithogenic effects of oxalate and methionine.

Lupeol, isolated from *C. nurvala* stem bark in doses 40 and 80 mg/kg body weight, p.o., for 10 days, decreased the concentration of BUN, creatinine and lipid peroxidation and increased GSH and CAT activities in cisplatin-induced nephrotoxicity in rats. The increased GSH and CAT activities are indicative of antioxidant properties of lupeol [245]

Shirwaikar *et al*. [246] evaluated the possible effect of the alcohol extract of *C. nurvala* on cisplatin-induced dysfunction model of renal proximal tubule cells by oxidative stress. The plant extract (250 and 500 mg/kg) was effective in significantly altering the indices of cisplatin induced dysfunction of renal proximal tubule cells under oxidative stress by decreasing the concentration of BUN nitrogen, creatinine and lipid peroxidation. The increased GSH and CAT activity are indicative of the antioxidant properties of *C. nurvala* stem bark extract.

Agarwal *et al*. [247] investigated the urolithiatic property of *C. nurvala* in albino rats. In the control group there was a slight increase in the serum and urinary creatine, which might be due to obstructive uropathy or other pathology developed in urinary system of the rat. But in the treated group, the serum and urinary creatine were decreased. Therefore it was assumed that the drug was helpful in reducing or normalizing the serum and urinary creatine and restoring the normal metabolism of the urinary system.

Shelkea *et al*. [248] investigated nephroprotective effect of stem barks ethanolic extract of *C. nurvula* in Cisplatin-induced nephrotoxic rats. The extract significantly improved packed cell volume (PCV), hemoglobin (Hb), and total leukocyte count (TLC) levels but non-significant increase in the mean corpuscular volume (MCV), mean corpuscular hemoglobin (MCH), and mean corpuscular hemoglobin concentration (MCHC).

Meher *et al*. [249] investigated the renal protective effect of aqueous extract of *C. nurvala*. Aqueous extract of bark showed protection to kidney against GM–induced nephrotoxicity in rats.

Crinum scillifolium A.Chev. Family: Amaryllidaceae

Bienvenu *et al*. [250] evaluated the protective effect of water and hydroethanolic extracts of leaves *Crinum scillifolium* on GM induced nephrotoxicity using biochemical approaches in rat. The treatment of animals suffering from nephrotoxicity with hydroethanolic and aqueous extracts of *C. scillifolium* significantly reduced biochemical parameters considered as markers of nephrotoxicity.

Crocus sativus L. Family: Iridaceae

Hosseinzadeh *et al*. [251] assessed the effect of aqueous saffron (*Crocus sativus*) extract and its active constituent, crocin, on oxidative stress following renal ischemia-reperfusion injury (IRI) in rats. In crocin pretreated groups, a reduction in TBARS levels and elevation in antioxidant power (FRAP value) and total thiol concentrations as compared with control group, were observed. The aqueous extract also reduced lipid peroxidation products and increased antioxidant power in ischemia-reperfusion injured rat kidneys.

Ajami *et al*. [252] evaluated GM nephrotoxicity in saffron treated rats. Saffron at 40 mg/k/d significantly reduced GM-induced increases in BUN and histological scores. GM-induced increases in BUN, SCr and MDA and histological injury were significantly reduced by treatment with saffron 80 mg/k/d.

The protective effects of saffron extract and crocin was evaluated in chronic - stress induced oxidative stress damage of the brain, liver and kidneys in rats. In the stressed animals that receiving saline, the levels of MDA, and the activities of GPx, GR, and SOD were significantly higher and the TAR capacity was significantly lower than those of the non-stressed animals. Both saffron extract and crocin were able to reverse these changes in the stressed animals as compared with the control groups [253].

Protective effect of cysteine and vitamin E, *Crocus sativus* and *Nigella sativa* extracts on cisplatin-induced toxicity in rats was investigated by El Daly [254]. Concurrent administration of cysteine together with vitamin E, *Crocus sativus* and *Nigella sativa* reduced the toxicity of cisplatin in rats. When administered i.p. with 3 mg/kg cisplatin, cysteine (20 mg/kg) together with vitamin E (2 mg/rat) and extract of *Crocus sativus* stigmas (50 mg/kg) and *Nigella sativa* seed (50 mg/kg) significantly reduced BUN and serum creatinine levels as well as cisplatin-induced serum total lipids increased. In contrast, the protective agents given together with cisplatin led to an even greater decrease in blood glucose than that seen with cisplatin alone. Addition of cysteine and vitamin E, *Crocus sativus* and *Nigella sativa* in combination with cisplatin partially prevented many changes in the activities of serum enzymes. Administration of cysteine and vitamin E, *Crocus sativus* and *Nigella sativa* together with cisplatin partially reversed many of the kidney enzymes changes induced by cisplatin. Cysteine together with vitamin E, *Crocus sativus* and *Nigella sativa* tended to protect from cisplatin-induced falls in leucocyte counts, haemoglobin levels and mean osmotic fragility of erythrocytes and also prevented the increase in haematocrit.

Croton zambesicus Müll.-Arg. Family: Euphorbiaceae

Okokon *et al*. [255] evaluated the protective effect of ethanolic root extract of *Croton zambesicus* against GM-induced kidney injury in rats. Administration of the root extract significantly reduced histopathological changes in the kidneys of the extract-treated rats especially in the rats treated with lower doses of the extract (27 and 54 mg/kg). The levels of serum urea and creatinine were also reduced significantly at these doses with no observable effect on the levels of uric acid and ions.

Cucumis sativus L. Family: Cucurbitaceae

Pethakar *et al*. [256] evaluated lithotryptic effect using hydro-alcoholic extract of *Cucumis sativus* (HCS). Treatment with preventive and curative doses of HCS was found to exert dose dependent antiurolithiatic action. Increased urine volume in HCS treated groups as compared to diseased group was indicative of diuretic property. Elevated calcium, phosphate and oxalate levels in diseased group animal were found to be decreased in animals treated with HCS. Increased levels of serum creatinine, BUN and uric acid were considerably brought down towards normal values in proportion to HCS doses administered. Animals treated with HCS showed remarkable recovery, suggestive of prevention of nucleation and aggregation of stone forming components.

Cucumis trigonus Roxb. Family: Curcurbitaceae

Effect of ethanolic fruit extract of *Cucumis trigonus* on urolithiasis induced wistar albino rats was investigated by Balakrishnan *et al*. [257]. The extract also repairs the changes that happened in the enzymatic, non enzymatic antioxidants and lipid peroxidation in kidney of urolithiasis induced rats. The results show that the ethanolic fruit extract has repaired the levels of antioxidants and MDA to their normal levels.

Cucurbita pepo L. Family: Cucurbitaceae

Debnath *et al*. [173] investigated the nephroprotective evaluation of ethanolic extract of the pumpkin seed (PuSE). The ethanolic extract of exhibited protection against cisplatin-induced nephrotoxicity, which were proved by the gross behavioural studies, histopathological, renal function and biochemical studies. Antioxidant studies like nitric oxide scavenging activity, lipid peroxidation in kidney also supported the nephroprotective activity of these seeds.

Abdel-Hady *et al*. [258] evaluated the nephroprotective active activity of *C. pepo* in cisplatin induced nephrotoxicity in rats. The defatted methanolic extract of *C. pepo* showed improvement of renal parameters.

Shehzad *et al*. [259] evaluated the antiurolithic potential of methanol extract of *C. pepo* (MECP) seed against sodium oxalate-induced renal calculi using both *in vitro* and *in vivo* models. GC-MS fingerprints showed that beta-tocopherol, stigmasterol, and squalene are the major phytochemicals found in MECP. MECP significantly inhibited various steps of CaOx crystal formation such as nucleation, aggregation, growth, and dissolution in dose-dependent manner. MECP normalized the raised levels of oxalate, calcium, sodium, phosphate, uric acid, restored alterations in histopathology while elevated the reduced levels of magnesium, urine volume, and pH.

Cuminum cyminum L. Family: Apiaceae

Mahesh *et al*. [260] evaluated the effect of water extract of *Cuminum cyminum* (AEC) seeds on GM-induced nephrotoxicity in rats. GM treated group caused nephrotoxicity as evidenced by marked elevation of serum urea, creatinine and urine glucose. Decreased clearance of urea, creatinine and rise in lipid peroxidation level. The AEC 200 mg/kg showed a marked decrease in elevated levels of serum urea, creatinine, lipid peroxidation and increased clearance compare to the AEC 100 mg/kg.

Jayasuda [261] investigated the potential of *C. cyminum* in the treatment of renal calculi. The fruit juice of *C. cyminum* (CC) was evaluated for antiurolithiatic and antioxidant activities. Supplementation with aqueous and alcoholic extract of *C. cyminum* fruits significantly reduced the elevated urinary oxalate, showing a regulatory action on endogenous oxalate synthesis. The increased deposition of stone forming constituents in the serum and urine of calculogenic rats was also significantly lowered by preventive and curative treatment using aqueous and alcoholic extracts.

The effect of *C. cyminum* on kidney exposed to profenofos was evaluated in female swiss albino mice. The results showed that cumin was effective in normalizing the uric acid and creatinine level [262].

Kumar *et al.* [263] evaluated nephroprotective potential of *C. cyminum* on chloropyrifos induced kidney of mice. Degeneration was observed in glomerulus and bowmen's capsule. PCT and DCT were also degenerated to greater extent in chloropyrifos administered group of mice. Effective restoration was observed in urea, uric acid and creatinine in *C. cyminum* administered group of mice. Glomerulus, proximal convoluted tubule, distal convoluted tubules and bowmens capsule was also restored effectively in *C. cyminum* administered group of mice.

In rats given the mixture of paracetamol 500 mg/kg plus 6% *C. cyminum* fruit for 4 weeks, the recovery of paracetamol hepatotoxicity was evidenced by increase in body weight, absence of hepatocellular fatty vacuolation and significant improvement of serbiochemical and hematological parameters [264].

Venu *et al.* [265] evaluated the antiurolithiatic effect of the methanolic extracts of the fruit of *C. cyminum* on ethylene glycol induced urolithiasis in rats. Methanolic extract of *C. cyminum*, significantly reduced the elevated levels of calcium, phosphorous, BUN, uric acid and serum creatinine in curative and preventive treatment groups. The histopathological findings also show sign of improvement after treatment with the methanolic extract of *C. cyminum*.

Curcuma longa L. Family: Zingiberaceae

Khorsandi and Orazizadeh [266] evaluated the protective effect of *Curcuma longa* extract on acetaminophen induced nephrotoxicity. BUN, Cr and uric acid reduced significantly in the T3 group. Necrosis of kidney reduced in test groups, especially in T3 group.

Thuawaini *et al.* [267] investigated the effect of aqueous extract of turmeric in nephrotoxicity induced in rats by tetracycline. Co-administrated of turmeric extracts with tetracycline appeared to ameliorate the adverse effects of tetracycline in renal function tests. All the toxic effects of the tetracycline were improved by administration of turmeric extract, but didn't bring them to the control limits.

Thuawaini *et al.* [268] estimated the effect of aqueous extract of turmeric (*Curcuma longa*) in nephrotoxicity induced in rats by isoniazid and rifampicin (RIF). The aqueous extract of turmeric (at a dose of 100 and 200 mg/kg bw, p.o. daily) showed reno-protective effects in reno-toxicity induced by RIF and INH in rats. Significant elevation of serum ALT, AST, ALP, total bilirubin, creatinine, urea, and total protein, due to RIF and INH treatment, were significantly decreased. The histopathological study further confirmed the biochemical results.

Pathak *et al.* [269] investigated the effects of carvedilol (5 mg/kg, p.o), aqueous and methanolic extract of *Curcuma longa* (500mg/kg, p.o) against cisplatin-induced nephrotoxicity in Wistar rats. Post treated rats with carvedilol and aqueous and methanolic extracts of *Curcuma longa* for 15 days significantly increased body weight, decreased cisplatin induced abnormalities and mortality and decreased all the kidney marker such as serum urea nitrogen (SUN), serum creatinine (SCr), total proteins (TP), and uric acid (UA) increased by cisplatin, however, no appreciable improvement in hematological parameters were observed when compared with cisplatin control.

Curcuma longa L. and *Zingiber officinale* Family: Zingiberaceae

Ademiluyi *et al.* [270] investigated the modulatory effects of dietary inclusion of ginger (*Zingiber officinale*) and turmeric (*Curcuma longa*) rhizomes on antioxidant status and renal damage induced by GM in rats. Renal damage was induced in albino rats pretreated with dietary inclusion of ginger and turmeric (2% and 4%) by intraperitoneal administration of GM (100 mg/kg body weight) for three days. Pretreatment with ginger and turmeric rhizome prior to GM administration significantly protected the kidney and attenuated oxidative stress by modulating renal damage and antioxidant indices.

Curcuma mangga Val. Family: Zingiberaceae

Rosita *et al.* [271] evaluated the nephroprotective activity of *Curcuma mangga* in paracetamol-induced male mice. *C. mangga* extract was able to inhibit the increase of creatinine level and showed a significant difference from negative control and did not differ significantly from the positive control. The result was supported by histopathology examination which did not show any cell damage. The nephroprotective effect of *C. mangga* was in a dose-dependent manner. *C. mangga* extract at dose of 400 mg/kg bw depicted the strongest nephroprotective effect.

Cyanotis fasciculata (B.Heyne ex Roth) Schult. & Schult.f. var. *fasciculata* Family: Commelinaceae

Murthy *et al.* [272] evaluated the nephroprotective activity of 70% hydroalcoholic extract of *Cyanotis fasciculata* var. *fasciculata* (CFEE) in cisplatin-induced nephrotoxicity. CFEE demonstrated dose-dependent decrement of elevated biochemical biochemical markers of nephrotoxicity along with significant restoration of protective GSH levels and suppression of LPO levels in tissues.

Further, the remarkable renal cellular rejuvenation found in histopathological studies also enunciated the organ protective activity of CFEE.

Cyclea peltata Lam. Family: Menispermaceae

The inhibitory effect of the root of *Cyclea peltata* on nephrolithiasis induced in was investigated by Christina *et al*. [273]. Simultaneous administration of the powdered root of *C. peltata* resulted in decreased urinary oxalate and calcium. Likewise, serum potassium was lowered and magnesium was elevated.

Vijayan *et al*. [274] evaluated the protective effect of a 70% methanolic leaf extract of *C. peltata* on cisplatin-induced nephrotoxicity. *C. peltata* extract significantly changed the increased MDA level and decreased GSH levels found in rats treated with cisplatin alone. The reduced activities of GSH-Px, SOD, and CAT in groups treated with cisplatin alone were significantly increased by the extract. The protective effect was greater in the post-treated than in the pre-treated group of animals.

Cymbopogon citratus (DC.) Stapf Family: Poaceae

Ullah *et al*. [275] investigated the protective activity of *Cymbopogon citratus* in GM-induced nephrotoxicity. Simultaneous administration of *C. citratus* and GM significantly protected alteration in body weight, BUN, serum creatinine, creatinine clearance, serum uric acid, serum electrolytes, urinary volume, urinary protein, urinary LDH and urinary alkaline phosphatase induced by GM. Histological examination of the kidney also suggested the same.

Cymbopogon schoenanthus (L.) Spreng. Family: Poaceae

Al Haznawi *et al*. [276] evaluated the effects of *Cymbopogon schoenanthus* in urolithiasis in male Wistar albino rats. Daily oral treatment with the *C. schoenanthus* (1 ml of the extract) significantly corrected the incidence of nephrotoxicity (BUN, creatinine and calcium level differences). Moreover, a highly potent diuretic activity was recorded for *C. schoenanthus*.

Cynodon dactylon (L.) Pers. Family: Poaceae

Atmani *et al*. [277] evaluated the effect of *Cynodon dactylon* aqueous extract as a preventive and curative agent in experimentally induced nephrolithiasis in a rat model. In both preventive and curative protocols, all measured variables were similar for both the rat groups. Nevertheless, urinary biochemical analysis was apparently unaffected by the extract except oxalate in preventive protocol, and calcium, sodium, and potassium in curative protocol which were significantly highly excreted in treated rats compared to untreated animals. The most apparent beneficial effect of Cynodon extract was seen in kidney tissues where reduced levels of CaOx deposition have been noticed especially in medullary and papillary sections from treated rats.

Methanolic extract of *C. dactylon* was tested by Patel *et al.* [109] for its *in vitro* antilithiatic/anticalcification activity. Extract of *C. dactylon* showed less activity than standard drug cystone. The effect of hydroalcoholic extract of *C. dactylon* was evaluated Mousa-Al-Reza *et al.* [278] in ethylene glycol-induced nephrolithiasis in a rat model. *C. dactylon* extract reduced the levels of CaOx deposition especially in medullary and papillary sections from of the kidney of the treated rats.

Rad *et al.* [279] evaluated the effect of different fractions of *C. dactylon* in ethylene glycol-induced nephrolithiasis in rats. In curative protocol, treatment of rats with *C. dactylon* n-butanol fraction, significantly reduced the number of the kidney CaOx deposits compared to ethylene glycol group. In preventive protocol, treatment of rats with *C. dactylon* ethyl acetate fraction significantly decreased the number of CaOx deposits compared to ethylene glycol group [279].

Cyperus rotundus L. Family: Cyperaceae

Pinakin *et al.* [280] investigated the antiurolithiatic activity of ethanolic extract of *Cyperus rotundus* (EECR) rhizome in male Wistar rats. In ethylene glycol induced urolithiatic model, EECR showed significant decrease in excretion and deposition of various urolithiatic promoters (calcium, oxalate, phosphate and uric acid) as compared to urolithiatic control. EECR also decreased serum concentration of urea, uric acid and cratine as compared to urolithiatic control.

Dalbergia sissoo DC. Family: Fabaceae

The aqueous extract of *Dalbergia sissoo* bark was screened by Narware *et al.* [281] for its nephroprotective activities against paracetamol (300 mg/kg i.p) and CCl_4 (1.0 ml/kg, i.p) induced kidney damage in albino rats. The aqueous extract of *D. sissoo* bark significantly decreased the serum enzyme ALT, AST, ALP, total bilirubin (TB) and significantly increased the total protein (TP) level and significantly increased the levels of SOD, GSH, LPO, CAT.

Daucus carota L. Family: Apiaceae

Mital *et al.* [282] evaluated the nephroprotective activity of *Daucus carota* root extract in renal ischemia reperfusion injury in rats. Renal ischemia reperfusion caused significant impairment of kidney function. Six day administration of *D. carota*, minimized this effect. Rats with renal I/R only showed significantly decreased activity of SOD, CAT, and reduced GSH compared with the sham operated rats. These declining trends were significantly less in the group treated with petroleum ether, fractional methanolic and direct methanolic extract of *Daucus carota* root compared with those in I/R group. Renal I/R produced a significant increase in MDA level, while pretreatment with *D. carota* extracts was associated with a significantly lower MDA level [282].

Afzal *et al*. [283] evaluated the protective and curative potential of *D. carota* root extract on renal ischemia reperfusion injury in rats. Petroleum ether extract (PEE) at a dose of 500 mg/kg significantly reduced the levels of serum creatinine, uric acid and urea compared to disease control. Fractional methanol extract at a dose of 500 mg/kg body weight significantly reduced the levels of serum creatinine, uric acid and urea compared to disease control. DME at a dose of 500 mg/kg body weight significantly reduced the levels of serum creatinine (1.173-3.090 mg/dl), uric acid (2.267-3.500 mg/dl) and urea (84.75-132.00 mg/dl) compared to disease control.

Sodimbaku *et al*. [284] investigated the nephroprotective effects of ethanolic root extract of *D. carota* against GM-induced nephrotoxicity in Albino Wistar rats. GM intoxication induced elevated serum urea, BUN, uric acid, and creatinine levels which were found to be significantly decreased in a dose-dependent manner in groups received *D. carota* which was also evidenced by the histological observations.

Pullaiah *et al*. [285] evaluated the antiurolithiatic activity of *D. carota* extract against ethylene glycol (EG) and Vitamin D 3 induced urolithiasis rats. Serum and urinary levels of calcium, creatinine, oxalate, blood urea and BUN level were found to be decreased significantly in groups pre-treated with test drug. The animals treated with *D. carota* extract showed much improvement in physical parameters like body weight, urine volume and pH of urine. Histopathology of kidney showed almost normal kidney architecture in treated groups compared to disease control rats. The biochemical and histopathological parameters studied in rats have revealed the presence of antiurolithiatic property in the roots of *D. carota*. This property was dose-dependent.

Dendropanax morbifera H.Lév. Family: Araliaceae

Kim *et al*. [286] evaluated the protective effect of *Dendropanax morbifera* (DP) on acute kidney injury (AKI) using cisplatin-induced nephropathic models. Methanolic extract from DP significantly reduced cisplatin-induced toxicity in renal tubular cells. Among different fractions the chlroform fraction (DPCF) was found to be most potent. The protective activity of DPCF was found to be mediated through anti-oxidant, mitochondrial protective, and anti-apoptotic activities. In *in vivo* rat models of AKI, treatment with DPCF significantly reversed the cisplatin-induced increase in BUN and serum creatinine and histopathologic damage, recovered the level of anti-oxidant enzymes, and inhibited renal apoptosis.

Desmodium styracifolium (Osbeck) Merr. Family: Fabaceae

Hiarayama *et al.* [287] have studied the inhibitory effects of *Desmodium styracifolium*-triterpenoid (Ds-t) on the formation of CaOx renal stones induced experimentally by ethylene glycol (EG) and 1 alpha (OH)D3 (1 alpha D3) in rats. The findings suggest that Ds-t inhibits the formation of Ca oxalate stones in rat kidneys by increasing the output of urine, decreasing the excretion of calcium and increasing the urinary excretion of citrate..

Xiang *et al.* [288] investigated the antilithic effects of the extracts from different polarity fractions of *D. styracifolium*. Among the four polarity fractions of *D. styracifolium* extracts, the petroleum ether (Fr. PE) and n-butyl alcohol fraction (Fr. NB) treatment significantly reduced the CaOx crystal deposition in kidneys, prevented the renal toxic changes like pH, Cr, and BUN. In addition, Fr. PE and Fr. NB treatment significantly decreased urinary excretion of oxalate along with an increase of citrate excretion. The increased amounts of MDA and decreased activities of SOD, CAT, and GPx were detected in lithogenic group, *D. styracifolium* extracts treatment prevented the oxidative stress changes especially for the Fr. PE and Fr. NB extracts.

In study of Zhou *et al.* [289] evaluated the antiurolithiatic effect in rats. After 4-week gavage, reduce of MDA content, increase of CAT and GSH-Px activities in renal homogenate as well as attenuation in the expression of MCP-1, OPN and TGF-β proteins of two extract groups (100 and 400 mg/kg BW) could be observed.

Dichrostachys cinerea Wight & Arn. Family: Fabaceae

Ethanolic extract of the root of *Dichrostachys cinerea* was evaluated by Jayakumari *et al.* [290] for its anti-urolithiatic effect in male Wistar albino rats. Supplementation with ethanolic extract of the plant (200mg/kg and 400mg/kg) significantly reduced the elevated urinary oxalate, showing a regulatory action on endogenous oxalate synthesis. Both the dose levels showed significant urolithiatic activity.

The alcoholic extract of roots of *D. cinerea* (200 and 400 mg/kg, p.o.) was studied by Sreedevi *et al.* [291] for its protective effect against cisplatin-induced renal injury in rats.. In curative regimen, the alcoholic extract exhibited dose dependent protection. Animals which received prophylactic treatment also showed partial protection against cisplatin-induced effects. Histopathological studies substantiated the above results.

Digera muricata (L.) Mart. Family: Amaranthaceae

Khan *et al.* [292] evaluated the protective effect of *Digera muricata* on CCl_4-induced nephrotoxicity. Treatment with n-hexane (HDMP) and methanolic (MDMP) extracts of *D. muricata* (200 and 250 mg/kg body wt., oral, respectively) effectively attenuated the alterations in the biochemical markers, telomerase activity was inhibited and confirms the restoration of normalcy and accredits the protective role of *D. muricata* against CCl_4-induced nephrotoxicity.

Diospyros lotus L. Family: Ebenaceae

Moghaddam *et al.* [293] evaluated the nephroprotective effects of *Diospyros lotus* seeds extract in GM-induced nephrotoxicity in *in vitro* and *in vivo* models. Extracts administrated i.p. in doses 200 and 400 mg/kg attenuated the GM-induced increase in level of serum creatinine and BUN.

Dolichos biflorus L. Family: Fabaceae

Peshin and Singla [294] evaluated *in vitro* effect of *Dolichos biflorus* seeds on crystallization of calcium phosphate. There was a marked decrease in anticalcifying activity with the maturation of seeds or post-harvest storage for 6 months. The results suggested that the inhibitors of crystallization present in seed extract of *D. biflorus* were water soluble, heat stable, polar, non-tannin and non-protein in nature.

Soxhlet extracts of seeds of *D. biflorus* and rhizomes of *Bergenia ligulata* were tested by Garimella *et al.* [295] for their *in vitro* antilithiatic/anticalcification activity by the homogeneous precipitation method. Also a combination of the extracts of the two plants was tested. Extracts of *D. biflorus* showed activity almost equivalent to cystone while *Bergenia ligulata* showed less activity and the combination was not as active as the individual extracts.

A novel dimeric antilithiatic protein (98 kDa) from seeds of *D. biflorus* was purified by Bijarnia *et al.* [296] based on its ability to inhibit CaOx crystallization *in vitro*. Amino acid analysis of *D. biflorus* antilithiatic protein showed abundant acidic amino acids.

Atodariya *et al.* [297] evaluated the antiurolithiatic property of aqueous, chloroform, benzene extracts of *D. biflorus* and standard for dissolving kidney stones- CaOx by an *in-vitro* model. Phenolic compounds were isolated from the benzene and aqueous extract, while flavanoids and steroids from aqueous fraction of the seed. Aqueous fractions showed highest dissolution of stones as compared to others.

Saha and Verma [298] evaluated the preventive effect of hydro-alcoholic extract of *D. biflorus* seeds (DBE) in ethylene glycol induced nephrolithiasis. Ethylene glycol also caused a significant increase in lipid peroxidation and concurrent decrease in activities of antioxidant enzymes in kidney. However, the seed extract of *D. biflorus* caused significant restoration of all these parameters. Histopathological and histochemical studies also showed the reduced calcifications in kidney of seed extract treated rats.

Mukundan [235] evaluated the *in vitro* antiurolithiatic activity of *D. biflorus* seeds. Both alcoholic and aqueous extracts of *D. biflorus* showed their maximum efficiencies in the dissolution of CaOx crystals. Alcoholic extract was more efficient than aqueous extracts in dissolution of CaOx crystals.

Dolichos lablab L. Family: Fabaceae

The antilithiatic study revealed that the methanolic extract of white and black seeds of *Dolichos lablab* possessed antilithiatic activity [299].

Drynaria fortunei (Kunze ex Mett.) J. Sm. Family: Polypodiaceae

The flavonoid fraction (FF) from *Drynaria fortunei* was investigated by Long *et al.* [300] to determine its biological activity expression in three acute renal failure animal models. The BUN and creatinine levels were found to be significantly higher in the GM group than in the GMFF group, the FF group and the saline group. Mice were treated once with 6 mg/kg of mercuric chloride, followed by 10 mg/kg of FF or saline. On days 3, 4 and 5, BUN and creatinine levels were found to be significantly higher in the $HgCl_2$-saline group than in the $HgCl_2$-FF group. After surgery for 5/6-nephrectomy, ten mice received FF at a dose of 10 mg/kg/day and eight received saline for 42 days. The saline group survived for 12-62 days and the FF group survived for 20-320 days. The FF group had a significantly longer survival time than the saline group. Regeneration of kidney tubular cells and significantly enlarged convoluted tubules were noted in the pathology study of the FF group.

Drynaria quercifolia (L.) J.Sm. Family: Polypodiaceae

Srinivas and Arun Kumar [145] assessed the effects of *Drynaria quercifolia* rhizomes on urolithiatic rats. From the study, it was found that the alcoholic extract of plant parts was effective in *in vivo* anti-urolithiatic activity on induced CaOx crystals in rats.

Echinacea pallida Nutt. Family: Asteraceae

Mustea *et al*. [301] evaluated the nephroprotective activity of *Echinacea pallida* in cisplatin-induced nephrotoxicity in Swiss mice. Preliminary assays proved that i.p. administration of Cisplatin to mice caused body weight loss and mortality depending on dose. The hydroalcohol extract of *E. pallida* given to mice p.o. along with with the i.p. administration of cisplatin exhibited protective effects expressed by a diminished loss and a faster recovery of the animal's body weight. Pretreatment with *E. pallida* also decreased cisplatin nephrotoxicity estimated from the level of kidney homogenate oxygen consumption.

Echinodorus macrophyllus (Kunthh) Micheli Family: Alismataceae

The diuretic and nephroprotective activities of crude extracts of *Echinodorus macrophyllus* (EM) were evaluated by Portella *et al*. [302]. EM was effective in reversing all GM-induced alterations such as polyuria and glomerular filtration rate reduction. The GM-induced morphological alterations were not observed when EM was given concomitantly with GM.

Eclipta prostrata (L.) L. [Syn.: *Eclipta alba* (L.) Hassk.] Family: Asteraceae

Dungca [303] evaluated the protective effect of the methanolic leaf extract of *Eclipta prostrata* on GM-induced nephrotoxicity in rats. The extract protected the rat kidneys against GM-induced renal tubular alterations and rises in BUN, serum creatinine, and microprotein levels. Lipid peroxidation and decrement in CAT levels were also ameliorated.

Ahmad *et al*. [304] evaluated the nephroprotective activity of *E. prostrata* hydroalcoholic leaves extracts against GM-induced nephrotoxicity in wistar rats. The oral administration of hydroalcoholic leaves extracts of *E. prostrata* (250mg/kg and 500mg/kg,p.o) along with GM reversed altered parameters to normal level when compared with standard cystone. The histopathological investigation of kidney was also supported nephroprotective activity of *E. prostrata.*

Elaeocarpus ganitrus Roxb. ex G. Don Family: Elaeocarpaceae

Kakalij *et al*. [305] evaluated the ameliorative effect of *Elaeocarpus ganitrus* on GM-induced nephrotoxicity in rats. The results revealed that coadministration of *E. ganitrus* significantly reduced the elevated level of serum creatinine, BUN, uric acid, and albuminuria with considerable increase in the serum albumin and urine creatinine. Furthermore, *E. ganitrus* noticeably increased serum total protein and antioxidant enzyme levels with significant alteration in phagocytic index and neutrophil adhesion assay when compared with GM-treated group in a dose-dependent manner.

Elephantopus scaber L. Family: Asteraceae

Sahoo *et al.* [306] evaluated the nephroprotective activty of *Elephantopus scaber* in GM-induced nephrotoxicity in male Wistar rats. Tested extract at 200–600 mg/kg/day decreased the levels of serum creatinine, total protein and serum urea but showed slight increase in the electrolyte levels in dose dependent manner.

Elettaria cardamomum (L.) Maton Family: Zingiberaceae

Kumari *et al.* [307] investigated the protective effect of cardamon on renal tissue damage caused by pan masala. Male Swiss mice were given orally pan masala at a dose of 2% of the feed which caused acute tubular necrosis along with dilation and atrophied glomerulus seen in its light microscopic structures, whereas ultrastructural changes showed pyknotic nucleus, swollen mitochondria and loss of membrane integrity. When cardamom was given at a dose of 0.2% along with pan masala or alone, damages were less showing normal glomerulus with less inflammation, and normal nucleus.

Sanjuna *et al.* [308] evaluated *in vitro* antiurolithiatic activity of *Elettaria cardamomum* seeds. It was observed that the highest CaOx crystals dissolution was observed in the ethanolic extract of seeds of *E. cardamomum*.

Eleusine coracana L. Family: Poaceae

The effect of *Eleusine coracana* grains on CaOx nephrolithiasis has been studied in male albino rats by Bahuguna *et al.* [309]. Supplementation with aqueous and alcohol extracts of *E. coracana* grains significantly reduced the elevated urinary oxalate, showing a regulatory action on endogenous oxalate synthesis. The increased deposition of stone forming constituents in the kidneys of calculogenic rats was significantly lowered by curative and preventive treatment using aqueous and alcohol extracts.

Elymus repens (L.) Gould. (Syn.: *Agropyron repens* L.) Family: Poaceae

Grases *et al.* [310] found that *Agropyron repens* exerted no effect on urolithiasis risk factors when given to the rats in combination with different diets.

Enicostemma littorale Blume Family: Gentianaceae

Bhatt *et al.* [311] investigated the role of *Enicostemma littorale* (EL) extract in GM-induced nephrotoxicity. GM treated animals showed high oxidative stress in mitochondrial as well as post-mitochondrial fractions of renal tissue. GM-induced nephrotoxicity was further corroborated by an increase in serum creatine and BUN levels and altered kidney histopathological observations. Treatment with EL ameliorates antioxidant defense system of mitochondrial as well as post-mitochondrial fraction, with better improvement seen in mitochondrial fraction.

Entandrophragma angolense (Welw.) C.DC. Family: Meliaceae

Evaluation of nephroprotective properties of aqueous and ethanolic extracts of *Entendrophragma angolense* against GM-induced renal dysfunction in the albino rats was carried out by Abou *et al.* [223]. The results showed that intra-peritoneal injection of GM causes a significant decrease of total serum rate of protein and a significant raise in serum rate of creatinine and urea. The results also show a significant increase in total protein and albumin in the urine of animals. However, changes in biochemical parameters measured were attenuated in co-treated rats with the extracts of *E. angolense*. Treatment with the extracts significantly attenueated levels of serum creatinine, serum urea, serum protein, proteinuria and albuminuria.

Equisetum arvense L. Family: Equisetaceae

Grases *et al.* [96] studied the effects of *Equisetum arvense* to prevent and treat stone kidney formation in female Wistar rats. The infusion does not affect calciuria and citraturia values, they do not diminish calcinuria or increase the crystallization inhibitory capacity of the urine.

The diuretic effect of *E. arvense* dried extract (EADE) was assessed clinically by monitoring the volunteers' water balance over a 24 h period. The dried extract (EADE, 900mg/day) produced a diuretic effect that was stronger than that of the negative control and was equivalent to that of hydrochlorothiazide without causing significant changes in the elimination of electrolytes [312].

Erica arborea L. Family: Ericaceae

Inhibition of CaOx monohydrate crystal growth using aqueous extract of leaved branch of *Erica arborea* was investigated by Beghalia *et al.* [61]. Activity was tested in bioassays. In the presence of plants extract, the length and the width of the crystals were reduced. It was found that extract of *E. arborea* inhibited potently the nucleation and aggregation phases. Inhibition was 94.51% at 25%

concentration, 93.91% at 50% concentration, 93.91% at 75% concentration and 97.61 at 100% concentration.

Erica multiflora L. Family: Ericaceae

Inhibition of calcium oxalate monohydrate crystal growth using aqueous extract of leaved branch of *Erica multiflora* was investigated by Beghalia *et al.* [61]. Activity was tested in bioassays. In the presence of plants extract, the length and the width of the crystals were reduced. It was found that *E. multiflora* extract inhibited potently the nucleation and growth phases. Inhibition was 95.58% at 25% concentration, 98.09% at 50% concentration, 98.09% at 75% concentration and 96.77 at 100% concentration.

Eruca sativa Mill. Family: Brassicaceae

The protective effect of ethanolic extract of *Eruca sativa* seeds was investigated by Alam *et al.* [313] on $HgCl_2$ induced renal toxicity. Feeding of the extract to rats afforded a significant protection against $HgCl_2$ induced renal toxicity. Oxidative modulation of renal tissues following $HgCl_2$ exposure was evident from a significant elevation in lipid peroxidation and attenuation in GSH contents and activities of antioxidant enzymes *viz.*, CAT, GPx, SOD and GR. Oral administration of *E. sativa* extract to rats at a dose regimen: 50-200 mg/kg body weight for 7 days prior to $HgCl_2$ treatment significantly and dose dependently protected against alterations in all these diagnostic parameters.

Euclea divinorum Hierns Family: Ebenaceae

Feyissa *et al.* [314] assessed the protective effects of the crude extract and solvent fractions of *Euclea divinorum* leaves against GM-induced nephrotoxicity in rats. Pre- and co-treatment with the crude extract and solvent fractions of *Euclea divinorum* leaves reversed GM-induced alterations as evidenced by a decrease in tubular necrosis, serum and oxidant markers as well as by an increase in antioxidant molecules. Effect was found to decrease with dose when the crude extract was used and maximum protection was conferred by 100mg/kg of the methanolic fraction in both *in vivo* and *in vitro* studies.

Euphorbia hirta L. Family: Euphorbiaceae

Suganya *et al.* [315] evaluated the nephrotoxicity properties of ethanolic extract (400 mg/kg) of *Euphorbia hirta*. The levels of non-protein nitrogenous compounds (urea, creatinine) were decreased and the level of uric acid was increased when compared with carcinogen induced rats. The level of tumor marker enzymes (ALP, ACP, LDH, γ-GT, xanthine oxidase) and total protein were decreased when compared with carcinogen induced rats.

Suganya *et al.* [316] evaluated the protective effect of *E. hirta* against nitrobenzene-induced nephrotoxicity in albino rats. Treatment with the ethanol extract of *E. hirta* significantly normalized the antioxidant levels. The nephroprotective activity was also supported by histopathologic studies of kidney tissue.

The diuretic effect of the *E. hirta* leaf extracts was evaluated in rats. The water and ethanol extracts (50 and 100 mg/kg) of the plant produced time-dependent increase in urine output. The water extract increased the urine excretion of Na+, K+ and HCO_3-, while, the ethanol extract increased the excretion of HCO_3-, decreased the loss of K+ and had little effect on renal removal of Na+ [317].

Euphorbia neriifolia L. Family: Euphorbiaceae

Pracheta *et al.* [318] investigated the preventive effects of hydro-ethanolic extract of *Euphorbia neriifolia* (EN) on N-nitrosodiethylamine (DENA) induced renal cancer in male Swiss albino mice. DENA increased oxidative stress through increase in LPO and decrease in antioxidant enzymes (SOD, and CAT). The EN extract significantly restored the antioxidant enzyme level in the kidney and exhibited significant dose dependant protective effect against DENA induced nephrotoxicity.

Eurycoma longifolia Jack Family: Simaroubaceae

Chinnappan *et al.* [319] evaluated the protective effect of the extract *Eurycoma longifolia* (EL) against Paracetamol (PCM)-induced nephrotoxicity rat model. In the treatment groups, there was a dose-dependent protection against PCM-induced changes observed in serum total protein, albumin, urea, and creatinine. Significant drop was seen in serum creatinine and blood urea content in treatment groups. Creatinine clearance, serum total protein and serum albumin content were significantly increased in treatment groups compared to PCM alone group. Histopathological examination of the rat kidneys revealed severe degeneration in the PCM alone group, while there was evidence of significant dose-dependent protection in the treatment groups against PCM-induced changes, the serum and urine biochemical results and histopathology.

Exacum lawii C.B.Clarke Family: Gentianaceae

Sharma *et al.* [320] explored the protective effect of the ethanolic extract of *E. lawii* against cisplatin-induced renal toxicity in the rat. Administration of *E. lawii* extract (ELE) restored the biochemical parameters. It also decreased the elevated proinflammatory cytokines level in kidney tissues and protected rat kidneys from oxidative stress in rats. The histological architecture was also conserved.

Eysenhardtia polystachya (Ortega) Sarg. Family: Fabaceae

The water extract of the bark of *Eysenhardtia polystachya* was assessed for its antilithiatic and diuretic activity. A significant decrease in the weight of stones was observed after treatment in animals that received aqueous extract compared with control groups. This extract showed an increase in the 24 h urine volume compared with the control [321].

Ficus carica L. Family: Moraceae

Kore *et al.* [322] assessed the protective effect of hydroalcohalic extract of *Ficus carica* (HEFC) on GM-induced renal proximal tubular damage. HEFC alone increased CAT concentration, GSH content and decreased MDA level. HEFC supplementation ameliorated GM-induced specific metabolic alterations and oxidative damage due to its intrinsic biochemical/antioxidant properties.

Ficus exasperata Vahl Family: Moraceae

Irene and Iheanacho [323] evaluated the nephroportective activity of *Ficus exasperata*. Administration of ethanol extracts *F. exasperata* at doses 50, 200, 500 mg/kg body weight resulted in body weight gain in all extract-administered groups over a 3-day period. Mean relative kidney weight increased in the control group. Serum urea concentration also increased in a dose dependent manner. Serum sodium concentration also increased from $44.95 + 10.94$ in the control group to $98.85 + 0.0$, 123 ± 1.95 and 152.0 ± 35.70 in groups II, III, and IV respectively.

Ficus hispida L.f. Family: Moraceae

The protective effect of fruits of *Ficus hispida* was assessed by Swathi *et al.* [324]. Methanolic extract showed significant nephroprotective activity than nephrocuration on cispaltin induced nephrotoxicity.

Ficus mucuso Welw. ex Ficalho Family: Moraceae

Komolafe *et al.* [205] evaluated the effect of extract of *Ficus mucoso* and its efficacy on the histomorphometry of the kidney in STZ induced diabetic rats. The glomeruli of the diabetic group were atrophied which is validated by significant decrease in its density, shrinkage and increased bowman's space. These observations were also characterized by diminished cellular proliferation, decreased cellular volume and ischemia. The histology and morphometric analysis revealed that the kidney in the group treated with *Ficus mucuso* showed significant increase in density compared to control.

Ficus racemosa L. Family: Moraceae

Khan and Sultana [325] evaluated the preventive effect of *Ficus racemosa* extract against Fe-NTA-induced renal oxidative stress, hyperproliferative response and renal carcinogenesis in rats. Treatment of rats orally with *F. racemosa* extract (200 and 400 mg/kg body weight) resulted in significant decrease in gamma-glutamyl transpeptidase, lipid peroxidation, xanthine oxidase, H_2O_2 generation, BUN, serum creatinine, renal ODC activity, DNA synthesis and incidence of tumors. Renal GSH content, glutathione metabolizing enzymes and antioxidant enzymes were also recovered to significant level.

The histopathological changes and nephroprotective effect of water extract of stem bark of *F. racemosa* (ARF) in albino Wistar rats were studied by Gowda and Swamy [326]. The sign of nephrotoxicity in rats was significantly alleviated by ARF. The results of histopathological examinations also confirmed the nephroprotective effect of ARF.

Ficus religiosa L. Family: Moraceae

Yadav *et al.* [16] and Yadav and Srivastava [327] determined the possible nephroprotective and curative effects of *F. religiosa* latex methanol extract against cisplatin induced acute nephrotixicity. The IC_{50} values of the extract were 31.75 ± 0.12 and 18.35 ± 0.48 µg/ml, respectively. The cisplatin-treated group showed significant changes; renal functions, biochemical parameters and histopathology were significantly recovered by 200 mg/kg curative and protective groups.

Hashmi *et al.* [328] evaluated the nephroprotective effects of *F. religiosa* stem bark against the toxic effects induced by rifampicin (RIF) and isoniazid (INH). The administration of alcohol extract of *F. religiosa* reduced this BUN level, almost close to normal value while its hydro extract also reduced the BUN level significantly but less than alcoholic extract of *F. religiosa*. Similar findings were found with creatinine. Kidney of RIF + INH treated rabbits showed severe degree of infiltration in the glomerulas without renal tubular space between the glomerulas when compared to normal group.

Ficus thonningii Blume Family: Moraceae

Study of its stem-bark ethanolic extract on blood glucose, cardiovascular and kidney functions of rats, and on kidney cell lines of the proximal (LLC-PK1) and distal tubules (MDBK) revealed remarkable renoprotective activities and presented the plant as a source of probable lead compound in the management of kidney diseases [329].

Foeniculum vulgare Mill. Family: Apiaceae

The ethanol extract of the dried ripe fruit of *Foeniculum vulgare* (500 mg/kg) showed diuretic activity [Tanira *et al.*, 330]. Shaheen *et al.* [331] evaluated the protective effects of different doses of aqueous extract of *Foeniculum vulgare* seeds, *Solanum nigrum* fruit and their mixture on GM-induced nephrotoxicity in albino rabbits. The aqueous extract of *Foeniculum vulgare* seeds, *Solanum nigrum* fruit and their mixture significantly prevented renal damage by normalizing increased levels of renal markers. Mixture of both plants at high doses exhibited improved nephroprotective and antioxidant activities. The correction of oxidative stress biomarkers was consistent with amelioration of the histopathological changes induced by GM.

The diuretic activity of aqueous and 80% methanol extracts of *F. vulgare* leaf was evaluated in rats using different doses of aqueous or 80% methanol extract orally. Rats treated with 200 and 400 mg/kg doses of aqueous and 80% methanol extract of *F. vulgare* showed an increased urine volume. However, 100 mg/kg dose of both extracts failed to produce significant increase in 24 h urine volume compared to control groups. Both extracts increased natriuresis, kaliuresis and chloriuresis at the middle and higher doses [332].

The renoprotective effect of the aqueous extract of *F. vulgare* (150 mg/kg bw) was studied in experimental PCOS female rats. The mean values of BUN in PCOS rats treated with low dose of extract of *F. vulgare* and estradiolvalerate and non-treated, was significantly increased compared with non-PCOS and PCOS rats treated with high dose of extract of *F. vulgare*. Moreover, histopathological changes of kidney samples were comparable in PCOS rats with respect to treated groups with extract of *F. vulgare* [333]. The protective effect of fennel essential oil (250, 500, and 1000 mg/kg/day, for 10 days) as a phytoestrogen source was studied against cisplatin -induced nephrotoxicity in rats. Fennel essential oil did not reduce the levels of BUN and Cr, KTDS, and KW and body weight changes. Also, the serum and tissue levels of nitrite were not altered significantly by fennel essential oil [334].

Garcinia kola Heckel Family: Clusiaceae

Komolafe *et al.* [335] investigated the protective effect of methanolic extract of root-bark and dichloromethane fraction of *Garcinia kola* on GM-induced nephrotoxicity in rats. The extract and DCMF did not elicit any adverse effect and a dose of 250 mg/kg bwt of ME and DCMF was selected for further studies. The administration of GM (80 mg/kg bwt) caused elevated levels of plasma renal biomarkers, reduction in AciPase activities. Moreover, administration of GM (80 mg/kg bwt) resulted in damage to kidney structures. Rats treated with 250 mg/kg extract and fraction reversed alterations of biochemical parameters and these were supported by low levels of tubular and glomerular injuries induced by GM treatment.

Ginkgo biloba L. Family: Ginkgoaceae

Inselmann *et al*. [336] examined the effects of *Ginkgo biloba* extract on cisplatin-induced lipid peroxidation and PAH accumulation changes in rat renal cortical slices *G. biloba* extract inhibited cisplatin-induced lipid peroxidation; however, at a cisplatin concentration of 1.0 mg/ml, extract did not prevent the decline of cisplatin-induced PAH uptake.

Naidu *et al*. [337] evaluated the effect of *G. bloba* on GM-induced nephrotoxicity in male Wistar rats. Changes in blood urea, serum creatinine and creatinine clearance induced by GM were significantly prevented by *G. biloba* extract and thus protected rats from GM-induced nephrotoxicity. There was a rise in plasma and kidney tissue MDA with GM, which was significantly reduced to normal with *G. biloba* extract. Histomorphology showed necrosis and desquamation of tubular epithelial cells in renal cortex with GM, while it was normal and comparable to control with *G. biloba* extract.

Okuyan *et al*. [338] investigated the protective effects of *G. biloba* on nephrotoxicity induced by cisplatin in rats. The serum creatinine and kidney MDA levels increased as a result of cisplatin administration and *G. biloba* extract significantly decreased them and also improved the depletion of kidney GSH levels. Histopathologic observations of the kidney tissues also supported these results.

EGb761 (EGb), a standardized extract from the leaves of the *G. biloba* trees, has been available on the market and Song *et al*. [339] investigated the nephroprotectve ability of EGb. The levels of creatinine, BUN, MDA, NO, SOD, CAT, GPx, and GSSG/GSH ratio in kidneys after cisplatin injection were restored withEGb treatment. The elevated NF-κB translocation and caspase-3 protein levels in cisplatin-treated kidneys were decreased by EGb. In porcine kidney proximal tubular epithelial (LLC-PK1) cell line authors found that EGb inhibited ROS accumulation and iNOS increase induced by cisplatin *in vitro*. EGb also attenuated IκB degradation and p65 NF-κB phosphorylation triggered by cisplatin in LLC-PK1 cells. But EGb failed to influence cisplatin-stimulated caspase cascade. Song *et al* [339] suggested that EGb's nephroprotective effect might be mediated by not only its well-known antioxidant activity but also the anti-inflammatory activity.

Glechoma longituba Family: Lamiaceae

Liang *et al.* [340] evaluated the antiurolithc activity of *Glechoma longituba* extract. Compared with the positive control group treatment with *G. longituba* extract significantly decreased CaOx-induced OPN expression, KIM-1 expression, and OS. *in vivo* rats that received *G. longituba* extract exhibited significantly decreased CaOx deposits and pathological alterations compared with urolithic rats. Significantly lower levels of oxalate, creatinine, and urea and increased citrate levels were observed among rats that received *G. longituba* compared with urolithic rats.

Globularia alypum L. Family: Globulariaceae

Inhibition of CaOx monohydrate crystal growth using aqueous extract of flowers and roots of *Globularia alypum* was investigated by Beghalia *et al.* [61]. Activity was tested in bioassays. In the presence of plants extract, the length and the width of the crystals were reduced. It was found that extract of the plant inhibited potently the nucleation and growth phases. Inhibition of the crystal formation of flower extract was 75.53% at 25% concentration, 90.45% at 50% concentration, 89.73% at 75% concentration and 96.09 at 100% concentration, while inhibition of the crystal formation of root extract was 88.78% at 25% concentration, 95.58% at 50% concentration, 96.77% at 75% concentration and 95.22 at 100% concentration.

Glochidion velutinium Wight Family: Phyllanthaceae

Vijaya *et al.* [341] assessed the effects of dried leaves of *Glochidion velutinium* (GV) as a preventive agent in experimentally induced urolithiasis model in rats. The urinary excretion of calcium, phosphate and oxalate are significantly increased in calculi-induced rats when compared with normal control (saline) rats. The increased levels of stone forming constituents in the kidneys of calculogenic rats was significantly reduced by using methanolic extract of dried leaves (250 and 500 mg/kg, p.o) of GV.

Glossostemon bruguieri Desf. Family: Malvaceae

Glossostemon bruguieri powder and its alcoholic extract together with four of the purified compounds (takakin 7-0-glucoside, isosctullarien, its 7-0–glucoside and takakin 8-0-glucoside) were shown to increase urine volume but not sodium on albino rats, being more pronounced and equipotent with that of the standard drug, furosemide [342].

Glycine max (L.) Merr. Family: Fabaceae

Ekor *et al.* [343] evaluated the protective effect of phenolic extract of soybean (PESB) on GM-induced nephrotoxicity rat model. The decrease in the activities of SOD, CAT, GST as well as GSH depletion observed in GM-treated rats was prevented in the rats pretreated with PESB. The activities of gamma-GT, AST and G6Pase were also increased in the kidney. These protective effects were dose dependent except for G6Pase activity and GSH levels that were preserved only at 500 mg/kg dose of PESB, and 5'-NTD activity that was dose dependently decreased. The extent of tubular damage induced by GM was reduced in rats that also received PESB. The lower dose of 500 mg/kg of the extract appeared to provide better histological protection.

Ekor *et al.* [344] evaluated the protective role of phenolic extract of soybean (PESB) in a rat model against cisplatin-induced nephrotoxicity. Following treatment with 250- and 500-mg/kg doses of the extract BUN was reduced by 49.8% and 59.0%, serum creatinine by 34.7% and 62.1% and urinary N-acety--beta-D-glucosaminidase also decreased by 37.7% and 49.2% respectively in the cisplatin-treated rats and renal myeloperoxidase activity by 26.8% and 40.6% at these doses. In the cisplatin-treated rats PESB also decreased renal xanthine oxidase activity and serum nitrate/nitrite. PESB significantly attenuated the marked renal oxidative damage that accompanied cisplatin treatment. The extract significantly increased the activities of the antioxidant enzymes measured [SOD, CAT, GST], prevented GSH depletion and decreased MDA level following cisplatin treatment. Furthermore, cisplatin-induced decrease in the activities of glucose-6-phosphatase and 5'-nucleotidase in these rats was attenuated only at 250 mg/kg dose of the extract.

Ramasamy *et al.* [345] evaluated the protective effect of *G. max* seed extract (soybean oil) against GM and rifampicin induced nephrotoxicity in Sprague-Dawley rats and to compare its effects with those of vitamin E. Soybean oil significantly decreased serum BUN, creatinine, urea, uric acid and urine volume, kidney weight, urinary sodium, urinary potassium, and total protein and significantly increased serum total protein and urine creatinine in GM- and rifampicin-treated animals, exhibiting nephroprotective effects. Soybean oil also showed strong antioxidant effects, causing significant increase in kidney homogenate CAT, GPx, and SOD and significant decrease in lipid peroxidase in GM- and rifampicin-treated animals.

Gomphrena celosioides Mart. Family: Amaranthaceae

Evaluation of nephroprotective properties of aqueous and ethanolic extracts of *Gomphrena celosioides*, against GM-induced renal dysfunction in the albino rats was carried out by Abou *et al.* [223]. The results showed that intra-peritoneal injection of GM causes a significant decrease of total serum rate of protein and a significant raise in serum rate of creatinine and urea. The results also show a significant increase in total protein and albumin in the urine of animals. However, changes in biochemical parameters measured were significantly attenuated in co-treated rats with the extracts of *G. celosioides*. Treatment with the extracts significantly attenuated levels of serum creatinine, serum urea, serum protein, proteinuria and albuminuria.

Gossypium herbaceum L. Family: Malvaceae

The diuretic activity of ethyl acetate and alcohol extract of leaves of *Gossypium herbaceum* (100 and 200 mg/kg body weight) was investigated in male Wistar albino rats. Compared with the control the total urine volumes of the both extracts (200mg/kg) treated rats were elevated nearly two folds. Compared with control group excretion of sodium, potassium and chloride ions were increased significantly. Alcoholic extract showed more significant diuretic activity compared with the ethyl acetate extract as a diuretic. The diuretic effect was comparable with that of the standard drug Furosemide The increase of sodium and potassium in the urine of the group treated with both extracts was dose dependent [346].

Grewia asiatica L. Family: Malvaceae

Babu *et al.* [347] evaluated the antilithiatic activity of an ethanolic leaf extract of *Grewia asiatica* (EEGA). Supplementation with EEGA significantly restored urea, uric acid, and creatinine, volume of urine and pH levels. The preventive regimen was found to be better than the curative regimen. The antilithiatic or nephoprotective activity of the extract was further corraborated by the histopathological examination.

Gymnema sylvestre R.Br. Family: Apocynaceae

Sree Lakshmi *et al.* [348] evaluated the antilithiatic effect of ethanolic extract of leaves of *Gymnema sylvestre* (EEGS). Treatment with ethanolic extract of *G. sylvestre* at both the doses (200 mg/kg and 400 mg/kg b.wt) showed a significant restoration of urinary and serum parameters on EG&AC induction. The extracts at doses 200 mg/kg and 400 mg/kg b.wt showed significant increase in antioxidant enzymes activity and decrease in MDA levels.

Harungana madagascariensis Lam. ex Poir. Family: Hypericaceae

Adeneye *et al.* [349] evaluated the nephroprotective effects of the root aqueous extract of *Harungana madagascariensis* in acute and repeated dose acetaminophen nephrotoxic rats. Pretreatments with graded oral doses of the extract attenuated elevations in the serum concentrations of UR, UA and CR, and improved diffuse tubular necrosis in both models of acetaminophen nephrotoxicity. The extract also significantly improved packed cell volume, hemoglobin, and total leucocyte count levels but non-significant increase in the mean corpuscular volume, mean corpuscular hemoglobin, and mean corpuscular haemoglobin concentration, in the repeated acetaminophen model.

Hedychium coronarium J. Koenig Family: Zingiberacee

Ethanolic and aqueous extracts of roots and rhizomes of *Hedychium coronarium* plant were evaluated by Tailor and Goyal [350] for their potential to dissolve experimentally prepared kidney stones like CaOx by titrimetic method with an *in vitro* model. Ethanolic roots and rhizomes extract of this plant produced highest dissolution of stones when compared to standard drug cystone and at 10 mg concentration.

Helianthus annuus L. Family: Asteraceae

Khan *et al.* [351] evaluated the urolithiatic effect of aqueous and ethanolic extracts of leaves of *Helianthus annuus* (Sunflower) in male Albino Wistar rats. By treatment using aqueous and ethanolic extracts the increased deposition of stone forming constituents in the kidneys of calculogenic rats was significantly lowered.

Helichrysum ceres S. Moore Family: Asteraceae

Musabayane *et al.* [352] evaluated the effects of *Helichrysum ceres* root and leaf extracts on renal fluid and electrolyte handling in anesthetized male Sprague-Dawley rats. Infusion of graded doses of aqueous leaf extracts of *H. ceres* provoked an increase in urine flow rates. The extracts produced dose dependent decrease in potassium excretion as well as increases in urinary Na^+ outputs and diuresis. Administration of the various doses of aqueous root extracts of *H. ceres* significantly increased urine flow rate and urinary Na^+ excretion in all groups.

Helichrysum graveolens (M. Bieb.) Sweet and *H. stoechas* ssp. *barellieri* (Ten.) Nyman Family: Asteraceae

In Turkey *Helichrysum* flowers are used to remove kidney stones and for their diuretic properties. Onaran *et al.* [353] determined the curative effect of infusions prepared from capitula of *Helichrysum graveolens* (HG) and *H. stoechas* ssp. *barellieri* (HS) on sodium oxalate induced kidney stones. *H. stoechas* extract showed prominent effect at 156 mg/kg dose, whereas number of kidney stones was maximum in sodium oxalate group. The reduction in the uric acid and oxalate levels of urine samples and the elevation in the urine citrate levels are significant and promising in extract groups.

Helichrysum plicatum DC. subsp. *plicatum* Family: Asteraceae

Bayir *et al*. [354] assessed the antilithiatic effects of *Helichrysum plicatum* subsp. *plicatum* (HP) in rats. The rats' weights were higher in HP groups than urolithiasis group. HP extract decreased levels of serum and urine biochemical parameters. Urine CaOx level was high in urolithiasis rats, whereas it was decreased by HP extract. Histopathological examinations revealed extensive intratubular crystal depositions and degenerative tubular structures in urolithiasis group, but not in HP treatment groups.

Heliotropium eichwaldii Steud. Family: Boraginaceae

Sharma and Goyal [355] evaluated the protective effect of methanolic extract of *Heliotropium eichwaldii* (MHE) in mice with cisplatin-induced acute renal damage. MHE treatment significantly reduced BUN and serum CRE levels elevated by cisplatin administration. Also, it significantly attenuated cisplatin-induced increase in MDA level and improved the decreased CAT and SOD activities in renal cortical homogenates. Histopathological examination and scoring showed that MHE markedly ameliorated cisplatin-induced renal tubular necrosis.

Hemidesmus indicus L. Family: Apocynaceae

Kotnis *et al*. [356] evaluated the efficacy of *Hemidesmus indicus* in the management of GM-induced nephrotoxicity in albino Wister rats. The treatment with *H. indicus* helped in the management of renal impairment, which was induced by GM in rats. This was evident from the results obtained for various kidney function tests for GM, along with the results from the plant treated group, and is in comparison with the results found for the GM recovery group. A histological examination of kidneys also supports the findings from haematological evaluations.

The ethanolic extract of the roots of *H. indicus* was investigated by Kaur *et al*. [357] for its protective activity in cisplatin-induced nephrotoxicity in rats. In the curative regimen, the ethanolic extract at dose levels of 250 and 500 mg/kg showed dose-dependent reduction in the elevated blood urea and serum creatinine.

There was increase in the GSH and GST enzyme level after treating rats with ethanolic extract of *H. indicus*. The ethanolic extract also showed inhibition of cisplatin-induced lipid peroxidation.

Sandeep and Nair [43] evaluated the protective activity of *H. indicus* against cisplatin-induced nephrotoxicity. Treatment of cisplatin-administered animals with the plant extracts could prevent the drug-induced oxidative damage in the renal tissue as evidenced from the decreased levels of lipid peroxidation and enhanced activities of the antioxidants in the renal tissue. Cisplatin treatment increased serum urea level and administration of the extracts of *H. indicus* brought down the level. Serum creatinine levels were increased following cisplatin administration, and treatment with extracts of *H. indicus* brought this. The histopathological observations indicated that treatment with the *H. indicus* extract restored the cisplatin-induced structural alterations in the renal tissue.

Herniaria hirsuta L. Family: Caryophyllaceae

Grases *et al*. [310] found that *Herniaria hirsuta* exerted no effect on urolithiasis risk factors when given to the rats in combination with different diets.

Atmani and Khan [358] evaluated the effectiveness of *Herniaria hirsuta* extract on CaOx crystallization *in vitro*. The *H. hirsuta* extract promoted the precipitation of CaOx particles in whole urine. There were more crystals with increasing concentration of extract but that they were proportionally smaller. The presence of herb extract favoured the formation of CaOx dihydrate rather than monohydrate crystals. The extract inhibited CaOx crystal aggregation. In an independent experiment, the herb extract was dialysed and filtered before inducing crystallization, to eliminate any fibrous particles and oxalate.

Atmani *et al*. [359] assessed the effect of aqueous extract from *H. hirsuta* on the adhesion of CaOx monohydrate (COM) crystals to cultured renal cells. COM crystal binding to cells was inhibited by extract in a concentration dependent manner. Prior exposure of crystals but not cells to extract blocked crystal binding, suggesting that plant molecules can coat and exert their effect at the crystal surface. Crystal attachment appeared related to membrane fluidity since crystal adhesion increased at higher *vs* lower temperatures (37 °C *vs* 0 °C) and Herniaria extract altered crystal adhesion only under conditions of increased fluidity (increased temperature). Extract also displaced a significant portion of prebound crystals without apparent effects on cell function or the morphology of preexisting CaOx crystals. *Herniaria* extract exerted no adverse or toxic effect on cells, which proliferated normally in its presence even at relatively high concentrations.

Atmani *et al*. [360] looked for an alternative treatment by using *H. hirsuta* on nephrolithiasic rats as a preventive agent against the development of kidney stones. The experiment was conducted in normal and CaOx nephrolithiasic rats during 3 weeks. Water intake and urinary volume increased in nephrolithiasic rats, but their urinary pH decreased especially in the third week of treatment. Urinary oxalate increased significantly during the second week for untreated rats and remained constant in rats treated with *Herniaria* decoction. However, urinary calcium decreased significantly in week 2 in untreated rats and remained constant in treated rats. Qualitative analysis of crystalluria showed that untreated rats excreted large CaOx monohydrate and few dihydrate crystals while treated animals excreted mostly small CaOx dihydrate crystals. The examination of kidney sections revealed that CaOx deposition was limited in treated rats when compared to untreated ones.

The prophylactic effect of oral administration of *H. hirsuta* decoction was investigated in experimentally induced CaOx nephrolithiasis in rats. *H. hirsuta* has an impressive prophylactic effect on CaOx stones in nephrolithic rats, the effect is not mediated by biochemical or diuretic changes [361].

Atmani *et al*. [362] attempted an initial fractionation of the methanol extract of the plant bio-guided by *in vitro* and *in vivo* crystallization assays to determine the nature of compound responsible for the beneficial effect of the plant. In the whole human urine, only the fraction eluted with ethanol/water was associated to formation of smaller crystals composed of calcium oxalate dihydrate, similarly to the aqueous extract. When tested at 5 mg/day, it reduced significantly crystal deposition in lithiasic rats. Preliminary identification of plant compound found in that fraction showed the presence of saponins.

The effect of *Herniaria hirsuta* extract on the disolution of cystine stones was studied *in vitro*. The results revealed that the studied herbal extracts were efficient for dissolving cystine stones, probably by formation of complexes between cystine and polyhydroxylated molecules present in the extracts [363].

Hibiscus platanifolius (Willd.) Sweet Family: Malvaceae

The nephroprotective effects of the ethanol extract of the *Hibiscus platanifolius* root were evaluated by Reddy *et al*. [364] using Wistar albino rats as experimental animal model. The nephrotoxicity has been induced by GM. The ethanol extract of *H. platanifolius* showed a significant protective effect on nephrotoxicity, this high dose (500mg/kg) significantly reduced the urea, uric acid, creatinine levels which is a broad spectrum antibiotic used to treat many ailments.

Hibiscus rosa-sinensis L. Family: Malvaceae

The water extract of flowers of *Hibiscus rosa-sinensis* was evaluated for antilithatic potential *in vitro*. The presence of CaOx crystals was evaluated immediately and after 24 hrs of stone induction. Crystal aggregation after 24 hrs was inhibited by *H. rosa-sinensis* extract. The extract interfered with early stages of stone formation [365].

The effect of water extract of *H. rosa-sinensis* on urinary volume and electrolyte extraction was studied in albino rats. Water extract of *H. rosa-sinensis* increased the urinary volume of the 5th and 24th hr samples. Na+ and Cl- excretion were also significantly increased in 200 and 400 mg/kg doses [366].

Hibiscus sabdariffa L. Family: Malvaceae

Kirdpon *et al.* [367] evaluated the changes of urine in normal subjects after consuming roselle (*Hibiscus sabdariffa)* juice in different concentrations and durations which may help the treatment and prevention of renal stone disease. 36 healthy men participated in the study. The urine after consumption of roselle juice showed a decrease of creatinine, uric acid citrate, tartrate, calcium, sodium, potassium and phosphate but not oxalate in urinary excretion. The CPR values of the majority of each individual increased and means PI values decreased in phase 1. Contrarily, the CPR value of the majority of volunteers decreased and means PI values increase in phase 2. In conclusion a low dose of roselle juice (16g/day) caused more significant decrease in salt output in the urine than a high dose (24g/day). The urinary changes were similar to the observations on villagers with and without stones in northeastern Thailand.

The Roselle (*H. sabdariffa*) was investigated by Prasongwatana *et al.* [368] for its uricosuric effect. A human model with nine subjects with no history of renal stones (non-renal stone, NS) and nine with a history of renal stones (RS) was used in this study. All analyzed serum parameters were within normal ranges and similar; between the two groups of subjects and among the three periods. Vis-à-vis the urinary parameters, most of the baseline values for both groups were similar. After taking the tea, the trend was an increase in oxalate and citrate in both groups and uric acid excretion and clearance in the NS group. In the RS group, both uric acid excretion and clearance were significantly increased. When the fractional excretion of uric acid (FEUa) was calculated, the values were clearly increased in both the NS and SF groups after the intake of tea and returned to baseline values in the washout period. These changes were more clearly observed when the data for each subject was presented individually.

Woottisin *et al.* [369] fed the rats with tablets containing the extracts from leaves of *H. sabdariffa* instead of adding in the drinking water. Four weeks later, the serum oxalate and glycolate level in group received a 3% glycolate diet and tablets containing the extracts from leaves of *H. sabdariffa* (3.5 mg extract per tablet) significantly decreased, while urinary citrate and oxalate levels of the group were higher than the group only received a 3% glycoside diet. Alternatively, the extracts from leaves of both *H. sabdariffa* decreased calcium crystal deposition in the kidneys of rats.

The ethanolic extract of *H. sabdariffa* leaves (EEHS) was evaluated by Betanabhatala *et al.* [370] for its antilithiatic activity in rats. The EEHS, however, significantly reduced the elevated level of crucial ions in urine. Also, it elevated concentration of urinary magnesium, which is considered as one of the inhibitors of crystallization.

Kunworarath *et al.* [371] evaluated the protective effect of *H. sabdariffa* aqueous extract (HSE) in ARF rat caused by cisplatin using renal clearance and renal lipid peroxidation study. It was found that the acute treatment with HSE was able to attenuate cisplatin-induced ARF by improving both renal plasma flow and glomerular filtration rate and reducing renal MDA level.

The diuretic, natriuretic, and potassium sparing effects of *H. sabdariffa* are due in part to the modulation of aldosterone activity by the presence of compounds potentially responsible for this modulation [372].

Holarrhena antidysenterica (L.) Wall. ex A.DC. Family Apocynaceae

Khan *et al.* [373] evaluated the possible antiurolithiatic effect of crude aqueous-methanolic extract *Holarrhena antidysenterica*. In the *in vitro* experiments, Ha.Cr demonstrated a concentration-dependent (0.25-4 mg/ml) inhibitory effect on the slope of aggregation. It decreased the size of crystals and transformed the CaOx monohydrate (COM) to CaOx dihydrate (COD) crystals, in CaOx metastable solutions. Ha.Cr (0.3 mg/ml) reduced the cell toxicity and LDH release in renal epithelial cells (MDCK) exposed to oxalate (0.5 mM) and COM (66 µg/cm(2) crystals. In male Wistar rats, receiving 0.75% ethylene glycol (EG) for 21 days along with 1% ammonium chloride (AC) in drinking water, Ha.Cr treatment (30-100 mg/kg) prevented the toxic changes caused by lithogenic agents; EG and AC, like loss of body weight, polyurea, oxaluria, raised serum urea and creatinine levels and crystal deposition in kidneys compared to their respective controls.

Homonoia riparia Lour. Family: Euphorbiaceae

Ethanol extract of the roots of *Homonoia riparia* was assessed by Prasad *et al.*

[374] for its antiurolithiatic activity against CaOx and magnesium ammonium phosphate stones in male albino rats. The ethanol extract of *H. riparia* (2 g/kg/day, orally) was found to be effective in reducing deposition of calcium in the kidney of both prophylactic and curative group animals. The extract did not show any significant effect on the activity of the liver enzyme glycolic acid oxidase and on the deposition of oxalate in the kidney. The extract was found to be effective in reducing the formation and also in dissolving the pre-formed magnesium ammonium phosphate type of stones.

Hordeum vulgare L. Family: Poaceae

Shah *et al.* [375] investigated the antiurolithiatic activity of ethanolic extract of *Hordeum vulgare* seeds (EHV) on ethylene glycol-induced urolithiasis in Wistar albino rats. The EHV treatment (both preventive and curative) increased the urine output significantly compared to the control. The EHV treatment significantly reduced the urinary excretion of the calcium, phosphate, uric acid, magnesium, urea, and oxalate and increased the excretion of citrate compared to EG control. The increased deposition of stone forming constituents in the kidneys of calculogenic rats were significantly lowered by curative and preventive treatment with EHV. It was also observed that the treatment with EHV produced significant decrease in lipid peroxidation, and increased levels of SOD and CAT.

Houttuynia cordata Thunb. Family: Saururaceae

Kang *et al.* [376] investigated the protective effects of *Houttuynia cordata* (HC) against GM sulfate-induced renal damage in rats. Treatment of rats with HC showed significant improvement in renal function, presumably as a result of decreased biochemical indices and oxidative stress parameters associated with GS-induced nephrotoxicity. Histopathological examination of the rat kidneys confirmed these observations.

Hygrophila auriculata (Shumach.) Heine (Syn.: *H. spinosa* T. Anderson) Family: Acanthaceae

Therapeutic effect of ethanolic extract of *Hygrophila auriculata* in GM-induced nephrotoxic model of kidney injury in male Sprague-Dawley rats was studied by Bibu *et al.* [377]. *H. auriculata* extract showed free radical scavenging activities at doses of 50 and 250 mg/kg with a predominant activity at 250 mg/kg. The ethanolic extract also caused a reduction in serum creatinine and urea levels. Histopathological studies were conducted to confirm the therapeutic action of the plant extract. The results demonstrated that the ethanolic extract of whole plant of *H. auriculata* evinced the therapeutic effect and inhibited GM-induced proximal tubular necrosis.

The antilithiatic effect of *H. aurculata* (Syn.: *H. spinosa*) was determined by Sathish *et al*. [378] on ethylene glycol induced lithiasis in male albino rats. Aqueous extract of *H. auriculata* (200 mg/kg) was administered orally from 1st day for preventive regimen and from 15th day for curative regimen. The *H. auriculata* significantly reduced the elevated levels calcium, oxalate, inorganic phosphate, protein concentration in urine. Also the extract significantly elevated the urinary concentration of magnesium. The elevated serum creatinine levels of lithiatic rats were reduced by prophylactic and curative regimen of extract treatment. The histological findings also showed improvement after treatment with the extract.

Ingale *et al*. [379] evaluated the antiurolithiatic activity of methanolic extract of *H. auriculata* (HAME) in ethylene glycol induced nephrolithiasic rats. Treatment with HAME significantly reduced the elevated urinary oxalate, urinary calcium and serum uric acid with increase in reduced urinary magnesium. Ethylene glycol feeding also resulted in increased levels of calcium and oxalate in kidney which was decreased after the treatment with HAME. The increased deposition of stone forming constituents in the kidneys of ethylene glycol treated rats was significantly lowered by treatment with HAME.

Ingale *et al*. [380] evaluated the protective effect of methanolic extract of *H. auriculata* (HAME) in cisplatin (CP)-induced nephrotoxicity in male Wistar rats. HAME pretreatment signficantly reduced blood urea and serum creatinine levels elevated by CP administration. Furthermore, HAME significantly attenuated CP-induced increase in MDA and decrease in reduced GSH, and CAT and SOD and GSH peroxidase activities in renal cortical homogenates. Additionally, histopathological examination showed that HAME markedly ameliorated CP-induced renal tubular necrosis.

Hypericum perforatum L. Family: Hypericaceae

Khalili *et al*. [381] investigated the effects of the hydroalcoholic extract of *Hypericum perforatum* leaves on urolithiasis in rats. Urine level of free calcium in groups EG and EG + *H. perforatum* (300 mg/kg) and phosphorous in EG + *H. perforatum* (500 mg/kg) significantly decreased compared to controls. Treatment of the rats with high dose of *H. perforatum* (500 mg/kg) markedly reduced decrementing effect of EG on serum level of free calcium. Histological experiments showed that chronic feeding of *H. perforatum* (300 and 500 mg/kg, orally) could significantly reduce the size and number of CaOx deposits in EG group.

Hyptis suaveolens (L.) Poit. Family: Lamiaceae

The inhibition of *in vitro* CaOx crystal formation by various extracts of *Hyptis suaveolens* was investigated by Agarwal and Varma [382] by titrimetric method. The inhibitor potency of alcohol extracts of *H. suaveolens* was found to be comparable to that of cystone (a proprietory drug for dissolving kidney stones).

Ichnocarpus frutescens (L.) W.T.Aiton Family: Apocynaceae

The inhibitory effect of the root of *Ichnocarpus frutescens* on nephrolithiasis induced in rats with ethylene glycol was investigated by Anbu *et al.* [383]. Supplementation with ethyle acetate extract of root of *I. frutescens* significantly reduced the elevated urinary oxalate, showing a regulatory action on endogenous oxalate synthesis. The increased deposition of stone forming constituents in the kidneys of calculogenic rats was also significantly lowered by the extract treated groups.

Indigofera tinctoria L. Family: Fabaceae

Priyadarsini *et al.* [384] evaluated for nephroprotective activity of decoction of *Indigofera tinctoria* in Cisplatin-induced nephrotoxicity in rats. Effect of concurrent administration of extract of leaves and extract of roots and leaves at a dose of 500 mg/kg and 1000mg/kg were given for respective animal groups by oral route was determined using serum creatinine and blood urea and change in body weight as indicators of kidney damage. The decoctions significantly decreased the cisplatin induced nephrotoxicity. Remarkable changes were observed in body weight, serum creatinine and urea levels. It was observed that the extract of roots and leaves significantly protected the kidneys from injury than the extract of leaves.

Ipomoea aquatica Forssk. Family: Convolvulaceae

Sharmin *et al.* [385] evaluated the protective effect of *Ipomoea aquatica* ethanol extract of leaves on GM-induced nephrotoxic rats. Pre and concomitant administration of IA ethanol extract on GM induced nephrotoxic rats significantly decreased the elevated serum creatinine and urea levels when compared to those of GM treated group. The comparative histopathological study of kidney exhibited almost normal architecture as compared to control group.

Ipomoea batatas (L.) Lam. Family: Convolvulaceae

Sathish and Jeyabalan [386] demonstrated the *in vitro* anti-lithiatic effect of ethanolic and aqueous extracts of *I. batatas* leaves and tuberous roots. In the estimation of CaOx by titrimetry method, the *I. batatas* leaves and roots have very significant capability to dissolve CaOx. The *I. batatas* leaves and roots significantly dissolved calcium phosphate also. The results clearly shown that *I. batatas* extracts significantly inhibited both nucleation and aggregation of CaOx crystals by concentration-dependent manner.

Ipomoea digitata L. Family: Convolvulaceae

Kalaiselvan *et al.* [387] assessed the renoprotectve activity of *Ipomoea digitata* in GM-induced nephrotoxicity in rats. Supplementation of *I. digitatata* GM intoxicated rats restored the altered parameters.

Ipomoea eriocarpa R.Br. Family: Convolvulaceae

Das and Malipeddi [388] investigated the preventive and curative effect of the ethanol leaf extract of *Ipomoea eriocarpa* (IEE) in ethylene glycol-induced urolithiasis in rats. The IEE treatment significantly restored the parameters in urine, serum, and kidney homogenate to near-normal level. The histopathological examinations revealed that CaOx crystal deposits in the renal tubules and congestion and dilation of the parenchymal blood vessels were significantly reverted after IEE treatment.

Ipomoea obscura (L.) Ker-Gawl. Family: Convolvulaceae

Hamsa and Kuttan [389] evaluated the protective effect of *Ipomoea obscura* against Cisplatin (CP)-induced uro- and nephrotoxicities in Swiss albino mice. The toxicities caused by CP were reversed by the extract administration as evident from the decrease in BUN, serum creatinine levels as well as an increase in body weight. A significant increase in kidney antioxidant system such as, GSH, SOD, CAT, and GPx was also observed in extract-treated animals. Histopathological analysis of urinary bladder and kidney indicated that CP-induced tissue damage was significantly reduced in animals treated with *I. obscura*. The lowered levels of cytokines IFN-γ and IL-2, after CP treatment were found to be increased in treated animals. At the same time the level of proinflammatory cytokine TNF-α, which was elevated during CP administration, was significantly reduced by extract administration.

Ipomoea staphylina Roem. & Schult. Family: Convolvulaceae

Bag and Mumtaz [390] investigated the protective effect of hydroalcoholic extract of leaves of *Ipomoea staphylina* against GM-induced nephrotoxicity in rats. The extract showed nephroprotective activity against GM-induced nephrotoxicity by significantly reducing the levels of blood urea, BUN, serum creatinine and significantly increasing the serum total protein. The extract also improved the histology of the kidney.

Jasminum auriculatum Vahl Family: Oleaceae

The effect of aqueous and alcohol extracts of *Jasminum auriculatum* flowers on CaOx nephrolithiasis has been studied in male albino rats by Bahuguna *et al.* [391]. Supplementation with aqueous and alcohol extract of *J. auriculatum* flowers significantly reduced the elevated urinary oxalate, showing a regulatory action on endogenous oxalate synthesis. The increased deposition of stone forming constituents in the kidneys of calculogenic rats was significantly lowered by curative and preventive treatment using aqueous and alcohol extracts.

Juglans regia L. Family: Juglandaceae

The modulatory effect of walnut extract on the toxicity of cyclophosphamide (CP) was evaluated in mice. Plant extract + CP group animals showed restoration in the level of cytochrome P450 (CYP) content and in the activities of GST, GPx and CAT in both liver and kidneys. But plant extract restored the activity of SOD and the level of reduced GSH in the kidneys only when compared with CP-treated animals. Plant extract treatment alone caused significant reduction in the content of CYP in the kidneys mainly. The extract showed a significant increase in the level of GSH and in the activities of GP in both the tissues and CAT in liver only, whereas no significant change was observed in the activities of GST and SOD. The extract+CP showed a significant decrease in the LPO in liver and kidneys when compared with the CP-treated group [392].

Juniperus communis L. Family: Cupressaceae

A 10% aqueous infusion of juniper, 0.1% aqueous solution of juniper oil (with 0.2% of Tween 20 solubilizer) and 0.01% aqueous solution of terpinen-4-ol were orally administered to rats at 5ml/100g bw to determine the effect on urine output. Compared to water, the 10% aqueous infusion of juniper and the 0.1% aqueous solution of juniper oil caused reductions of only 6% in diuresis over a 24-hour period, equivalent to the effect of 0.004 IU/100g of ADH, while the 0.01% solution of terpinen-4-ol caused a reduction of 30% in diuresis, equivalent to 0.4 IU/100g intraperitoneal of ADH. Continued daily administration at the same daily dose level, the two juniper preparations and terpinen-4-ol stimulated diuresis on days two and three, although only the 10% aqueous infusion of juniper exerted significant diuretic activity (+ 43% on day two; +44% on day three), suggesting that the diuretic effect is partly due to the essential oil and partly to hydrophilic constituents [393].

However, oral administration of lyophilized aqueous extract of juniper at 1000 mg/kg bw to rats, it didn't increase urine volume or excretion of Na^+, K^+ or Cl^- ions over a six-hour period compared to the effect of the same volume of water [394].

Justicia adhatoda L. (Syn.: *Adhatoda zeylanica* Medik.) Family: Acanthaceae

Kumar *et al.* [395] presented the scientific evidence for the use of common herb *Justicia adhatoda* as supplementary in the GM treated acute renal failure (ARF) subjects. The beneficial effect of *J. adhatoda* against GM nephrotoxicity possibly depends on its ability to scavenge the GM-induced free radicals. This study demonstrates the effectiveness of the extract improved with the polarity of the solvents over a period of 10 days and the plant has the potential to ameliorate GM-nephrotoxicity.

Kelussia odoratissima Mozaff. Family: Apiaceae

Torki *et al.* [396] investigated *in vitro* effect of crude extract and fractions of *K. odoratissima* on kidney stones (CaOx and calcium phosphate). Total extract and its fractions had significant potency to dissolve CaOx and calcium phosphate crystals. Higher potency of fractions containing nonpolar compounds to dissolve calcium phosphate and CaOx stones compared to the fractions containing polar compounds. *n*-butanolic fraction had the least effect and hexane fraction had the greatest effect on the calcium phosphate stones. Furthermore, the total extract has less dissolution ability, compared to the fractions.

Khaya senegalensis (Desv.) A.Juss. Family: Meliaceae

The effects of water extract of *Khaya senegalensis* were tested by El Badwi *et al.* [397] against GM-induced nephrotoxicity in Wistar rats. Oral administration of *K. senegalensis* at 250 and 500 mg/kg to rats significantly ameliorated the increase in serum urea, creatinine, total protein and albumin and similarly ameliored the damage in the kidney tubules.

Kigelia africana (Lam.) Benth. [Syn.: *Kigelia pinnata* (Jacq.) DC.] Family: Bignoniaceae

The protective effect of methanolic extract of *Kigelia africana* fruit against cisplatin-induced nephrotoxicity in male rats was studied by Azu *et al.* [398]. The fruit extract alone and as a prophylaxis significantly increased the altered parameters. Though post-treatment of animals with fruit extract after cisplatin did not restore serum CAT activity it was lower than those receiving cisplatin alone.

Kumar *et al.* [399] studied the effect of oral administration of ethanolic extract of *K. africana* fruit on CaOx urolithiasis in male Wistar albino rats. Supplementation with ethanolic extract of *K. africana* fruit significantly reduced the elevated urinary oxalate, uric acid and phosphate. The increased deposition of stone forming constituents in the kidneys of caulogenic rats was also significantly lowered by ethanolic extract of *K. africana* fruit.

Lagenaria siceraria (Molina) Standl. Family: Cucurbitaceae

Mahurkar *et al.* [400] evaluated the nephroprotective activity of methanolic and watr extracts of *Lagenaria siceraria* seeds. The extract was found to be potent diuretic which causes excretion of sodium and potassium. The increased levels of biochemical parameters and extent of renal damage due to GM administration were decreased by the methanolic and water extracts of *L. siceraria* seeds at a dose of 250 mg/kg.

Takawale *et al.* [401] determined anti-urolithiatic effect of *L. siceraria* fruit powder (LSFP) against sodium oxalate (NaOx) induced urolithiasis in rats. The increased severity of microscopic CaOx crystals deposition along with increased concentration in the kidney was seen after 7 days of NaOx (70 mg/kg, i.p.) pre-treatment. LSFP (500 mg/kg, p.o.) and standard marketed formulation Cystone (500 mg/kg, p.o.) caused a significant reversal of NaOx-induced changes in ion excretion and urinary CaOx concentration in 7 days treatment.

Evaluation of *in vitro* antiurolithiatic activity of *L. siceraria* seeds was carried out by Prasad *et al.* [402]. Titrimetric method was used to assess the antiurolithiatic activity of methanolic extract of *L. siceraria* seeds. It was observed that the highest CaOx crystals dissolution was observed in the methanolic extract of *L. siceraria*. It was found that methanolic extract of *L. siceraria* seeds was more efficient to dissolve CaOx.

Lantana camara L. Family: Verbenaceae

Ethanolic extract of *Lantana camara* leaves were evaluated by Mayee and Thosar [403] for antiurolithiatic activity against ethylene glycol and ammonium chloride induced CaOx urolithiasis in male albino rats. On treatment with the extract, a significant reduction in the deposition of calcium, oxalate and also urinary excretion of calcium, oxalate and creatinine was observed, indicating its antiurolithiatic effect. The extract administration also decreased the extent of lipid peroxidation and hence enhanced the levels of antioxidant enzymes in the kidneys of urolithic rats, reflecting its antioxidant efficacy against hyperoxaluria induced renal oxidative stress.

Chatterjee *et al.* [404] explored the protective effect of methanol extract of *L. camara* (MELC) against acetaminophen and cisplatin induced nephrotoxicity in rats. In the acetaminophen nephrotoxic rats, 200 and 400 mg/kg/day significantly attenuated elevations in the serum creatinine, total protein and BUN levels in dose related fashion, as well as, attenuation of acetaminophen induced tubulonephrosis. Similar effects were also recorded in the Cisplatin model of acute renal injury.

Khalid *et al.* [405] explored the protective effect of the ethanolic extract of *L. camara* flowers against cisplatin induced acute renal toxicity in rats. The extract significantly decreased the levels of serum creatinine, serum urea and BUN and improved morphological parameters and the histoarchitecture revealed improved protection against the acute kidney damage as dose dependent effect with respect to the normal group. The nephroprotective effect was due to proanthocyanidins, a flavonoid is known for its high antioxidant property, present in flower ethanolic extract of *L. camara*.

Vyas and Argal [406] evaluated the antiurolithiatic activity of ethanolic extract of roots (ELC 200 mg/kg) and oleanolic acid isolated from roots of *L. camara* in albino Wistar male rats. Treatment with OA and ELC significantly reduced the calcium output as compared with zinc disc implanted group. The rats which received OA and ELC showed reduced formation of depositions around the zinc disc. The X-ray images of rats also showed significant effect of OA and ELC on urolitiasis.

Abdel-Hady *et al.* [258] assessed the protective active activity of *L. camara* in cisplatin-induced nephrotoxicity in rats. The defatted methanolic extract and ethyl acetate fraction of *L. camara* showed highest improvement of renal parameters.

Launaea procumbens (Roxb.) Ramayya & Rajagopal Family: Asteraceae

Methanolic, chloroform, ethyl acetate, and n-hexane fractions of *Launaea procumbens* were evaluated by Khan *et al.* [407] against CCl_4-induced nephrotoxicity in rat. CCl_4 exposure led to a significant oxidative stress in kidneys which was remarkably attenuated with co-administration of various fractions and rutin thereby increased the level of CAT, POD, SOD, GSH, GSR, GST, GSH-Px, quinone reductase, while reduced the xanthine oxidase, gamma-GT, TBARS, H_2O_2, nitrite, tissue proteins and DNA fragmentation%. Ameliorated effects of fractions and rutin were also recorded for the function of kidneys and the level of urobilinogen, urea, albumin, creatinine, RBC and WBC in urine were decreased. Serum level of creatinine, urobilinogen, BUN, direct bilirubin, total bilirubin and globulin were decreased while total proteins, albumin and creatinine clearance were increased with fractions and rutin. Protective effects of rutin and fractions were also evident on histopathology by reducing glomerular atrophy, tubular degeneration, congestion of blood capillaries, necrosis of epithelium and edema. Similarly body weight was increased while kidney and relative kidney weight was decreased with co-administration of fractions and rutin.

Makasana *et al.* [408] investigated the anti-urolithiatic activity of *L. procumbens* against ethylene glycol-induced urolithiasis and its possible underlying mechanisms. The crude methanolic extract of *L. procumbens* leaves was studied using ethylene glycol-induced renal calculi in rat model. Supplementation with methanolic extract of *L. procumbens* leaves (MELP) significantly prevented changes in urinary calcium, oxalate and phosphate excretion dose-dependently. The increased calcium and oxalate level and number of CaOx crystal in the kidney tissue of calculogenic rats were significantly reverted by supplementation with MELP. The MELP supplementation also prevents the impairment of renal functions.

L. procumbens has been investigated for its anti-urolithiatic activity by Bansode *et al.* [409] by constructing an *in-vitro* model. Various crude extracts of *L. procumbens* were evaluated for their potential to dissolve experimentally prepared kidney stones of CaOx, calcium phosphate. Chloroform, alcoholic and acetone fractions of plant leaves showed highest dissolution of CaOx stones as compared to others while ethyl acetate, pet ether, acetone fractions of plant leaves were more effective in dissolving calcium phosphate compared to reference standard-formulation Cystone.

Launaea taraxacifolia (Willd.) Amin. ex C. Jeffrey Family: Asteraceae

The protective effect of leaf water extract of *Launaea taraxacifolia* against Cisplatin-induced renal injury in Wistar rats was investigated by Adejuwon *et al.* [410]. Hepatorenal histological toxicities were observed in rats exclusively exposed to cisplatin while dose-dependent ameliorations of these histopathologies were seen in those with combined exposure with the aqueous extract of *L. taraxacifolia* and virtually normal histoarchitecture was seen in extract alone treated rats. The renal (BUN and CREAT) injury markers significantly increased in groups exclusively exposed to cisplatin with less severity in cotreated groups. The oxidative stress markers, LPO, SOD and CAT levels which were significantly elevated in cisplatin exclusively exposed Group B, were not altered in other groups when compared with control. However, GSH levels significantly decrease in kidney tissue of cisplatin alone relative to control.

Laurus nobilis L. Family: Lauraceae

Sanjuna *et al.* [411] evaluated the *in vitro* antiurolithiatic activity of *Laurus nobilis* leaves. Water extract of leaves showed their maximum efficiencies in the dissolution of CaOx crystals.

Lawsonia inermis L. Family: Lythraceae

Sreedevi *et al.* [412] evaluated the protective potential of ethanol extract of leaves of *Lawsonia inermis* in cisplatin-induced renal injury in male albino rats. Treatment with extract significantly attenuated drug-induced nephrotoxicity in cisplatin model by restoring the biochemical and oxidative stress markers in dose dependent passion in both regimens. Histological studies also substantiated the biochemical parameters.

Leea macrophylla Roxb. Family: Leeaceae

Nizami *et al.* [413] evaluate the antilithiatic effect of the whole *Leea macrophylla* ethanol extract in ethylene glycol-induced urolithiasis model of rats. Significant difference on recovery was observed between preventive and therapeutic interventional trials.

Lens culinaris Medik. Family: Fabaceae

Sreedevi and Saisruthi [414] evaluated the potential role of ethanol extract of seeds of *Lens culinaris* in attenuation of Cisplatin-induced renal injury in male albino rats. The administration of extract significantly attenuated the cisplatin-induced nephrotoxicity remarkably by restoring the biochemical and oxidative stress markers in both curative and prophylactic regimens in a dose dependent manner. Histological and immunohistochemical studies also substantiated the biochemical studies.

Lepidium sativum L. Family: Brassicaceae

Shinde *et al.* [415] investigated the effects of the water extract of *Lepidium sativum* against nephrotoxicity-induced by doxorubicin (DXN). The elevated serum urea and creatine levels due to DXN treatment were reduced in the *L. sativum* (200 and 400mg/kg, p.o) treated groups. The activities of SOD, CAT and level of GSH were elevated and level of MDA declined significantly in the *L. sativum* plus DXN. Histological studies also substantiated the biochemical parameters.

Yadav *et al.* [416, 417] investigated the possible potential curative and protective activity of 400mg/kg ethanolic extract of *L. sativum* against cisplatin-induced nephrotoxicity. A single dose of cisplatin induced loss in body weight, increase urine excretion, increased urea and creatinine level in serum; it was significantly recovered by 400mg/kg in curative and protective groups. In the enzyme estimation in kidney tissue, it was found that there was an increase in MDA, SOD, CAT and reduced GSH level, it was significantly monitored by 400mg/kg in curative and protective groups. The level of enzymes like Na^+/K^+ ATPase, Ca^{++} ATPase and Mg++ATPase were found significantly reduced after single dose cisplatin injection. It was overcome by treatment of same extract in curative and protective groups.

Balgoon [418] assessed the protective and curative effects of *L. sativum* (LS) against Al-induced impairment of kidney in albino rat. Administration of LS after or along with $AlCl_3$ signifcantly restored the serum biomarkers of liver and kidney functions to their near-normal levels and had the ability to overcome Al-induced oxidative stress and preserved, to some extent, the normal hepatic and renal structure. The coadministration of LS had a superior effect in alleviating Al-induced changes.

Lithospermum officinale L. Family: Boraginaceae

Grases *et al.* [96] studied the effects of *Silene saxifraga* to prevent and treat kidney stone formation in female Wistar rats. The infusion does not affect calciuria and citraturia values, they do not diminish calcinuria or increase the crystallization inhibitory capacity of the urine.

Lygodium japonicum (Thunb.) Sw. Family: Lygodiaceae

Cho *et al.* [419] assessed the effect of an ethanol extract of Lygodii spora (LS) as a preventive and therapeutic agent for experimentally induced CaOx nephrolithiasis in rats. Treatment with the LS preventive protocol significantly decreased the levels of urinary calcium, oxalate and uric acid, and increased the levels of urinary citrate as compared to those in the EG control. No significant changes in the urinary parameters except oxalate and citrate levels were observed in the rats in the therapeutic protocol. In both preventive and therapeutic protocols, the extract significantly decreased kidney peroxides, renal calcium, oxalate content, and the number of kidney oxalate deposits as compared to those in the EG group.

Macrothelypteris oligophlebia (Bak.) Ching Family: Thelypteridaceae

Wu *et al.* [420] evaluated the protective effect of ethanol extract of *Macrothelypteris oligophlebia* rhizomes (EMO) on GM-induced renal injury. Pre-treatment with EMO (500 mg/kg) significantly decreased the levels of BUN, Cr, MDA and NO, and also restored the activities of renal antioxidant enzymes (SOD, CAT, and GSH-Px).

Macrotyloma uniflorum (Lam.) Verdc. Family: Fabaceae

The effect of aqueous and alcohol extracts of *Macrotyloma uniflorum* seeds on

CaOx urolithiasis has been studied in male albino Wistar rats [421]. Supplementation with aqueous and alcohol extract of *M. uniflorum* seeds significantly reduced the elevated urinary oxalate showing a regulatory action on endogenous oxalate synthesis. The increased deposition of stone forming constituents in the kidneys of calculogenic rats was significantly lowered by curative and preventive treatment using aqueous and alcohol extracts. The results indicate that the alcoholic extract of *M. uniflorum* shows better anti urolithiatic activity than aqueous extract.

Madhuca longifolia (J.Koenig ex L.) J.F.Macbr. Family: Sapotaceae

Palani *et al.* [422] investigated the protective activity of the ethanol extract of *Madhuca longifolia* (EEML) on APAP induced nephrotoxicity in rats. Biochemical studies show that there is an increase in the levels of serum urea, hemoglobin (Hb), total leukocyte count, creatinine, packed cell volume, DLC, mean corpuscular volume and raised body weight along with reduced levels of neutrophils, mean corpuscular Hb content, mean corpuscular hematocrit, granulocytes, uric acid, and platelet concentrations. These values were retrieved significantly by the treatment with extracts at two different doses. The antioxidant studies revealed that the levels of renal SOD, CAT, reduced GSH and GPx in the APAP treated animals were increased significantly along with decreased MDA content in EEML treated groups. Apart from these, histopathological changes also reveal the protective nature of the *M. longifolia* extract against APAP induced necrotic damage of renal tissues.

Madhuca neriifolia (Moon) H.J.Lam. (Syn.: *Bassia malabarica* Bedd.) Family: Sapotaceae

Sushma *et al.* [423, 424] investigated the prophylactic and curative effect of ethanolic extract of *Madhuca neriifolia (Syn.: Bassia malabarica)* bark (EBBM) and leaves (EBML) against cisplatin induced nephrotoxicity in male albino Wistar rats. On administration of cisplatin there was a rise in weight of the kidney, creatinine, urea, uric acid, BUN, LPO and a decrease in bwt, urine volume, total protein, GSH and CAT indicating the role of oxidants to induce nephrotoxicity. EBBM and EBML has significantly restored the urinary parameters, serum parameters of cisplatin-induced nephrotoxic rats, Authors concluded that prophylactic and curative groups were found to ameliorate the cisplatin induced alterations in the kidney in a dose-dependent manner.

Mahonia leschenaultii Takeda Family: Berberidaceae

Palani *et al.* [425] investigated the protective activity of the ethanol extract of *Mahonia leschenaultii* on APAP-induced nephrotoxicity in rats. *M. leschenaultii* extract inhibited the hematological effects of APAP. *M. leschenaultii* extract increased activities of renal SOD, CAT, GSH, and GPx and decreased MDA content of APAP-treated rats. Histopathological changes also showed the protective nature of the *M. leschenaultii* extract.

Mallotus philippinensis Muell.-Arg. Family: Euphorbiaceae

Antiurolithiatic activity of alcoholic leaf extract of *M. philippinensis* against ethylene glycol-induced urolithiasis in Wistar rats. The calcium, oxalate and phosphate concentration were significantly increased in disease control animals as compared to the normal control animals. However, the tested extracts (250 and 500 mg/kg) and Cystone (750 mg/kg) significantly reduced calcium, oxalate and phosphate concentration in urine as compared to disease control animals [426].

Malva sylvestris L. Family: Malvaceae

Gazwi and Mahmoud [427] evaluated the potential effect of *Malva sylvestris* extract on nephrotoxicity caused by CCl_4 in rats. Results appeared that rats treated with CCl_4 showed a significant increment in WBCs, kidney function (urea and creatinine), total lipid, cholesterol, triglycerides, glucose, MDA, and nitric oxide (NO) levels, but a significant decline in the mean values of weight gain, RBCs, PCV, Hb, uric acid, and CAT as compared with the control group. The treatment with *M. sylvestris* (150 and 300 mg/kg b.w) improved the hematological and biochemical parameters. These protective effects were dose dependent. The histological results confirmed these parameters that enhanced by CCl_4.

Mangifera indica L. Family: Anacardiaceae

Rad *et al.* [428] evaluated the effects of hydroalcoholic extract of Mango (*Mangifera indica*) on GM-induced renal injury in rat. Hydroalcoholic extract of Mango at 200mg/kg was able to reduce plasma Cr and urea concentrations significantly as well as kidney tissue necrosis.

Manilkara zapota (L.) P.Royen Family: Sapotaceae

Sanjuna *et al.* [429] evaluated the *in vitro* antiurolithiatic activity of the seeds of *Manilkara zapota*. Methanolic extracts showed their maximum efficiencies in the dissolution of CaOx crystals.

Matricaria chamomilla L. Family: Asteraceae

Thuwaini *et al.* [431] investigated the influences of water extract of *M. chamomilla* in nephrotoxicity induced in rats by tetracyclines. Co-administration of *M. chamomile* extract with tetracycline appeared to be ameliorate the adverse effects of tetracycline in renal function tests. Histopathological examination of kidney sections of tetracycline-induced neprotoxic non treated animals showed marked attenuated the severity of tetracycline nephrotoxicity. However, all these toxic effects were improved by administration of *M. chamomilla* extract, but didn't bring them to the control limits.

Matricaria chamomilla L. Family: Asteraceae and ***Nigella sativa*** L. Ranunculaceae

Salama *et al.* [430] evaluated the protective effects of supportive treatments (*Nigella sativa, Matricaria chamomilla* and vitamin E) in cisplatin-induced nephrotoxicity in rat model. *M. chamomilla* followed by *N. sativa* and vitamin E improved the biochemical and pathological renal injury, as determined by increasing the body weight, normalizing the kidney functions, decreasing the oxidative stress markers, improving the apoptotic markers, minimizing the pathological changes.

Melia azedarach L. Family: Meliaceae

The effect of the water extract of *Melia azedarach* against ethylene glycol–induced nephrolithiasis in male Wistar albino rats was evaluated by Christina *et al.* [432]. Simultaneous administration of aqueous extract of *M. azedarach* orally for 28 days along with ethylene glycol reduced urinary calcium, oxalate, phosphate, and elevated urinary magnesium level. It also increased the urine volume, thereby reducing the tendency for crystallization. Histological studies also substantiated the biochemical parameters.

Bahuguna *et al.* [433] assessed antiurolithiatic activity of *M. azedarach* in rats. From their observations helped Bahuguna *et al.* [433] concluded that the alcoholic leaf extracts were endowed with antiurolithiatic activity.

Dharmalingam *et al.* [434] investigated the anti-urolithiatic activity of the aqueous and alcoholic extracts of *M. azedarach* leaves in CaOx urolithiasis in male albino rats. Treatment with aqueous or ethanol extract (250 mg/kg, p.o.) significantly reduced the elevated levels of calcium, oxalate and phosphate excretion in urine. Following treatment with the ethanol extract serum creatinine excretion was restored to the normal level. Histopathological data for the kidney supported the foregoing results.

Mentha arvensis L. Family: Lamiaceae

Singh *et al.* [435] evaluated the effect of *Mentha arvensis* on cisplatin-induced nephrotoxicity in Sprague-Dawley rats. *M. arvensis* hydroalcoholic extract

(MAHE) was found effective at both (200 mg/kg and 400 mg/kg) doses, although high dose was found more effective, which was evidenced by decrease in serum creatinine, total protein, BUN, urea, and LPO and increased in SOD activity. Histopathological studies were also confirmed the nephroprotective action of MAHE.

Mentha piperita L. Family: Lamiaceae

Ullah *et al*. [436] evaluated the protective effect of *Mentha piperita* against GM-induced nephrotoxicity in male rabbits. Derangements in serum and urinary biochemical parameters were reversed by treatment with *M. piperita* extract. The histological changes showed in GM group were also reverted by treatment with the extract.

Akdogan *et al*. [437] investigated the biochemical and histological effects of *M. piperita* and *M. spicata* on rat kidney tissue. The results indicate that *M. piperita* does not show nephrotoxicity but *M. spicata* presents markedly nephrotoxic changes in rats.

Manasa Reddy *et al*. [438] evaluated the *in vitro* antiurolithiatic activity of leaf extracts of *Mentha piperita*. Methanolic extract showed their maximum efficiencies in the dissolution of CaOx crystals.

Michelia champaca L. Family: Magnoliaceae

Satyavati *et al*. [439] evaluated the protective effect of *Michelia champaca* flowers ethanolic extract in cisplatin-induced renotoxicity. Administration of *M. champaca* flowers ethanolic extract produced significant nephroprotective activity in cisplatin induced renal injury model as evident by decrease in elevated serum creatinine, urea, BUN, uric acid and total protein levels, which was further confirmed by histopathological study.

Mimosa pudica L. Family: Fabaceae

Antiurolithiatic effects of *Mimosa pudica* on experimental kidney renal calculi in rats was invesitagated by Joyamma *et al*. [440]. According to them *M. pudica* was not effective in either preventing stone deposition or dissolving preformed stones.

Mimusops elengi L. Family: Sapotaceae

Ashok *et al*. [441] evaluated the potential of *Mimusops elengi* in the treatment of urolithiasis. The increased deposition of stone forming constituents in the kidneys of calculogenic rats were significantly lowered by curative and preventive treatment with alcohol extract (AlE) of *M. elengi*. It was also observed that alcoholic extract of *M. elengi* produced significant decrease in MDA, and increased GSH, SOD, and CAT.

Momordica dioica Roxb. Family: Cucurbitaceae

The ethanolic extract of the fruits of *Momordica dioica* was assessed by Jain and Singhai [442, 443] for its prophylactiv and curative effect against GM- and cisplatin-indued nephrotoxicity in albino rats. In the preventive regimen, the extract at dose levels of 200 mg/kg showed significant reduction in the elevated blood urea and serum creatinine. This treatment normalised the histopathological changes compared to the intoxicated group. In the curative regimen at 200 mg/kg blood urea was found to be 48.21 +/- 2.36 and serum creatinine level was 2.050 +/- 0.183, which revealed significant curative effect. Reduced GSH level was significantly increased in the extract treated groups whereas MDA was reduced significantly.

Monochoria vaginalis (Burm.f.) C.Presl. Family: Pontederiaceae

Palani *et al.* [444] evaluated the nephroprotective activity of the ethanol extract of *Monochoria vaginalis* on acetaminophen induced toxicity in rats. The altered values of biochemical parameters- were retrieved significantly by treatment with *M. vaginalis* extracts at two different doses. The antioxidant studies revealed that the levels of renal SOD, CAT, GSH and GPx in the APAP treated animals are increased significantly along with a reduced MDA content in ethanol extract of *M. vaginalis* treated groups. Histopathological changes also revealed the protective nature of the *M. vaginalis* extract.

Monotheca buxifolia (Falc.) A.DC. Family: Sapotaceae

Jan and Khan [445] investigated the protective potential of the methanol extract of *Monotheca buxifolia* (MBM) in rat exposed to CCl_4 toxicity. MBM administration significantly alleviated the toxic effect of CCl_4 in rat and decreased the elevated level of RBCs, pus and epithelial cells, specific gravity, creatinine, urobilinogen, urea and albumin while increased the pH and urinary protein. Increase in the level of urobilinogen, BUN, urea and total bilirubin while decrease of albumin and total protein in serum was restored by the administration of MBM to CCl_4 fed rat. Administration of MBM to CCl_4 exposed rats significantly increased the activity level of phase I and phase II enzymes and GSH while decreased the level of TBARS, H_2O_2, nitrite and DNA damages in renal tissues of rat. Furthermore, histopathological alterations induced with CCl_4 in renal tissues of rat were also diminished with the administration of MBM.

Morinda citrifolia L. Family: Rubiaceae

The effect of Noni (*Morinda citrifolia*) against nephrolithiasis in albino Wistar rats was evaluated by Verma *et al*. [446]. Simultaneous administration of 1ml (1 in 10) Noni formulation orally for 28 days along with ethylene glycol (0.75% v/v) reduced urinary calcium, phosphate, oxalate and elevated urinary magnesium level. It also increased urinary volume thereby reducing the tendency for crystallization. The histopathological studies confirmed the induction as degenerated glomeruli, necrotic tubule and inflammatory cells was observed in section of kidney from animals treated with ethylene glycol. This was reduced; however after treatment with Noni formulation.

Morinda citrifolia (Noni fruit) juice was evaluated by Shenoy *et al*. [447] for its diuretic potential in Wistar albino rats. Noni fruit juice increased the volume of in a dose dependent manner increasing the diuretic index to 2.04 and 2.36 for 5ml.kg and 10ml/kg dose ranges respectively. However, there was a significant decrease in sodium ion excretion when compared to the control. Though there was a similar decrease in potassium excretion.

Effect of noni (*Morinda citrifolia*) extract on treatment of ethylene glycol and ammonium chloride induced nephrotoxicity was investigated by Bhavani *et al*. [448]. After the treatment with Noni the urinary parameters like creatinine, protein, calcium, oxalate, phosphate are decreased except magnesium, its level is increased and serum creatinine level is decreased.

Karamcheti *et al*. [449] assessed the ethanolic extract of *Morinda citrifolia (EEMC)* fruits for chemoprotective effect in cisplatin-induced nephrotoxicity in rats. Extract at 100 and 200 mg/kg b.w. doses produced significant protective activity in cisplatin-induced nephrotoxicity models as evident by decrease in serum creatinine, serum urea, serum protein in extract treated groups which was elevated by cisplatin, which was further confirmed by histopathological study. Cisplatin induced glomerular atropy, infiltration of cells and tubular congestion of the kidney cells were found to be reduced in the groups receiving EEMC along with cisplatin.

Moringa oleifera Lam. (Syn.: *M. pterygosperma*) Family: Moringaceae

The effect of of water and alcoholic extract of *Moringa oleifera* (Syn.: *M. pterygosperma*) root-wood on CaOx urolithiasis has been investigated by Karadi *et al*. [450] in male Wistar albino rats. Supplementation with aqueous and alcoholic extract of *M. oleifera* root-wood significantly reduced the elevated urinary oxalate, showing a regulatory action on endogenous oxalate synthesis. The increased deposition of stone forming constituents in the kidneys of calculogenic rats was also significantly lowered by curative and preventive treatment using aqueous and alcoholic extracts.

Aqueous extract of bark of *M. oleifera* was evaluated by Fahad *et al*. [451] for its antiurolithiatic potential in albino rats of Wistar rats. Two doses of extract for prophylactic and curative groups were used. The oral administration of the extract of bark of *M. oleifera* has resulted in significant reduction in the weight of bladder stones compared to the control group.

The ethanolic extract of whole part of *M. oleifera* plant in ethylene glycol induced lithiatic albino rats showed marked increase in renal excretion of calcium and phosphate in two different doses of curative regimen of 250 mg/kg and 300 mg/kg as well as preventive regimen of 250 mg/kg for 28 days and the effect was compared with standerd drug *i.e.* allopurinol [452]. The increased deposition of stone forming constituents in the kidney of calculogenic rats was also significantly lowered by curative and preventive treatement using alcohol extract.

Lakshmana *et al*. [453] investigated the protective activity of ethanolic leaf extract of *M. oleifera* against paracetamol-induced nephrotoxicity in rats. The extract showed nephroprotective activity by significantly reducing the levels of blood urea, serum creatine, increasing the red blood cell count and haemoglobin content.

The protective effect of water-ethanolic extract of *M. oleifera* leaves was investigated by Ouédraogo *et al*. [454] against GM-induced renal injury in rabbits. Serum urea and creatinine levels were reduced in the *M. oleifera* (150 and 300 mg/kg) plus GM treated groups. On histological examinations, kidney of intoxicated rabbits groups which received *M. oleifera* extract showed reparative tendencies. A highly significant elevation was observed in lipid peroxidation (LPO) level in the kidneys of GM-intoxicated rabbits whereas combined treatment of *M. oleifera* and GM group showed a highly significant depletion in LPO.

Christi and Senthamarai [39] evaluated the antiurolithiatic activity of water and alcoholic extract of leaves *M. oleifera* in rats. The drug treated group animals showed a significant reduction in the bladder stones compared to the control. The herbal drug exerted its antilithogenic property by altering the ionic composition of urine *viz*.; decreasing the calcium and oxalate ion concentration or increasing magnesium and citrate excretion. The extract at a dose of 200mg/kg produced reduction in MDA and increased GSH and antioxidant enzyme likes SOD and CAT.

Nafiu *et al*. [455] evaluated the protective effect of fatty acids from ethanolic extract of *M. oleifera* seeds (EEMOS) against GM-induced nephrotoxicity in rats. Treatment with EEMOS significantly ameliorated the alterations caused by GM in the plasma, urine and kidney homogenate of the rats.

Morus alba L. Family: Moraceae

Nematbakhsh *et al.* [456] investigated the protective effect of hydroalcoholic extract and flavonoid fraction of *Morus alba* leaves on cisplatin-induced nephrotoxicity in rat. Hydroalcoholic extract was ineffective in reversing these alterations but flavonoid fraction (50 and 100 mg/kg) significantly inhibited CP-induced increases of BUN and Cr. None of the treatments could affect serum concentration of nitric oxide. Flavonoid fraction could also prevent CP-induced pathological damage of the kidney.

The effect of the ethanolic leaf extract of *M. alba* against nephrolithiasis in Wistar rats was evaluated by Maya and Pramod [457]. The extract of *M. alba* showed a potent percentage inhibition in different *in vitro* models. The treatment with plant extract exhibited a significant effect in preventing CaOx formation and also in dissolving the preformed stones. Significant effect was exhibited by the treatmet groups with 1000mg/kg/day. Histopathological evaluation also supported the protective effect of *M. alba*.

Ullah *et al.* [458] explored the renal protective effects of *M. alba*. Ethanol extract of *M. alba* prevented alterations in serum creatinine, BUN, and serum uric acid levels. However, a decrease in creatinine clearance and urinary volume was observed in experimental groups. Histopathological examination and urinary enzymes excretion also suggested the protective role of the extract.

Hashim and Asker [459] invetigated the ameliorating effect of methanolic extract of *M. alba* leaves on nephrotoxicity induced by intramuscular injection of GM. The results showed significant increase in serum levels of creatinine, BUN, uric acid, MDA oxidative enzyme and significant decrease at the serum levels of GSH antioxidant enzyme in the group (G2) in the periods of treatment 5, 10 and 20 days recovery, while there were significant decrease in serum levels of creatinine, BUN, uric acid, MDA and increase in GSH antioxidant enzyme in the groups G3, G4 and G5 which return to normal levels. The co-administration of gentanicin + methanolic extract of *M. alba* leaves has exhibited more activity as antioxidant in treating of nephrotoxicity induced by GM and indicate that the methanolic leaves extract of *M. alba* displays a good therapy against nephrotoxicity and nephrotoxicant agents.

Mucuna pruriens (L.) DC. Family: Fabaceae

Modi *et al.* [460] evaluated the protective effects of water extract of *Mucuna pruriens* on GM-induced nephrotoxicity in rats. Use of *M. pruriens* extract along with GM caused a dose dependant decrease in serum creatinine and urea levels and an increase in creatinine clearance. There was a significant increase in the urinary sodium levels by *M. pruriens* extract at a dose of 400 mg/kg but not at the dose of 200 mg/kg when compared with GM control rats. Treatment with *M. pruriens* extract at a dose of 400 mg mg/kg further increased the urine volume as compared to GM control rats. However, further increase in urine volume by *M. pruriens* extract at a dose of 200 mg/kg was not significant. *M. pruriens* extract significantly and dose-dependently reduced lipid peroxidation and enhanced GSH levels and SOD and CAT activities

Murraya koenigii (L.) Spreng. Family: Rutaceae

Mahipal and Pawar [461] investigated the nephroprotective effect of defatted methanolic extract and aqueous extract of *Murraya koenigii* against cyclophasphamide drug. The renal function markers like BUN and creatinine level were found to be decreased significantly by *M. koenigii* extract treatment.

Musa paradisiaca L. Family: Musaceae

The fresh juice of *Musa* stem (Puttubale) was evaluated by Prasad *et al.* [462] for its antilithiatic activity. *Musa* stem juice (3 mL/rat/day orally) was found to be effective in reducing the formation and also in dissolving the pre-formed stones.

Poonguzhali and Chegu [463] investigated the effect of banana stem extract on urinary risk factors in male rats of hyperoxaluria. In the rats treated with banana stem water extract, urinary oxalate excretion was significantly reduced when compared with the controls. The extract reduced urinary oxalate, glycollic and glyoxylic acid and phosphorus excretion in the hyperoxaluric rats. The extract appeared to have no effect on urinary calcium excretion.

The effect of ethanol extract of dried roots of *M. paradisiaca* against ethylene glycol induced renal calculi in albino wistar rats was studied by Jha *et al.* [464]. Simultaneous administration of 1 ml *M. paradisiaca* for 28 days along with ethylene glycol reduced urinary calcium, oxalate and elevated magnesium level. It also increased urinary volume thereby reducing the tendency for crystallization. The histopathological studies confirmed the protective role of *M. paradisiaca*.

Prasobh and Revikumar [465] evaluated the effectiveness of Musa tablet on albino Wistar rats as a preventive agent against the development of kidney stones. Administration of Musa to rats with ethylene glycol-induced lithiasis significantly reduced and prevented the growth of urinary stones. The treatment of lithiasis-induced rats by Musa tablet also restored all the elevated biochemical parameters (creatine, BUN and uric acid), restored the urine pH of normal and increased urine volume significantly when compared to the model control drug.

The effect of banana cultivar Monthan corm extract for its antilithiatic potential under *in vitro* condition has been investigated by Kalpana *et al.* [466]. The results of the *in vitro* assays performed indicate that ethanol extract of Monthan readily prevented crystal nucleation, growth and aggregation.

The anti-urolithiatic activity of the aqueous extract of the stem core of *Musa paradisiaca* was investigated by Thirumala *et al.* [467] on ethylene glycol and ammonium chloride induced on albino rats. Oral administration of extract of *Musa paradisiaca* for 28 days resulted in significant reduction in urine level. All rats in the lithiatic groups had urine and serum levels well within the lithiatic range, at the initial stage of the experiment but after four weeks of treatment with extracts or cystone the urine, serum significantly dropped in dose-dependent manner.

Panigrahi *et al.* [468] evaluated the efficacy and possible mechanism of antiurolithiatic effect of *M. paradisiaca* pseudostem to rationalize its medicinal use. Administration of ethylene glycol and ammonium chloride resulted in increased crystalluria and oxaluria, hypercalciuria, polyuria, crystal deposition in urine, raised serum urea, and creatinine as well as nitric oxide concentration and erythrocytic lipid peroxidation in lithiatic group. However, aqueous-ethnol extract of *M. paradisiaca* pseudostem treatment significantly restored the impairment in above kidney function test as that of standard treatment, cystone in a dose-dependent manner.

Myristica fragrans Houtt. Family: Myristicaceae

Nivetha and Prasanna [469] evaluated the nephroprotective effect of an aqueous extract of *Myristica fragrans* against GM induced experimental animal models. Serum urea, uric acid and creatinine and lipid peroxides were significantly increased in GM alone treated group compared to the normal group. Also GM induced decline of body weight, kidney weight, protein and renal antioxidants such as GSH, SOD, and CAT levels. *Myristica fragrans* 150 and 300mg/kg treatment to GM treated rats significantly altered the above all parameters to near normal with dose depended fashion. The maximum nephroprotection was offered by the extract at 300 mg/kg.

Neolamarckia cadamba (Roxb.) Bosser Family: Rubiacaeae

Prathibhakumari and Prasad [470] evaluated the antiurolithiatic potential of aqueous fruit extract of *Neolamarckia cadamba* (AFENC) on ethylene glycol induced urolithiasis in wistar albino rats at 200 and 400 mg/kg of fruit extract. The oral administration of ethylene glycol (EG) and ammonium chloride (AC) for 28 days in all experimental animals resulted in increased deposition of CaOx stones in kidney and were served as control. Animals received the fruit extract along with EG/AC were served as curative regimes (CR) and that treated with fruit extract after 28 days of EG/AC administration were taken as preventive regimes (PR). An increased deposition of stone forming constituents was observed in calculogenic rats. Supplementation with the fruit extract significantly lowered the elevated protein, calcium and phosphorus in urine. Blood urea, BUN, uric acid and creatinine were decreased in serum. Kidney parameter such as phosphorus and calcium was also lowered in treatment groups.

Nigella sativa L. Family: Ranunculaceae

Ali [471] evaluated the protective effect of *N. sativa* oil against GM-induced nephrotoxicity. Treatment with *N. sativa* oil produced a dose-dependent amelioration of the biochemical and histological indices of GM nephrotoxicity. Compared to controls, treatments of rats with *N. sativa* did not cause any overt toxicity, and it increased GSH and TAS concentrations in renal cortex and enhanced growth.

Hadjzadesh *et al.* [472] investigated the effects of the ethanolic extract of *Nigella sativa* (NS) seeds on ethylene-glycol-induced kidney calculi in Wistar rats. Treatment of rats with ethanolic extract of NS reduced the number of CaOx deposits in a group of rats that received ethanolic extract of NS. The NS could also lower the urine concentration of CaOx.

Bayrak *et al.* [473] investigated the possible effects of *N. sativa* oil (NSO) in Ischaemia/Reperfusion-induced renal injury in rats. Pre- and post-treatment with NSO produced reduction in serum levels of BUN and creatinine caused by I/R and significantly improved serum enzymatic activities of SOD and GPx and also tissue enzymatic activities of CAT, SOD and GPx. NSO treatment resulted in lower total oxidant status (TOS) and higher total antioxidant capacity (TAC) levels and also significant reduction in serum and tissue MDA, nitric oxide (NO) and protein carbonyl content (PCC) that were increased by renal I/R injury. The kidneys of untreated ischaemic rats had a higher histopathological score, while treatment with NSO nearly preserved the normal morphology of the kidney.

Begum *et al.* [474] evaluated the protective effect of the n-hexane extract of the *N. sativa* (kalajira) on GM-induced nephrotoxicity in rats. Significant amelioration in all the biochemical parameters supported by significantly improved renal cortical histology was observed in the n-hexane extract of *N. sativa* treated nephrotoxic rats, which was more evident in the post-treatment group than the pre- treatment and the concomitantly-treated group.

Yildiz *et al.* [475] examined the effect of *N. sativa* in modulating inflammation and apoptosis after renal ischemia/reperfusion (I/R) injury. *N. sativa* was effective in reducing serum urea and creatinine levels as well as decreasing the tubular necrosis score. *N. sativa* treatment significantly reduced Oxidative Stress index and Total Oxidant Status levels and increased Total Antioxidant Capacity levels in both kidney tissue and blood.

Yaman and Balicki [476] investigated the possible protective effect of *N. sativa* against GM-induced nephrotoxicity. Creatinine and urea levels significantly decreased in NSL+GS and NSH+GS groups. In the GS group, plasma MDA and NO levels increased significantly and erythrocyte SOD and GSH-Px activities decreased significantly when compared with control group. NS administration with GS injection resulted in significantly decreased MDA and NO generation and increased SOD and GSH-Px activities when compared with GS group. Co-treatments with NS (low and high dose) considerably decreased the renal damage when compared with the GS group.

Abdelaziz and Kandeel [73] evaluated the effect of *N. sativa* oil in ameliorating amikacin-induced nephrotoxicity in rats. *N. sativa* oil significantly decreased the levels of NO, MDA and total antioxidant capacity. Furthermore, they increased the level of reduced GSH. These results were coinciding with the lower levels of urea, uric acid and creatinine (which were significantly elevated in amikacin treated groups). Semi-quantitative analysis of cellular infiltration, necrosis of tubular cells and tubular cellular damage indicated the protective effect of the used plant materials in reducing renal damage induced by amikacin.

Hadjizadeh *et al.* [477] tested whether *N. sativa* (NS) seeds can reduce cisplatin-induced toxicity. BUN increased in the cisplatin and NS groups on days 14 and 42 compared to day 0. Serum creatinine had a similar profile in the cisplatin and NS groups as BUN. Serum triglyceride increased in the cisplatin and NS groups on day 14, but it decreased on day 42. Urine glucose concentration decreased in the cisplatin group on days 14 and 42 compared to day 0, and the same trend was seen in the NS group. Histology of the kidneys exposed to cisplatin showed significant kidney injury, but the rats treated with NS showed a relatively well-preserved architecture.

Saleem *et al.* [478] investigated the nephroprotective effect of *N. sativa* oil. *N. sativa* oil had nephroprotective effect as they lowered the values of nephrotoxicity indicators (serum creatinine, BUN, and antioxidant activity) as compared to GM control group values. When these two antioxidants were given as combination, they proved to have synergistic nephroprotective effect.

The effect of water extracts of dried seeds powder of *N. sativa* against ethylene glycol induced renal calculi in albino Wistar rats has been studied by Sikandari *et al.* [162]. Oral administration of *N. sativa* aqueous suspension to ethylene glycol induced urolithic rats had reduced the concentration of calcium, oxalate, BUN, Creatinine, phosphorous, and diminished the crystals deposition in the kidneys.

Benhelima *et al.* [479] investigated the influences, preventive and diuretic, of *Nigella sativa* seeds oil (*NSSO*) on CaOx urolithiasis induced in Wistar male rats. Administration of (*NSSO*) at 5 ml/kg body weight/dose/day for 28 days exerts a protective effect by reducing significantly urinary and serum rates of calcium, phosphate and oxalate. This preventive diet could increase the volume of urine excreted.

Hosseinian *et al.* [480] investigated the protective effect of *N. sativa* against cisplatin-induced nephrotoxicity in rats. Serum urea and creatinine concentration in preventive+treatment *N. sativa* (100 mg/kg, BW) group significantly decreased compared with cisplatin group. Urine glucose concentration in preventive and preventive + treatment. *N. sativa* groups and urine output in preventive and preventive+treatment *N. sativa* (200 mg/kg, BW) groups significantly decreased compared with cisplatin group.

Canayakin *et al.* [481] tested the effects of *N. sativa* seeds ethanol extract in paracetamol-induced acute nephrotoxicity in rats. NS administration increased SOD and GSH and decreased MDA levels in the kidneys. Kidney histopathological examinations showed that NS administration antagonized paracetamol-induced kidney pathological damage.

Hosseinian *et al.* [482] evaluated the protective effects of aqueous-ethanolic extract of *N. sativa* on cisplatin-induced nephrotoxicity in rats. Tissue damage in all groups that received *N. sativa* extract showed a significant improvement compared with the cisplatin group. In addition, serum and tissue total thiol content in preventive and preventive + treatment. *N. sativa* groups showed significant increase compared with cisplatin group. There was no significant difference in serum MDA concentration of the control rats compared with the preventive and preventive + treatment. *N. sativa* groups. *N. sativa* extract improved the pathology and oxidative stress in the rat kidney.

Nothosaerva brachiata Wight Family: Amaranthaceae

Goswami and Srivastava [483] evaluated the protective effect of aqueous and alcoholic extract of root of *Nothosaerva brachiata* in ethylene glycol-induced urolithiasis in Wistar rats. Supplementation with aqueous and alcoholic extracts of *N. brachiata* root significantly reduced the elevated urinary oxalate, showing regulatory action on endogenous oxalate synthesis. The increased deposition of stone forming constituents in the kidneys of calculogenic rats was also significantly lowered by curative treatment using aqueous and alcoholic extracts.

Nymphaea alba L. Family: Nymphaeaceae

Shelke *et al.* [484] investigated the effect of ethanolic extract of *Nymphaea alba* on urolithiatc rats. Oral administration of the *N. alba* has resulted in significant reduction in the weight of bladder stones compared to the control group.

Ocimum basilicum L. Family: Lamiaceae

The hydroalcoholic extract of *Ocimum basilicum* was evaluated by Zaveri *et al.* [485] for its protective activity in cisplatin-induced nephrotoxicity in albino rats. In the curative regimen, the extract at dose levels of 100, 300 and 500 mg/kg showed dose-dependent reduction in the elevated blood urea and serum creatinine and normalized the histopathological changes in the curative regimen.

Sakr and Al-Amoudi [486] investigated the protective effect of *O. basilicum* extract on deltamethrin-induced nephrotoxicity in albino rats. Treating animals with deltamethrin and aqueous extract of basil led to an improvement in histological and biochemical alterations induced by deltamethrin. The biochemical results showed that creatinine and urea appeared within normal level. Reduction in the level of MDA and increase in the activities of SOD and CAT was recorded.

Ocimum gratissimum L. Family: Lamiaceae

The effect of aqueous leaf extract of *Ocimum gratissimum* (O.G.) on cisplatin-induced nephrotoxicity in male albino Wistar was evaluated by Arhoghro *et al.* [487]. Most of the changes due to cisplatin treatment were alleviated by prophylactic treatment with aqueous extract of *O. gratissimum* dose and time dependently. The ameliorating effect was further evident through decreased histopathological alterations of kidney tissues in the groups treated with aqueous extract of *O. gratissimum* (5% and 10%).

Antiurolithiatic activity of *O. gratissimum* extract was evaluated by Agarwal and Varma [488]. In nucleation assay, the aim was to evaluate the effectiveness of different concentrations of the extract (100-1000 mg/ml) on CaOx crystallization *in vitro* while in synthetic urine method the percentage inhibition and growth of the CaOx monohydrate crystals from synthetic urine at different % concentrations of extract (25-100%) was investigated. In both the assay percentage inhibition for CaOx crystal formation was found directly proportional to the increase in concentration of the plant extract with maximum inhibition of 66.08% at 1000 mg/ml, while in synthetic urine assay maximum inhibition was 62.07% at 100%

concentration of extract.

The effect of aqueous extract of *O. gratissimum* leaf (AOGL) on GM-induced nephrotoxicity in rats was investigated by Ogundipe *et al.* [489]. Post-treatment with graded doses of AOGL caused significant increase in food consumption, GSH, urine, and plasma creatinine, as well as significant decrease in relative kidney weight, TBARS, and urine total protein. There was an appreciable difference in the kidney histology of the AOGL-treated groups when compared with the toxic control.

Olea europaea L. Family: Oleaceae

Tavafi *et al.* [490] evaluated the inhibitory effect of Olive leaf extract on GM-induced nephrotoxicity in rats. Cotreatment of GM and olive leaf extract significantly decreased serum creatinine, MDA, tubular necrosis, and renal MDA, and increased renal GSH, CAT, SOD, volume density of proximal convoluted tubules, and creatinine clearance in comparison with GM-only treated group. Serum MDA, serum creatinine, tubular necrosis, and volume density of proximal convoluted tubules were maintained at the same level as that of the control group by cotreatment of GM and olive leaf extract.

Al-Sowayan and Mousa [491] investigated the protective effect of olive leaf extract (OLE) on CCl_4 induced nephrotoxicity in Wistar rats. Treatment with olive leaf extract (50 mg /kg body wt./d or 100 mg/kg body wt./d) significantly attenuated the biochemical and histopathological alterations induced by CCl_4 suggesting that OLE protected CCl_4-induced nephrotoxicity through enhancement of renal antioxidant system.

Alenzi *et al.* [492] assessed the antiurolithic effect of olive oil in a mouse model of ethylene glycol (EG)-induced urolithiasis. Administration of olive oil at different doses restored the elevated serum parameters compared with EG treated group. Urine and kidney calcium, oxalate, and phosphate levels were significantly lower in olive oil group than in animals with EG-induced urolithiasis. Olive oil treated mice showed a significant restoration effect on serum as well as urine and kidney parameters compared with EG group. Supplementation with olive oil (1.7 mL/kg body weight) reduced and prevented the growth of urinary stones, possibly by inhibiting renal tubular membrane damage due to peroxidative stress induced by hyperoxaluria.

Opuntia megacantha Salm-Dyck. Family: Cactaceae

Bwititi *et al.* [493] investigated the influence of the extracts on renal function in male diabetic Sprague-Dawley rats. *O. megacantha* leaves' extracts significantly increased urinary Na^+ output in diabetic and nondiabetic rats resulting in significantly low plasma concentration by comparison with untreated animals. Treatment with the extract significantly increased FE (Na^+) and GFR in all groups. The urinary K^+ outputs in nondiabetic were slightly lowered, but did not reach statistically significance.

Origanum vulgare L. Family: Lamiaceae

Khan *et al.* [494] evluated the crude aqueous-methanolic extract of *Origanum vulgare* (Ov.Cr) for antiurolithic effect. In the *in vitro* experiments, Ov.Cr exhibited a concentration-dependent (0.25-4 mg/ml) inhibitory effect on the slope of nucleation and aggregation and also decreased the number of CaOx monohydrate crystals (COM) produced in CaOx metastable solutions. Ov.Cr reduced the cell toxicity using MTT assay and LDH release in renal epithelial cells (MDCK) exposed to oxalate (0.5 mM) and COM (66 $\mu g/cm^2$) crystals. In male Wistar rats receiving lithogenic treatment Ov.Cr treatment (10-30 mg/kg) prevented as well as reversed toxic changes including loss of body weight, polyurea, crystalluria, oxaluria, raised serum urea and creatinine levels and crystal deposition in kidneys compared to their respective controls.

Oroxylum indicum (L.) Kurz Family: Bignoniaceae

Nephroprotective activity of extracts of *Oroxylum indicum* whole plant was investigated by Mishra *et al.* [111] against GM-induced acute renal injury in Wistar rats. The extracts of root significantly attenuated the nephrotoxicity by elevation of body weight, CAT, GPx and SOD or lowering urine LDH and creatinine, serum urea; serum creatinine and LPO respectively.

Orthosiphon grandiflorus Bold Family: Lamiaceae

Premgamone *et al.* [495] evaluated the efficacy of *Orthosiphon grandiflorus* (OG), in treatment of renal calculi in rural stone formers. This study indicates that treatment of renal calculi with OG tea is an alternative means of management. Woottisin *et al.* [369] evaluated the antilithic effect of *O. grandiflorus*, on known risk factors for CaOx stones in rats. They reported that there is no antilithic effect of the extract.

Orthosiphon stamineus Benth. Family: Lamiaceae

Kannappan *et al.* [496] investigated the neproprotective activity of *Orthosiphon stamineus* in rats in GM induced nephrotoxicity. The increased levels of serum creatinine, blood urea, urinary protein and extent of renal damage were decreased by the methanolic extract of *O. stamineus* at both dose levels that is 100 and 200 mg/kg body weight in rats. The drug was found to be potent diuretic which causes excretion of sodium and potassium.

Maheswari *et al*. [497] evaluated the protective effect of methanol leaf extract of *O. stamineus* against cisplatin induced nephrotoxicity in rats. Administration of *O. stamineus* methanol leaf extracts (100mg/kg and 200mg/kg) orally 1h before cisplatin (16 mg/kg bwt, i.p) protected the kidney as indicated by restoration of Blood urea, creatinine, urinary protein and GSH levels. Co-administration of the orthosiphon leaf extract with cisplatin significantly prevented renal toxicity both functionally and histologically.

Ramesh *et al*. [498] assessed the nephroprotective activity of the ethanolic extracts of *O. stamineus* leaves. Ethylene glycol was used to inducing the urolithiasis in albino rats. Ethanolic extracts of *O.stamineus* have good nephroprotective activity when compared with the standard drug. It was proved by analyzing the biomarkers and enzymes level.

Oryza sativa L. Family: Poaceae

Ohkawa *et al*. [499] conducted study to confirm the hypocalciuric effect of rice bran experimentally and clinically. Urinary calcium excretion and its absorption in the intestine were reduced significantly by rice bran or phytin in rats fed high calcium diets, while there were no significant decreases with a low calcium diet. For the clinical study 70 patients with idiopathic hypercalciuria were treated with rice bran (10 gm. twice daily) for 1 month to 3 years. In almost all patients rice bran caused a significant decrease in urinary calcium excretion, which was maintained during treatment. Evidence of stones has decreased clearly among patients treated with rice bran for 1 to 3 years, although this might be a halfway judgment of the long-term treatment.

The efficacy of rice-bran therapy was studied by Ebisuno *et al*. [500] in patients with hypercalciuria who were suffering from calcium stones. The frequency of stone episodes was reduced dramatically, especially in "active recurrent stone formers". Urinary calcium excretion was considerably reduced, while urinary phosphate and oxalate were slightly increased. Urinary magnesium, uric acid, serum calcium, phosphate, magnesium and uric acid were not affected. There were no changes in serum iron, copper and zinc even when patients were treated for long periods. The treatment was tolerated well and there were no serious side effects.

Ebisuno [501] from his study reported that although rice bran therapy should be effective in correcting absorptive hypercalciuria, there may be limits to the overall ability of rice bran monotherapy to prevent recurrence [501].

Paeonia lactiflora Pall Family: Paeoniaceae

Li *et al.* [502] carried out a study to estimate the possible effects of an aqueous extract of *Radix Paeoniae Alba* on the crystal formation *in vitro* and CaOx nephrolithiasis *in vivo*. *in vitro*, treatment with 64 mg/mL of the aqueous extracts remarkably dissolved formed crystals and inhibited crystal formation compared with the control. Reduced urinary and renal oxalate levels, decreased OPN expression, renal crystallization and pathological changes as well as increased urinary citrate and calcium levels were merely observed in preventive group as compared to the group treated with EG.

Panax ginseng C.A.Mey Family: Araliaceae

Qi *et al.* [503] evaluated the nephroprotective effects of anthocyanin from the fruits of *Panax ginseng* (GFA) in a murine model of cisplatin-induced acute kidney injury. Pretreatment with GFA attenuated cisplatin-induced elevations in BUN and creatinine levels and histopathological injury induced by cisplatin. The formation of kidney MDA, heme oxygenase-1, cytochrome P450 E1 and 4-hydroxynonenal with a concomitant reduction in reduced GSH was also inhibited by GFA, while the activities of kidney SOD and CAT were all increased. GFA also inhibited the increase in serum tumour necrosis factor-α and interleukin-1β induced by cisplatin. In addition, the levels of induced nitric oxide synthase and cyclooxygenase-2 were suppressed by GFA. Furthermore, GFA supplementation inhibited the activation of apoptotic pathways by increasing B cell lymphoma 2 and decreasing Bcl2-associated X protein expression.

Panax quinquefolius L. Family: Araliaceae

Ma *et al.* [504] tested the protective effect of American ginseng (*Panax quinquefolius*) berry extract (AGBE) on cisplatin-induced nephrotoxicity in mice. The histopathological changes and elevated levels of serum creatinine (CRE) and urea nitrogen (BUN) caused by cisplatin were significantly diminished by AGBE treatment. Oxidative stress caused by cisplatin, evidenced by increases in kidney tissues MDA content, cytochrome P450 E1 (CYP2E1), renal 4-hydroxynonenal (4-HNE) levels and decreases of GSH and SOD contents, was significantly ameliorated by AGBE pretreatment.

Paronychia argentea Lam. Family: Caryophyllaceae

Renal protection and antiurolithiasic effects of aqueous extract (APA) and the butanolic extract (BPA) of aerial parts of *Paronychia argentea* (PA) were evaluated by Bouanani *et al.* [505] in Wistar rats. The effect of the extracts could be advantageous in preventing urinary stone retention by reducing renal necrosis and thus inhibit crystal retention. In contradiction with APA, the two doses of BPA attenuated elevation in the serum creatinine and blood urea levels (nephroprotective effect).

Passiflora leschenaultii DC. Family: Passifloraceae

Farook *et al.* [36] investigated antiurolithiatic effect of *Passiflora leschenaultii*. Inhibition efficiencies of leaves, seeds and fruits of *P. leschenaultii* have been investigated in different models. Study suggests that the fruit juice and seed extract is moderate to good inhibitor of CaOx, calcium carbonate and calcium phosphate mineralization. Relatively poor inhibition of mineralization of CaOx, calcium phosphate and calcium carbonate precipitation by leaves extracts was reported.

Pedalium murex L. Family: Pedaliacee

Ethanolic extract of dried fruits of *Pedalium murex* was evaluated by Shelke *et al.* [506] for nephroprotective activity in cisplatin induced renal damage in rats. The extract significantly decreased the cisplatin induced nephrotoxicity. Remarkable changes were observed in body weight, serum creatinine and urea levels.

The ethanolic fruit extract of *P. murex* to ethylene glycol intoxicated rats reverted the levels of the kidney markers to near normal levels protecting renal tissues from damage and also prevents the crystal retention in tissues [507].

Pergularia daemia (Forssk.) Chiov. Family: Apocynaceae

The whole-plant, *Pergularia daemia* extract (50% alcohol) was investigated for its antiurolithiatic and diuretic activity by Vyas *et al.* [508]. Supplementation with extract significantly lowered the urinary excretion and kidney retention levels of oxalate, calcium and phosphate. Furthermore, high serum levels of urea nitrogen, creatinine and uric acid were significantly reduced by the extract. The results were comparable with the standard drug, cystone. The reduction of stone-forming constituents in urine and their decreased kidney retention reduces the solubility product of crystallizing salts such as CaOx and calcium phosphate, which could contribute to the antiurolithiatic property of the extract.

Petroselenium crispum (Mill.) Nyman Family: Apiaceae

Alyami and Rabah [509] investigated the effect of parsley (*Petroselenium crispum*) leaf tea on urolithiasis. Authors found no significant difference in the urine volume, pH, sodium, potassium, chloride, urea, creatinine, phosphorus, magnesium, uric acid, cystine, or citric acid.

Jassim [510] reported protective effect of parsley extract against kidney damage induced by sodium valproate in male rats. Gumaih *et al.* [511] evaluated the antiurolithiatic effect of parsley using experimental rats and ethylene glycol (EG) induced urolithiasis. Authors found significant decrease in parsley group in serum urea, creatinine, uric acid and electrolytes. Also a significant decrease in urinary calcium and proteins in this group compared to positive control.

Al-Yousofy *et al.* [512] evaluated the antiurolithiatic effect of parsley and its mechanism. The kidneys of parsley treated group appeared mostly to be calculi-free (less CaOx) even better than the cystone treated group. CaOx crystals were significantly lower both in histological sections and in urine samples in parsley treated group. Authors found significant increase in urine volume and pH in parsley treated rats compared to negative control. Parsley acts as antiurolithiatic drug through decreasing urinary calcium excretion, increasing urinary pH, dieresis, decreasing urinary protein excretion and its nephroprotective activity.

Petroselinum sativum Hoffm. Family: Apiaceae

Jafar *et al.* [513] investigated the therapeutic effects of the aqueous extract of *Petroselinum sativum* aerial parts and roots on kidney calculi. On the 14th and 30th days of the experiment, serum level of magnesium decreased significantly while serum level of calcium increased significantly in group B compared with the control group. In the treatment groups of C, D, E, and F, the number of deposits decreased significantly compared with group B on the 30th day. The weight of the kidneys increased significantly in group B compared with the control group and decreased significantly in treatment groups.

Peucedanum grande C.B.Clarke Family: Apiaceae

Aslam *et al.* [514] evaluated the protective effect of *P. grande* against nephrotoxic effects of potassium dichromate. *P. grande* pretreatment prevented deteriorative effects induced by Potassium dichromate through a protective mechanism that involved reduction of increased oxidative stress as well as by restoration of histopathological change against potassium dichromate administration.

Kumar *et al.* [515] evaluated the antiurolithiatic activity of *P. grande* in experimental model. Test drug reduced number of CaOx crystals in urine; levels of serum calcium, phosphorus, creatinine, urea; urinary calcium and sodium decreased significantly in standard and test groups. The urine volume increased significantly in both the test groups. Histopathology of kidney showed no CaOx crystal deposition in both the test groups.

Phaseolus radiatus L. Family: Fabaceae

Chaware [516] evaluated the preventive effect of aqueous extract of *Phaseolus radiatus* seeds on GM induced nephrotoxicity in albino Wistar rats. The protective effects were evidenced by complete inhibition of the GM-induced elevation of serum BUN and complete blockage of GM-induced elevation of serum creatine.

Phaseolus vulgaris L. Family: Fabaceae

Sree Lakshmi *et al.* [517] evaluated the antiurolithiatic potential of the ethanolic extract of the seed of *Phaseolus vulgaris* (EPV). In the preventive and curative disease-control groups, urinary excretion of calcium, oxalate, and their deposition in the kidney were significantly increased. Elevated levels of phosphate and uric acid in urine and uric acid, creatinine, and BUN in serum were observed in both the control groups. Creatinine clearance was reduced in the control groups. On treatment with cystone and EPV, all the urinary, serum biochemical, and oxidative stress parameters were reversed to almost normal values. Cystone and EPV significantly restored the *in vivo* antioxidant enzymes by decreasing the lipid peroxidation in the kidney.

Vinciya [518] evaluated the antiurolithiatic activity of ethanolic and aqueous extracts of *P. vulgaris* (EEPV and AEPV) seeds in rat models of preventive and curative lithiasis. In preventive and curative studies of AEPV and EEPV showed significant reduction in calcium, oxalate and phosphate levels in urine and an increase in the urinary magnesium and a restoration of normal urine volume. Serum levels of creatinine, uric acid and BUN were also brought down to normal values by the extracts. Histopathological observations also confirmed the same. These findings indicate the potential of the extracts in inhibiting kidney stone formation as well as a lithotripsic action on the formed renal stones. Aqueous extract is more potent than the ethanolic extract in the urolithiasis rat models.

Phlogacanthus thyrsiformis Nees Family: Acanthaceae

Das *et al.* [519] synthesized the biofabricated silver nanoparticles of aqueous extracts from flowers of *Phlogacanthus thyrsiformis* and evaluated its therapeutic activity against struvite urinary stones and CaOx kidney stones in rat models. It was demonstrated that treatment with the biofabricated silver nanoparticles remarkably reduced the size of struvite stones *in vitro* and eliminated CaOx stones in urolithiasis model rats *in vivo*.

Phoenix dactylifera L. Family: Arecaceae

Al-Qarawi *et al.* [520] evaluated the effect of an extract of the flesh and pits of dates (*Phoenix dactylifera*) on GM nephrotoxicity in rats. GM treatment significantly increased the plasma concentrations of creatinine and urea and induced a marked necrosis of the renal proximal tubules. The date flesh and pits were effective in significantly reducing the increases in plasma creatinine and urea concentrations induced by GM nephrotoxicity and ameliorating the proximal tubular damage.

Ali and Abdelaziz [521] evaluated the potential effect of date seeds against nephrotoxicity induced by CCl_4 in rats. The treatment with date seeds has preserved the kidney histology, kidney function close to control values. It significantly restored the activities of SOD and GST and decreased kidney MDA, GSH and NO levels. Dry date seeds confers an appealing nephroprotective effect which might be explained partially *via* diminishing the generation of MDA and NO and induction of antioxidant systems.

Al-Gamli *et al.* [522] evaluated the activity of anti-urolithiatic of the hydroalcoholic extracts of *Phoenix dactylifera* seeds (roasted and non-roasted) in CaOx urolithiasis in male albino rats. Treatment with both hydroalcoholic seed extracts restored urine volume, magnesium and kidney GSH, MDA and NO levels while treatment with non-roasted extracts reduced the elevated level of urinary calcium, serum creatinine and urea levels as compared to lithiatic group. Histopathological examination revealed tubular degeneration, dilatation, presence of CaOx crystals in the lumen of renal tubules and intense interstitial mononuclear cell infiltration in the lithiatic control group. These histopathological alterations were markedly regressed in other treated groups.

Phyla nodiflora (L.) Greene Family: Verbenaceae

Ethanolic extract of whole plant of *Phyla nodiflora* was studied by Sujatha *et al.* [523] for its antiurolithiatic activity. Ethanolic extract of *P. nodiflora* exhibited significant effect in preventing CaOx stone formation and also in dissolving the pre-formed CaOx stones in the kidney along with significant effect on both *in vitro* and *in vivo* antioxidant parameters.

Phyllanthus amarus Schum. & Thonn. Family: Phyllanthaceae

Protective effect of the leaf and seed aqueous extract of *Phyllanthus amarus* (PA) were studied by Adeneye and Benebo [524] for their protective effects in acetaminophen- and GM-induced nephrotoxic Wistar rats. Results suggest that the nephroprotective effect of PA could be due to the inherent antioxidant and free-radical-scavanging principle(s) contained in the extract.

The effects of the methanolic extracts of the leaves of *P. amarus* on some biochemical parameters of male Guinea pigs were investigated by Obianime and Uche [525]. The methanol extract of *P. amarus* leaves caused a significant decrease in the levels of total cholesterol, AST, ALT, urea, uric acid, total protein, prostatic, alkaline, and acid phosphatases. The highest reduction effect was obtained with uric acid at 400mg/kg of *P. amarus* extract while the least effect was observed in total cholesterol. These effects were dose- and time- dependent.

Woottisin *et al.* [369] fed the rats with tablets containing the extracts from leaves of *P. amarus*. Four weeks later, the serum oxalate and glycolate level in group received a 3% glycolate diet and tablets containing the extracts from leaves significantly decreased, while urinary citrate and oxalate levels of the group were higher than the group only received a 3% glycoside diet. Alternatively, the extracts from leaves of *P. amarus* decreased calcium crystal deposition in the kidneys of rats.

Bakhtiary *et al.* [526] evaluated the nephroprotective activity on *P. amarus* methanolic extracts of seeds in GM-induced nephrotoxicity in Wistar rats. Nephroprotection was assessed by measuring serum creatinine, BUN and kidney weight. *P. amarus* seed possesses a potent protective effect against GM-induced renal damage.

Phyllanthus fraternus G.L.Webster Family: Phyllanthaceae

Singh *et al.* [527] evaluated the protective effects of aqueous exrtact of *Phyllanthus fraternus* (AEPF) on the CPA-induced nephrotoxicity in mice. The KSI decreased while creatinine increased significantly after CPA treatment. These changes were almost restored following co-administration of AEPF. This might be due to decreased activity of oxidative stress.

Phyllanthus maderaspatensis L. Family: Phyllanthaceae

The protective effect of *Phyllanthus maderaspatensis* (PME) was studied by Chandrasekar *et al.* [528] on cisplatin-induced nephrotoxicity in male Swiss albino mice. The treatment of mice with different doses of PME before the administration of a single i.p. dose of cisplatin exhibited significant chemoprotective activity. A single dose of cisplatin significantly elevated the levels of BUN, serum creatinine, and the kidney to body weight ratio, but pretreatment with PME (600 mg kg^{-1} day^{-1}) for 7 days significantly attenuated the cisplatin-induced nephrotoxicity.

Phyllanthus niruri L. Family: Phyllanthaceae

Boim *et al.* [529] reviewed the work on treatment of urolthiasis with *Phyllanthus niruri*. Melo *et al.* [530] reported antiurolithiatic activity of *Phyllanthus niruri*. Campos and Schor [531] evaluated the *in vitro* effect of an aqueous extract of *P. niruri* on urolithiasis by Madin-Darby canine kidney cells. The extract exhibited a potent and effective non-concentration-dependent inhibitory effect on the CaOx crystal internalization. This response was present even at very high (pathologic) CaOx concentrations and no *P. niruri* -induced toxic effect could be detected.

Freitas *et al.* [532] evaluated the effect of an aqueous extract of *P. niruri* (Pn), on the urinary excretion of endogenous inhibitors of lithogenesis, citrate, magnesium and glycosaminoglycans (GAGs). The creatinine clearance or urinary and plasma concentrations of Na^+, K^+, Ca^{2+}, oxalate, phosphate and uric acid were unaffected by Pn or the induction of lithiasis. Treatment with Pn strongly inhibited the growth of the matrix calculus and reduced the number of stone satellites compared with the group receiving water. The calculi were eliminated or dissolved in some treated animals. The urinary excretion of citrate and magnesium was unaffected by Pn treatment. However, the mean (sd) urinary concentration of GAGs was significantly lower in rats treated. In contrast, the content of GAGs in the calculi was higher in the CaOx + Pn rats.

Barros *et al.* [533] investigated the effect of an aqueous extract of *P. niruri* on CaOx crystallization *in vitro*. The presence of *P. niruri* extract did not inhibit CaOx precipitation and even more crystals were obtained, although they were significantly smaller than those in the control urine. Crystal aggregation observed 24 h after crystallization was also inhibited by *P. niruri* extract.

Nishiura *et al.* [534] evaluated the effect of *P. niruri* intake on 24 h urinary biochemical parameters in an attempt to assess its *in vivo* effect in calcium stone forming (CSF) patients. Overall, there were no significant differences in the mean values of urinary parameters between the urine samples before and after *P. niruri* intake, except for a slight reduction in mean urinary magnesium after *P. niruri,* which was within the normal range. However, in the subset analysis, *P. niruri* induced a significant reduction in the mean urinary calcium in hypercalciuric patients. In this short-term follow-up, no significant differences in calculi voiding and/or pain relief between the groups taking *P. niruri* or the placebo were detected. *P. niruri* intake reduced urinary calcium based on the analysis of a subset of patients presenting with hypercalciuria.

Barros *et al.* [535] evaluated the effect of *P. niruri* (Pn) on the preformed calculus induced by introduction of a CaOx seed into the bladder of male Wistar rats. Precocious Pn treatment reduced the number (75%) and the weight (65%) of calculi that frequently exhibited a matrix-like material on its surface, compared to the untreated CaOx group. In contrast, Pn treatment in the presence of a preformed calculus did not prevent further calculus growth; rather, it caused an impressive modification in its appearance and texture. Calculi from Pn-treated animals had a smoother, homogeneous surface compared to the spicule shape of calculi found in the untreated CaOx group. XRD analysis revealed the precipitation of struvite crystals over the CaOx seed and Pn did not change the crystalline composition of the calculi.

Gaddam *et al*. [536] investigated the protective effects of mehanolic extractof *P. niruri* leaves on GM-induced renal injury in rats. Co-administration of methanolic extract of *P. niruri* leaves with GM have markedly improved all the physical parameters, urinary and blood parameters. There was a significant reduction in lipid peroxidation and rise in GSH levels with mehanolic extract of *P. niruri* leaves treatment. Histopathological reports showed reduction in the damage of kidneys when treated with the extract.

Physalis alkekengi L. Family: Solanaceae

Hydroalcoholic extract of *P. alkekengi* (PAHE) was studied by Sabatullah *et al*. [537] and Aslam *et al*. [538] for its nephroprotective activity against cisplatin induced acute renal injury in albino rats. Significant reduction in the elevated blood urea, serum creatinine, uric acid, TBARS level was observed and also normalized the histopathological changes. However, the results were comparatively better at 420mg/kg dose level. Incidentally the second publication is duplicate of the first paper.

Physalis peruviana L. Family: Solanaceae

Abdel-Moneim and El-Deib [539] evaluated the protective effect of *Physalis peruviana* extract against CCl_4-induced kidney injury. The combination (both physalis and CCl_4) group has preserved the kidney histology, kidney function near to control, exhibited a significant induction in the activities of CAT, SOD and GST, increased the kidney content of GSH and Bcl-2 and conversely showed significant decrease in kidney MDA and NO levels compared to CCl_4-treated rats.

Picrorhiza kurroa Royle ex Benth. Family: Scrophulariaceae

Yamgar *et al*. [540] evaluated protective and curative activity of rhizome of *Picrorhiza kurroa* in female Wistar rats against cisplatin induced nephrotoxicity. One of the Ayurvedic formulations *viz*. Arogyawardhini, containing *P. kurroa* as a major ingredient was also studied for the nephroprotective and nephrocurative effects against cisplatin induced nephrotoxicity. Treatments with the ethanolic extract of the rhizome in the dose of 600 mg/kg b.w.p.o. could significantly reduce the elevated serum levels of creatinine and blood urea. The formulation was found to have better activity as compared to the rhizome.

Pimpinella anisum L. Family: Apiaceae

Changizi-Ashtiyani *et al*. [541] explored protective effects of *Pimpinella anisum* on the alleviation of GM-induced damage. The plasma levels of creatinine, BUN, MDA and the absolute excretion of sodium and potassium were increased in the GM group, while FRAP level was reduced compared to the sham group. In addition, congestion of renal vessels and tubular cell necrosis was observed. They found that 300 mg/kg bw/day *P. anisum* significantly reduced the plasma concentrations of renal function markers in the group receiving GM. Additionally, GM-induced tubule damage was improved by *P. anisum*.

Aiswarya *et al*. [542] evaluated the protective activity of water extract of *P. anisum* seeds in a rodent model of GM-induced renal injury. Co-administration of *P. anisum* extract with GM decreased the rise in these parameters in a dose dependent manner. Histopathological analysis revealed epithelial loss with intense granular degeneration in GM treated rats, whereas aqueous extract of *P. anisum* mitigated the severity of GM-induced renal damage.

Pimpinella tirupatiensis N.P.Balakr. & Subram. Family: Apiaceae

Palani *et al*. [543] investigated the protective and antioxidant activities of the ethanol extract of *Pimpinella tirupatiensis* on APAP induced toxicity in rats. Altered values of the biochemical parameters are retrieved significantly by treatment with *P.tirupatiensis* extracts. The antioxidant studies reveal that the levels of renal SOD, CAT, GSH and GPx in the APAP treated animals are increased significantly along with a reduced MDA content in ethanol extract of *P.tirupatiensis* treated groups. Apart from these, histopathological changes also reveal the protective nature of the *P.tirupatiensis* extract against acetaminophen induced necrotic damage of renal tissues.

Pinus eldarica Medw. Family: Pinaceae

Hosseinzadeh *et al*. [544] evaluated the protective activity of *Pinus eldarica* cone on induced CaOx nephrolithiasis in rats. The aqueous extract prophylactic treatment (500 mg/kg/day) increased urinary calcium excretion. Qualitative analysis of crystalluria and histopathologic examination showed that the administered dose of extract prevented stone formation in the kidneys significantly. The prophylactic treatment did not increase urine volume in comparison with ethylene glycol. Stone formation did not decrease in the treatment group.

Piper cubeba L.f. Family: Piperaceae

Kabab chini (*Piper cubeba*) was studied by Ahmad *et al.* [545] for protective effect against cisplatin induced nephrotoxicity in Wistar rats. The test drug produced significant decrease in serum urea and creatinine and protected the histological structure of the kidney.

Ahmad *et al.* [546] evaluated the protective effect of *P. cubeba* against GM-induced renal injury in Wistar rats. The pre-treated and post-treated groups showed that *P. cubeba* produced a significant degree of nephroprotection based on the biochemical markers of kidney function and the histopathological features. In inter-group comparison, however, the effect in the pre-treated group was more significant.

Bano *et al.* [547] investigated the antilithiatic effect of hydroalcoholic extract of *P. cubeba* fruit in male Sprague Dawley rats. Urine analysis showed significant increase in magnesium while calcium, sodium, chloride and phosphorus significantly decreased along with histopathological improvement in kidney tissue in treated groups.

Pistacia atlantica Desf. Family: Anacardiaceae

Heidarian *et al.* [548] evaluated the protective effects of *Pistacia atlantica* leaf hydroethanolic extract against GM-induced nephrotoxicity in rats. Treatment with *P. atlantica* leaf hydroethanolic extract resulted in a significant increase in CAT, SOD, vitamin C, and high-density lipoprotein cholesterol, and significantly decreased the levels of Cr, urea, uric acid, MDA, PC, triglyceride, total cholesterol, low-density lipoprotein cholesterol, very low-density lipoprotein cholesterol, TNF-α protein, and the gene expression of TNF-α compared with the untreated group. Histopathological studies showed that in lymphocyte infiltration, remarkable reduction was observed in *P. atlantica* leaf hydroethanolic extract-treated groups, compared with the untreated group.

Pistacia khinjuk Stocks Family: Anacardiaceae

Ghaedi *et al.* [549] investigated the protective effects of *Pistacia khinjuk* against GM-induced nephrotoxicity in rats. Treatment with *P. khinjuk* produced amelioration in biochemical indices in plasma and renal tissue when compared with the GM treated group.

Pistacia vera L. Family Anacardiaceae

Ehsani *et al.* [550] evaluated the protective effect of the hydroalcoholic extract of *Pistacia vera* (pistachio) on GM-induced nephrotoxicity in rats. Co-administration with pistachio extract showed reduction in the levels of serum creatinine, urine volume, urine glucose and BUN and increase of creatinine clearance in all doses but the most significant alteration was observed in doses of 100 mg/kg. Also, the nephroprotective effect of the GA was confirmed by the histological examination of the kidneys.

Plantago major L. Family: Plantaginaceae

The *in vitro* effect of *Plantago major* extract on CaOx crystals was investigated. The concentrations of *P. major* extract used were from 100 ppm to 350 ppm. Extract of *P. major* has inhibitory effect on the number of crystals but it was not significant. However, extract of *P. major* was better than allopurinol and potassium citrate in inhibiting the size of the CaOx crystal *in vitro* [551].

Sharifa *et al.* [552] determined the inhibition effects of the terpenoid of *P. major* on CaOx crystals *in vitro* and to compare the effects of *P. major* with clinically used drugs like zyloric and potassium citrate for the treatment of urinary stone. Crude methanol extract of *P. major* contained the active compound terpenoid. Terpenoid, zyloric and potassium citrate at concentrations in the range of (100 μg/mL - 250 μg/mL) significantly inhibited the area of crystal formation in comparison to the negative control after 24 h. The Zyloric and terpenoid of *P. major* in the concentrations of (100 μg/mL-250 μg/mL) inhibited the sizes of crystals significantly. Potassium citrate was more effective, than terpenoid of *P. major* in inhibiting the size of crystals at two concentrations *i.e.* 100 μg/mL and 150 μg/mL respectively. The inhibition effect of the terpenoid of *P. major* extract on crystal size was much better than Zyloric and potassium citrate.

Plectranthus amboinicus (Lour.) Spreng. Family: Lamiaceae

Modulatory effect of *Plectranthus amboinicus* on ethylene glycol induced nephrolithiasis in male Wistar rats was investigated by Jose *et al.* [553]. Treated animals showed a significant reduction in all the parameters almost comparable with normal control. The urine and histopathological results clearly revealed the antilithiatic activity of *P. amboinicus*, particularly of CaOx origin.

Palani *et al.* [554] investigated the nephroprotective, diuretic, and antioxidant activities of the alcoholol extract of *P. amboinicus* (PA) at two doses of 250 and 500 mg/kg bw on acetaminophen-induced toxicity in rats. Ethanol extract of PA rescued these phenotypes by increasing anti-oxidative responses as assessed by biochemistry and histopathology. In addition, the ethanol extract of PA at two doses showed a significant diuretic activity by increased levels of total urine output and urinary elerolytes such as sodium and potassium.

Polygonum glabrum Will. Family: Polygonaceae

The nephroprotectic effect of methanolic extract of *Polygonum glabrum* was studied in cisplatin and GM-induced albino rats. Oral administration of extract to albino rats produced significant effect in animals treated with extract in dose dependent manner, when compared to control drugs. Treatment with extract 200mg/kg and 400mg/kg showed significant improvement in body weight and serum and urine urea, uric acid, total protein, creatinine, when compared to nephroprotective control. Histopathological studies also confirmed biochemical findings [555].

Pongamia pinnata (L.) Pierre Family: Fabaceae

Ethanolic extract of flowers of *Pongamia pinnata* was studied by Shirwaikar *et al.* [556] for its protective effect against cisplatin and GM-induced nephrotoxicity in rats. In the preventive regimen, co-administration of the extract with GM significantly prevented the renal injury both functionally and histologically. Ethanolic extract of flowers had a marked nitric oxide free radical scavenging effect, suggesting an antioxidative property.

Portulaca oleracea L. Family: Portulacaceae

The protective effect of aqueous and ethanolic extract of *Portulaca oleracea* against cisplatin-induced nephrotoxicity was studied in rats by Karimi *et al.* [557]. Treatment with aqueous and ethanolic extracts of *P. oleracea* in the highest dose (0.8 and 2 g/kg), 6 and 12 hr before cisplatin injection reduced BUN and Scr. Tubular necrotic damage was not observed either.

The effect of GM without or with oral administration of aqueous purslane (*P. oleracea*) extract and fish oil co-treatments was evaluated by Hozayen *et al.* [558] in rats. Co-administration of aqueous purslane extract and fish oil was found to improve the adverse changes in the kidney functions with an increase in antioxidant activities and reduction of peroxidation.

The protective activity of the ethanolic extract of aerial parts of *P. oleracea* was investigated using the ethylene glycol and ammonium chloride induced urolithiasis model in albino rats. Treatment with the extract restored all the elevated biochemical parameters including serum and urine (calcium, creatinine, urea, BUN), restored the urine pH to normal and increased the urine volume significantly when compared to disease control group. The histopathological studies confirmed the induction of lithiasis as microcrystal deposition was observed in section of kidney from animals treated with ethylene glycol and ammonium chloride. This was reduced, after treatment with the extract [559].

Prosthechea michuacana (Lex.) W.E.Higgins Family: Orchidaceae

Methanol, hexane, and chloroform extracts of bulbs of *P. michuacana* were studied by Gutierrez *et al.* [560] in the cisplatin-induced renal injury model in rats. Treatments with methanolic extract increased levels of biochemical markers of renal injury like reduced GSH, GST, and SPD and inhibited the increases in blood urea and serum creatinine concentrations and lipid peroxidation induced by cisplatin. Hexane and chloroform extracts did not show any effect.

Prunus avium (L.) L. [Syn.: *Cerasus avium* (L.) Moench.] Family: Rosaceae

Azaryan *et al.* [561] investigated the therapeutic effects of the aqueous extract of *Prunus avium* (Syn.: *Cerasus avium*) stem on urolithiasis. On the 30th day of the experiment, serum level of magnesium and potassium decreased significantly in EG group compared with A,C,D,E and F groups, while serum level of calcium, creatinine, uric acid, sodium and urine level of calcium, creatinine, uric acid, increased significantly in EG group compared with A,C,D,E and F groups. In the prevention and treatment groups, the number of deposits decreased significantly compared with EG group on the 30th day.

Prunus domestica L. Family: Rosaceae

Kessler *et al.* [562] evaluated the influence of plum (*Prunus domestica*) on urolithiasis. Investigations were carried out in 12 healthy male subject's aged 18-38 y. The plum juice had no significant effect on the urinary composition.

Pseudocedrela kotschyi (Schweinf.) Harms Family: Meliaceae

Ojewale *et al.* [563] evaluated the protective activities of ethanolic roots extract of *Pseudocedrela kotschyi* against nephrotoxicity in alloxan induced diabetic albino rats. The ethanolic roots extract of *P. kotschyi* exhibited significant reduction of blood glucose when compared with the standard drug Glibenclamide. Urea and creatinine levels were significantly increased in diabetic group without treatment as compared to control. In addition, the level of oxidative stress markers such as SOD, CAT, GPx, GSH were significantly decreased in diabetic rats as compared to normal rats while the lipid peroxidation (MDA) significantly increased in diabetic group without treatment as compared to control (normal) rat. Apart from these, histopathological changes also revealed the cytoprotective nature of the ethanolic roots extract of *P. kotschyi* against alloxan induced necrotic damage of renal tissues.

Psidium guajava L. Family: Myrtaceae

The protective effects of ethanolic extract of *Psidium guajava* (EEPG) on adriamycin-induced nephrotoxicity were investigated in rats by Adesia [564]. Renal dysfunction caused by 20mg/kg adriamycin (urea,-7.6 μmol/L, creatinine,-11.8 μmol/L) was prevented by pre-treatment with EEPG at 250 mg/kg (4.9 μmol/L, 7.9 μmol/L) while antioxidant status was improved significantly by reducing LPO (0.5 nmol) and increasing activities of SOD (3.6 units), GPx (0.3nmol), CAT (0.1 μmol), GST (0.3nmol), GR (0.6nmol) and GSH (16.0 μg/g) when compared with adriamycin-treated rats (0.9 nmol, 1.7 units, 0.1 nmol, 0.04 μmol, 0.2nmol, 0.4nmol and 13.9 μg/g), respectively. Increase in creatinine by 15mg/kg adriamycin (1.0mg/dL) was reduced by co-treatment with 250 and 500mg/kg EEPG (0.4mg/L, 0.3mg/dL). This reduction was accompanied by increase in GST activity (0.11nmol, 0.09nmol) when compared with adriamycin (0.08nmol) and inhibition of CYP3A4 activity (7.9±0.3, 8.2±0.2) when compared with adriamycin (9.0 ±0.1). Toxicity was profound when adriamycin was administered as cumulative dose. The EEPG (125, 250 and 500mg/kg) decreased the frequency of MPE (11.8, 8.8 and 3.4/1000 MPEs respectively) when compared with 20mg/kg adriamycin (19.3/1000 MPEs). The EEPG showed significant antioxidant activities *in vitro* through reduction of AAPH-induced LPO-65.3%, RSA in H_2O_2- 98.7%, nitric oxide-30.1%, DPPH.-70.4% and hydroxyl radicals-72.8% when compared with catechin (39.5%, 62.8%, 32.2%, 44.9% and 55.5%) respectively. Adriamycin induced renal tubular necrosis, while normal renal histology was maintained with EEPG at all doses. The purified compound from EEPG was found to be a triterpene [564].

Komolafe *et al*. [205] evaluated the effect of *P.guajava* extract and their efficacy on the histomorphometry of the kidney in STZ induced diabetic rats. The histology and morphometric analysis revealed that the kidney in the group treated with *P.guajava* showed significant increase in density compared to control.

Mohan *et al*. [565] investigated the protective effect of ethanolic extract of *P. guajava* leaves against doxorubicin-induced nephrotoxicity in rats. Treatment with *P. guajava* showed significant decrease in serum urea, BUN, creatinine, total protein, LPO and significant increase in CAT, SOD, GSH levels as compared to doxorubicin treated group. Histopathological examinations of kidney tissue showed that doxorubicin changed the renal architecture significantly which was less evident in *P. guajava* pre-treated rats.

Pterocarpus Indicus Willd. Family: Fabaceae

Saputri *et al.* [566] evaluated the protective effect water-boiled *Pterocarpus indicus* leaves against GM-induced nephrotoxicity in rats. The highest dose of 115.2 mg/kg water-boiled *P. indicus* decreased plasma urea and creatinine levels also significantly different compared induction group.

Pterocarpus santalinus L.f. Family: Fabaceae

Yadav *et al.* [158] explored the nephroprotection of water decoction of *Crataeva nurvala, Pueraria tuberosa, Pterocarpus santalinus, Albizzia lebbek, Boerhaavia diffusa* and *Tribulus terrestris* incisplatin-induced Acute Kidney Injury (AKI) in rats. Treated groups have reached the normal values of SOD and CAT. Antioxidant properties were further correlated with reducing potential, tannins, flavonoids and phenolic content of the fraction.

Punica granatum L. Family: Punicaceae

Tugcu *et al.* [567] studied the protective effects of pomegranate juice (PJ) on ethylene glycol (EG)-induced crystal deposition in renal tubules, renal toxicity, and inducible nitric oxide synthase (iNOS) and nuclear factor- B activities in rat kidneys. There was limited or no crystal formation in the EG + PJ-given groups. There were marked iNOS and p65 expressions in only the EG-given rats compared with control and PJ groups, immunohistochemically.

The protective effect of pomegranate peel ethanol extract against ferric nitrilotriacetate (Fe-NTA)-induced renal oxidative stress was studied by Ahmed and Ali [568]. Treatment of rats orally with pomegranate peel extract resulted in significant decrease in lipid peroxidation and serum urea and creatinine levels. Renal GSH content, GST and antioxidant enzymes were also recovered to a significant level.

The effect of pomegranate seed oil (PSO) on Hexachlorobutadiene (HCBD)-induced nephrotoxicity was investigated by Boroushaki *et al.* [569] in adult male rats. PSO pretreatment resulted in a significant and dose-dependent decrease in serum creatinine and urea levels as well as urine glucose and protein concentrations when compared with HCBD treated alone. PSO also significantly reversed the HCBD-induced depletion in total thiol content and elevation in TBARS in kidney homogenate samples.

Singh *et al.* [570] investigated the ameliorative potential of hydroalcoholic extract of flowers of *Punica granatum* in glycerol-induced acute renal failure (ARF) in rats. Pretreatment with hydroalcoholic extract of flowers of *P. granatum* significantly attenuated hypertonic glycerol-induced renal dysfunction in a dose-dependent manner.

The aqueous extract of *P. granatum* (AEPF) was investigated by Ali and Saeed [571] for its protective effects on GM-induced renal toxicity in rats. AEPF protected the rats from alteration in serum levels of urea, creatinine, uric acid, sodium, potassium and chloride better when co-administered with GM than when given after induced GM nephrotoxicity and also through reversing the mild tubular necrosis than severe tubular necrosis.

Boroushaki *et al*. [572] investigated the effect of pomegranate seed oil (PSO) on GM-induced nephrotoxicity in adult male rats. PSO pretreatment resulted in a significant and dose-dependent decrease in serum creatinine and urea levels as well as urine glucose and protein concentrations when compared with GM treated alone. PSO also significantly reversed the GM-induced depletion in total thiol content and elevation in TBARS in kidney homogenate samples.

An animal model of CaOx urolithiasis was used to evaluate the anti-urolithiatic effect of *P. granatum*. The treatment of Chloroform extract and methanol extract at 100, 200 and 400mg/kg doses, significantly decreased the urine oxalate, calcium and phosphate, renal tissue oxalates and serum creatinine, urea and uric acid after 28 days [573].

Cekmen *et al*. [574] investigated the protective effect of Pomegranate extract (PE) against GN-induced nephrotoxicity. Serum urea and creatinine levels were significantly higher in rats treated with GN alone than rats in the control and the GN and PE-treated groups. The GSH level in renal tissue of only GN-treated rats was significantly lower than those in the control group, and administration of PE to GN-treated rats significantly increased the level of GSH. The group that was given GN and PE had significantly lower MDA levels in kidney cortex tissue than those given GN alone. In rats treated with GN and PE, despite the presence of mild tubular degeneration and tubular necrosis is less severe, and glomeruli maintained a better morphology when compared with the GN-treated group.

Pomegranate flower extract (PFE) has been evaluated Motamedi *et al*. [575] against cisplatin-induced-renal toxicity. The results indicate that PFE ameliorated the deleterious effects of cisplatin in kidney.

Tracy *et al*. [576] examined the effects of the pomegranate extract on risk factors for nephrolithiasis in human beings. There was 10% increase in paraoxonase1 arylesterase (an anti-atherosclerotic component associated with high-density lipoprotein) activity in recurrent stone formers after 3-month treatment with the extract, which correlated with a trend toward decreasing values of supersaturation of CaOx and were in line with finding of previous animal experiments.

Mestry *et al.* [577] explored the possible mechanism of action of methanolic extract of *P. granatum* leaves (MPGL) in exerting a protective effect on GM-induced nephropathy. Simultaneous administration of MPGL and GM protected kidneys against nephrotoxic effects of GM as evidenced from normalization of renal function parameters and amelioration of histopathological changes.

Pyracantha crenulata (D.Don) Roem. Family: Rosaceae

Bahuguna *et al.* [578] investigated the effect of juice extract and alcohol extract of fruit of *Pyracantha crenulata* against ethylene glycol-induced urolithiasis in male albino rats. The increased deposition of stone forming constituents in the kidneys of calculogenic rats was significantly lowered by curative and preventive treatment using juice and alcohol extracts of *P. crenulata* fruit which showed a regulatory action on endogenous oxalate synthesis.

Quercus salicina Blume and *Quercus stenophylla* Makino Family: Fagaceae

The effects of *Quercus salicina* /*Quercus stenophylla* (QS) extract on oxalate-induced cell injury was investigated by Moriyama *et al.* [579]. When NRK-52E cells were injured by exposure to oxalate for 24 h, QS extract prevented the injury in a dose-dependent manner. In addition, QS extract suppressed the increase in NADPH-induced O_2^- production, or NADPH oxidase activity, in the homogenate of cells injured by oxalate exposure. These findings suggest that the reduction in oxalate-induced O_2^- production contributes to the cytoprotective effect of QS extract.

Moriyama *et al.* [580] investigated the mechanism of Urocalun, an extract of *Q. salicina* Blume/*Q. stenophylla* Makino (QS), in the treatment of urolithiasis. The increase in urinary MDA and renal calcium levels was significantly suppressed by the administration of QS extract, suggesting that the inhibition of renal calcium accumulation by QS extract is due to its antioxidative activity.

Randia echinocarpa Moc. & Sesse ex DC. Family: Rubiaceae

Vargas and Gutierrez [581] evaluated the diuretic and urolithiatic activities of *Randia echinocarpa*.

Raphanus sativus L. Family: Brassicaceae

The aqueous extract of the bark of *Raphanus sativus* was tested for its antiurolithiatic and diuretic activity. Significant decrease in the weight of stones was observed after treatment in animals which received aqueous extract in comparison with control groups. This extract showed an increase in the 24 h urine volume as compared to the control [582].

Rhazya stricta Decne Family: Apocynaceae

Ali [583] evaluated possible protective effect of crude water extract of leaves of *Rhazya stricta* on GM nephrotoxicity. The plant extract was ineffective in significantly altering the indices of GM-induced nephrotoxicity. However, a dose-related amelioration in the indices of toxicity was noted when the two higher doses of the plant extract were given.

Rheum emodi Wall. Family: Polygonaceae

The effect of rhubarb extract was examined by Yokozawa *et al.* [584] in rats with chronic renal failure. On treatment of the rats with the rhubarb extract, the level of urea nitrogen and creatinine in the serum was dose-dependently decreased. In addition, administration of the rhubarb extract to rats produced an increase in the serum calcium level, indicating an improvement of hypocalcemia. Improvement of hyperphosphatemia was also observed. Furthermore, rhubarb extract appeared to cause a gradual decrease of the taurocyamine, guanidinosuccinic acid, and methylguanidine levels in the serum with increasing dosage. Methylguanidine was not detectable in the serum or in the kidney of the rhubarb extract-treated group given 55 mg/rat/d. Treatment of chronically uremic rats with the rhubarb extract resulted in a normal or nearly normal serum level of branched-chain amino acids.

The renal effects of the alcoholic extract of *Rheum emodi* were investigated by Alam *et al.* [585] on cadmium chloride, mercuric chloride, potassium dichromate and GM-induced nephrotoxicity in rats. This investigation provide evidences that W-S fraction has nephroprotective effect on all the proximal tubule segments possibly through antioxidant action of the tannins present in the fraction. W-INS also improved the renal function by protecting S2 segment of proximal tubule nephrotoxicity induced by metals viz cadmium chloride and mercuric chloride in rat models, however, this fraction has been found to enhance GM nephrotoxicity.

Ribes nigrum L. Family: Glossulariaceae

Kessler *et al.* [562] evaluated the influence of blackcurrant (*Ribes nigrum*) juice on urinary stone risk factors in 12 male subjects. Blackcurrant juice increased the urinary pH and the excretion of citric acid. The excretion of oxalic acid was increased too.

Rivea hypocraterformis Family: Convolvulaceae

Ethanolic extracts of *Rivea hypocraterformis* was tested by Patel *et al*. [109] for its *in vitro* antilithiatic /anticalcification activity. Extract of *R. hypocraterformis* showed activity almost equivalent to standard drug cystone.

Rosa canina L. Family: Rosaceae

The effects on Magnesium chloride-induced urolithiasis urinary risk factors of *Rosa canina*, has been studied by Grases *et al*. [586] using female Wistar rats. The herb infusion did not cause any diuretic effect. Calciuria decreased and citraturia increased when taking the herb infusion. The same beneficial effects of the studied infusion herb on CaOx urolithiasis urinary risk factors can be clearly detected. Some possible effects depend on dietary components, thus, *i.e.*, an increase in the urinary pH was only detected when the intake of the herb infusion was studied in a magnesium chloride-supplemented diet.

Tayefi-Nasrabadi *et al*. [587] investigated the therapeutic potential of *R. canina* (RC) in experimentally induced CaOx nephrolithiasis with ethylene glycol in rats. The supplementation of the hydromethanol RC extract contributed to reducing the kidney and liver lipid peroxides to optimum levels in rats that had been treated with EG-induced CaOx lithiasis. The extract also decreased renal and urinary calcium contents, decreased the size and number of CaOx calculi in the kidneys, and significantly increased citrate excretion without changing the volume, pH, or urinary concentrations of oxalate in comparison with the control group.

Rotula aquatica Lour. Family: Boraginaceae

The decoction of *R. aquatica* was screened for antilithic activity in male Wistar rats by Christina *et al*. [588]. Simultaneous treatment with the decoction reduced calcium and oxalate ion concentration in urine, confirming the stone inhibitory effect. Histopathological studies of kidney tissue samples further substantiated the findings..

Raut *et al*. [138] screened anticrystal activity of *R. aquatica* against basic calcium phosphate (BCP), calcium pyrophosphate (CPPD) and monosodium urate monohydrate (MSUM). The aqueous extracts of *R. aquatica* have shown crystal dissolving activity against MSUM.

The inhibitory effect of aqueous extract of root of *R. aquatica* was investigated by Chauhan *et al*. [589] against struvite crystals grown *in vitro*. It was observed that the number, dimension, total mass, total volume, growth rate and depth of growth of struvite crystals decreased with the increasing extract concentrations in the supernatant solutions.

The effect of the alcoholic extract of *R. aquatica* against ethylene glycol-induced urolithiasis in albino rats was investiagated by Umesh *et al.* [590]. The deleterious effects of ethylene glycol were reduced after treatment with the extract.

Sasikala *et al.* [591] investigated the effectiveness of a different extracts obtained from *R. aquatica* on CaOx crystallization *in vitro*. A result obtained showed that aqueous extract of root has the higher capacity to inhibit the crystal formation and aggregation as compared to petroleum ether, chloroform and methanol extracts of leaf and stem.

In Ayurveda, *R.aquatica* is described as 'Paashanabhedha' meaning 'stone breaking'. Prashanthi *et al.* [592] evaluated the antiurolithiatic potential of the roots using *in vitro* model. The aqueous extract had high dissolving potential of 29.182% for Ca-Ox and 65.445% for CaPO4. A trend of dose dependent dissolution was identified with increasing the concentration of aqueous extract. 100% dissolution was found at 38 and 20 mg of aqueous extract for Ca-Ox and $CaPO_4$ respectively.

Vijayakumari *et al.* [593] assessed the antiurolithiatic activity of the aqueous root extract of *R. aquatica* in rats. The treatment with aqueous root extract of *R. aquatica* significantly decreased the urine protein, calcium, phosphate, uric acid, creatinine and oxalate, serum protein, calcium, phosphate, uric acid, creatinine, BUN and oxalate and renal tissues calcium, phosphate and oxalate, in EG induced urolithiasis. Aqueous root extract of *R. aquatica* at the dose of 200 mg/kg body weight was more effective in decreasing the urolithiasis and regeneration of renal tissues in male rats.

Vysakh *et al.* [594] evaluated the protective effect of ethyl acetate fraction from *R.aquatica* (EFRA) against GM induced nephrotoxicity. The changes in antioxidant parameters were restored by the treatment of EFRA at different. The serum parameters, ROS, MDA and nitrate level were decreased by administration of EFRA. The EFRA ameliorates histological changes associated with GM induced nephrotoxicity. The mRNA level expression of KIM-1, NF-κB, TNF- α, and IL-6 were downregulated in EFRA treated groups.

Rubia cordifolia L. Family: Rubiaceae

Divakar *et al.* [595] investigated the protective effect of the hydro-alcoholic extract of roots of *Rubia cordifolia* (HARC) against ethylene glycol induced urolithiasis in male Wistar albino rats. Supplementation with HARC significantly prevented change in urinary calcium, oxalate and phosphate excretion dose-dependently. The increased calcium and oxalate levels and number of CaOx crystals deposits in the kidney tissue of calculogenic rats were significantly reverted by HARC treatment. The HARC supplementation also prevents the impairment of renal functions..

Joy and Nair [596] investigated whether the hydro-alcoholic extract of *R. cordifolia* could decrease the intensity of toxicity in Swiss albino mice. The extract could significantly decrease the cisplatin induced nephrotoxicity as inferred from the tissue antioxidant status in the drug administered animals. Remarkable change was observed in serum creatinine and urea levels. Lipid peroxidation in the kidney and liver tissues was also considerably reduced in *R. cordifolia* extract treated animals.

Rubus ellipticus Sm. Family: Rosaceae

Sharma and Kumar [597] evaluated the protective effect of *Rubus ellipticus* fruits extracts on GM and cisplatin induced naphrotoxicity in rats. It was observed that pet.ether etahnolic and aqueous extracts of *R. ellipticus* significantly protect rat's kidney from GM and cisplatin induced damage by normalized the GM and cisplatin induced increase in serum creatinine, serum uric acid, BUN and serum urea levels.

Rudgea viburnoides (Cham.) Benth. Family: Rubiaceae

Galdino *et al.* [598] evaluated the nephron-protective effect of extract of *R. viburnoides* on GM-induced kidney injury using rats. *R. viburnoides* leaves extract improved renal function and impairments caused by GM-induced nephrotoxicity, as revealed by glomerular filtration rate, urine output and proteinurea.

Saccharum spontaneum L. Family: Poaceae

The effect of the alcoholic extract of *Saccharum spontaneum* against glycolic acid induced urolithiasis in albino rats was investigated by Sathya and Kokilavani [599]. Therapeutic treatment with plant extract has significantly ameliorated to near normalcy in the curative group. It also increased the urine volume, thereby reducing the tendency for crystallization.

Salacia oblonga Wall. Family: Celastaceae

Palani *et al.* [600] investigated the nephroprotective and antioxidant activities of the ethanol extract of *Salacia oblonga* (EESO) at the two dose levels of 250 and 500 mg/kg bw on APAP-induced toxicity in rats. APAP significantly increased the levels of serum urea, creatinine, and reduces levels of uric acid concentration. The EESO reduced these by increasing anti-oxidative responses as assessed by biochemical and histopathological parameters.

Salix caprea L. Family: Saliacaceae

Jabbar and Ali [601] evaluated the nephroprotctive activity of the alcoholic extract of flowers of *Salix caprea* in albino Wistar rats. The alcoholic extract inhibited 28.52% BUN in rats. Water soluble fraction exhibited significant reduction of the BUN in rat and it was up to 68.64%. The alcoholic extract presented 24.75% inhibition of creatine in rats. The water soluble and water insoluble fractions of the extracts showed significant reduction of the creatine in rats which were 50.97% and 39.67% respectively.

Salix taxifolia Kunth Family: Salicaceae

The aqueous extract of the bark of *Salix taxifolia* was tested by Vargas and Perez [602] for antilithiatic and diuretic activities. A significant decrease in the weight of the stones was observed after treatment in animals with the aqueous extract. This extract caused an increase in the 24 h urine volume.

Salvia miltiorhiza Bunge Family: Lamiaceae

Jeong *et al*. [603] determined the beneficial effect of salviae radix extract (SRE) against cisplatin-induced renal failure in rabbits. PAH uptake by renal cortical slices was inhibited by the administration of cisplatin. Such changes were prevented by SRE pretreatment. Cisplatin injection increased lipid peroxidation, which was prevented by SRE pretreatment. The protective effect of SRE was supported by morphological studies. Cisplatin injection reduced renal blood flow that was not affected by SRE pretreatment. Cisplatin treatment *in vitro* in renal cortical slices increased LDH release and lipid peroxidation, which were prevented by SRE.

Salvia officinalis L. Family: Lamiaceae

Dizaye [604] evaluated the protective effects of the aqueous extract of *Salvia officinalis* leaves against nephrotoxicity induced by cisplatin in rats. Aqueous extract of *S. officinalis* leaves significantly protected rat kidneys from cisplatin-induced histopathological changes. This extract also normalized cispaltin induced increases in serum creatinine and blood urea.

Samanea saman (Jacq.) Merr. Family: Fabaceae

Patel *et al*. [605] invesitageted the protective potential of hydroalcoholic extract of *Samanea saman* leaves on paracetamol induced renal damage in rats. Administration with hydroalcoholic extract of leaves of *S. saman* improved changes in physical, tissue and blood parameters. Even elevated LPO and reduced tissue GSH level were significantly reversed.

Sclerocarya birrea (A. Rich) Hochst. Family: Anacardiaceae

Treatments with stem-bark ethanolic extract of *Sclerocarya birrea* resulted in decreased plasma urea and creatinine concentrations of streptozotocin-diabetic rats with concomitant increase in glomerular filtration rate [606].

Scoparia dulcis L. Family: Plantaginaceae

Farook *et al.* [36] investigated inhibition of mineralization of urinary stone forming minerals by *Scoparia dulcis*. Inhibition efficiencies of leaves, seeds and fruits of *S. dulcis* have been investigated in different models. Study suggests that the fruit juice and seed extract is moderate to good inhibitor of CaOx, calcium carbonate and calcium phosphate mineralization. Relatively poor inhibition of mineralization of CaOx, calcium phosphate and calcium carbonate precipitation by leaves extracts was reported.

Christi and Senthamarai [39] evaluated the antiurolithiatic activity of aqueous and alcoholic extract of leaves *S. dulcis* using ethylene glycol induced hyperoxaluria model in rats. The drug treated group animals showed a significant reduction in the bladder stones compared to the control and standard cystone treated group and enzyme activity for antioxidant property and more in methanolic extract. The herbal drug exerted its antilithogenic property by altering the ionic composition of urine *viz.* decreasing the calcium and oxalate ion concentration or increasing magnesium and citrate excretion. The extract at a dose of 200mg/kg produced significant reduction in MDA and increased GSH and antioxidant enzyme likes SOD and CAT compared to standard group cystone.

Jose and Adikay [607] evaluated the protective potential of ethanolic extract of aerial parts of plant *S. dulcis* against cisplatin induced nephrotoxicity in Wistar rats. Supplementation of ethanolic extract of *S. dulcis* reduced the elevated serum creatinine, BUN levels, lipid peroxidation levels and improved the creatinine clearance. Supplementation of *S. dulcis* during cisplatin therapy reduces the risk of cisplatin induced nephrotoxicity in a dose dependent manner in curative regimen. The prophylactic regimen also possessed significant nephroprotection against cisplatin toxicity.

Scrophularia hypericifolia Wydler Family: Scrophulariaceae

The nephroprotective effects of the ethanol extract of the aerial parts of *Scrophularia hypericifolia* were evaluated by Alqasoumi [608] using Wistar albino rats as experimental animal model. The ethanol extract of the aerial parts of *S. hypericifolia* showed dose dependent moderate level of protection against paracetamol induced hepatrotoxicity and nephrotoxicity as indicated from the obtained results. The reduction of the sodium and potassium levels by the higher dose of the extract exceeded that obtained by silymarin.

Sechium edule (Jacq.) Sw. Family: Cucurbitaceae

The aqueous extract of leaves of *Sechium edule* was evaluated by Mumtaz *et al.* [609] for its protective activity against GM, potassium dichromate-induced nephrotoxicity and streptozotocin-induced diabetic nephropathy in experimental animals. In these three conditions, the extract of *S. edule* (200 mg/kg) has significantly decreased the level of blood urea, BUN and serum creatinine and also significantly increased the serum levels of total protein. The serum uric acid level was also significantly decreased in diabetic mice treated with the extract. The extract also improved the histology of the kidney.

Sesamum indicum L. Family: Pedaliaceae

Bhuvaneswari and Krishnakumari [610] evaluated the effect of ethanolic extract of *Sesamum indicum* on kidney function in Streptozotocin Nicotinamide induced diabetic rats. Decrease in the levels of serum total protein, albumin and globulin and significant increase in the levels of blood urea, serum creatinine and uric acid with STZ diabetic rats were reverted after the treatment regimen.

Sesbania grandiflora (L.) Pers. Family: Fabaceae

Sujatha *et al.* [611] investigated the potential of *S. grandiflora* in the treatment of renal calculi. The leaf juice of *S. grandiflora* was safe orally and exhibited no gross behavioral changes except for an increase in urination. The leaf juice of *S. grandiflora* showed significant antiurolithiatic activity against CaOx -type stones and also exhibited antioxidant properties.

Sida cordata (Burm.f.) Borrss.Waalk. Family: Malvaceae

Shah *et al.* [612] evaluated the protective effect of *Sida cordata* against CCl_4 induced nephrotoxicity. Decrease in the count of red blood cells, neutrophils, eosinophils and concentration of hemoglobin whereas increase in lymphocyte count and estimation of sedimentation rate (ESR) with CCl_4 administration was restored dose dependently with co-treatment of SCEE (150 and 300 mg/kg b.w.). Treatment of rats with CCl_4 markedly increased the count of urinary red blood cells and leucocytes, concentration of urea, creatinine and urobilinogen and specific gravity whereas creatinine clearance was reduced. Co-administration of SCEE, dose dependently, protected the alterations in the studied parameters of rats.

Sida cordifolia L. Family: Malvaceae

Lovkesh *et al.* [613] evaluated the ethanolic and aqueous extracts of leaves of *Sida cordifolia* for nephroprotective effect in GM-induced nephrotoxicity in rats. Extracts at dose of 200 and 400 mg/kg b.w. produced significant protective activity in GM-induced nephrotoxicity models as evident by decrease in serum creatinine, serum urea, urine creatinine and BUN levels in extract treated groups which was elevated by GM, which was further confirmed by histopathological study. GM induced glomerular congestion, blood vessel congestion, and epithelial desquamation, accumulation of inflammatory cells and necrosis of the kidney cells were found to be reduced in the groups receiving extracts of *S. cordifolia* along with GM.

Makwana *et al.* [614] evaluated nephroprotective activity of an aqueous extract of root of *S. cordifolia* (SCAE) against GM and cisplatin induced experimental animal models. The aqueous extract of *S. cordifolia* significantly prevents renal damage by normalizing increased levels of renal markers.

Sida rhomboidea Roxb. Family: Malvaceae

Thounaojam *et al.* [615] evaluated the protective potential of SR against GM induced nephrotoxicity and renal dysfunction. SR treatment to GM treated rats (GM+SR) recorded significant decrement in plasma and urine urea and creatinine, renal lipid peroxidation along with significant increment in renal enzymatic and non-enzymatic antioxidants.

Silene saxifraga L. Family: Caryophyllaceae

Grases *et al.* [96] studied the effects of *Silene saxifraga* to prevent and treat stone kidney formation in female Wistar rats. The infusion does not affect calciuria and citraturia values, they do not diminish calcinuria or increase the crystallization inhibitory capacity of the urine. The beneficial effect caused by this herb infusion on urolithiasis can be attributed to some disinfectant action, and tentatively to the presence of saponins.

Silene villosa Forssk. Family: Caryophyllacae

Yusufoglu *et al.* [616] evaluated the nephroprotectve activity of whole plant of *Silene villosa* against CCl_4-induced nephrotoxicity. Administration at two different doses of 250 and 500 mg/kg with CCl_4 showed a significant protective ability against CCl_4 intoxication by repairing kidney abnormalities. The protective ability was further confirmed by the histological study.

Smilax china L. Family: Smilacaceae

Chen *et al.* [617] investigated the effect of *Smilax china* on hyperuricemia and renal dysfunction in induced hyperuricemic animals. Ethyl Acetate Fraction (EAF) exhibited stronger anti-hyperuricemic activity in hyperuricemic mice compared with the other four fractions. Caffeic acid, resveratrol, rutin and oxyresveratrol isolated from EAF showed different inhibitory activities on xanthine oxidase *in vitro* and exhibited competitive or mixed inhibitory actions. Moreover, EAF markedly reversed the serum uric acid level, fractional excretion of urate and BUN to their normal states, and prevented the renal damage against tubulointerstitial pathologies in hyperuricemic rats..

Solanum nigrum L. Family: Solanaceae

The 50% ethanol extract of the whole plant of *Solanum nigrum* was tested by Kumar *et al*. [618] *in vitro* for its cytoprotection against GM-induced toxicity on Vero cells. Cytotoxicity was significantly inhibited. The test extract also exhibited significant hydroxyl radical scavenging potential, thus suggesting its probable mechanism of cytoprotection.

Kushwaha *et al*. [619] evaluated the nephroprotective and nephrocurative activity of *S. nigrum* on GM induced nephrotoxicity in experimental rats. There was significant decrease in BUN and serum creatinine values as compared to GT group in all test duration in phase-1. In phase two there was no significant difference of these markers in two groups.

Solanum virginianum L. Family: Solanaceae

Chinnala *et al*. [620] evaluted the antiurolithiatic activity of *Solanum virginianum* in ethylene glycol induced urolithiasis in male Spargue Dawley rats. Treatment with ethanolic extract of *S.virginianm* significantly reduced the elevated levels of ions in urine as well as BUN, serum creatinine and seum uric acid levels. The elevated calcium and phosphate levels in urine, serum creatinine, BUN and uric acid levels of urolithiasis induced rats were reduced with preventive and curative regimens of plant extract treatment. The histological findings also showed improvement in kidney architecture after treatment with the plant extract.

Solanum xanthocarpum Schrad & H. Wendl. Family: Solanaceae

Hussain *et al*. [621] evaluated the nephroprotective potential of *Solanum xanthocarpum* fruit extract (SXE) against GM induced nephrotoxicity. SXE 200 and 400 mg/kg treatment to GM treated rats recorded significant decrement in plasma and urine urea and creatinine, renal lipid peroxidation along with significant increment in renal enzymatic and non-enzymatic antioxidants. Histological observations of kidney tissues too correlated with the biochemical observations.

Patel *et al.* [622] investigated the aniurolithiatic effect of saponin rich fruit fraction of *S. xanthocarpum* (SXS) in kidney stone. *in vitro* CaOx crystal nucleation as well as aggregation was inhibited in artificial urine solution by SXS. The lithogenic treatment caused polyuria, damage renal function and oxidative stress, manifested as increased MDA, depleted reduced GSH and decreased antioxidant enzyme CAT activities of the kidneys, which were prevented by simultaneous administration with SXS. Co-administration of SXS had potential to prevent the pathological changes due to lithogenic treatment. Moreover, SXS raised level of glycosaminoglycan, a stone inhibitor macromolecule found in urine which decreased.

Alam and Vijayanarayana [623] evaluated the nephroprotective effect of alcoholic extracts of fruits of *S. xanthocarpum* against cisplatin-induced nephropathy in Wistar rats. The ethanolic extract 400 mg/kg treated rat group showed significant elevation in body weight with a significant increase in urine volume output. However, the urine creatinine and albumin decreased significantly when compared with the toxic control group. *S. xanthocarpum* showed nephroprotective activity in a dose dependent manner compared to cystone.

Solena amplexicaulis (Lam.) Gandhi Family: Cucurbitaceae

Farook *et al.* [36] investigated inhibition of mineralization of urinary stone forming minerals by *Solena amplexcaulis*. Inhibition efficiencies of leaves, seeds and fruits of *S. amplexcaulis* have been investigated in different models. Study suggests that the fruit juice and seed extract is moderate to good inhibitor of CaOx, calcium carbonate and calcium phosphate mineralization. Relatively poor inhibition of mineralization of CaOx, calcium phosphate and calcium carbonate precipitation by leaves extracts was reported.

Solidago virgaurea L. Family: Asteraceae

Melzig [624] reported that herbal remedies based on goldenrod (*Solidago virgaurea* L.) have been well-tried for centuries in the treatment of urinary tract diseases. Extracts prevent formation of kidney stones and help remove urinary gravel.

Sonchus asper (L.) Hill Family: Asteraceae

Khan *et al.* [625] investigated the effects of *Sonchus asper* methanolic extract (SAME) against CCl_4-induced nephrotoxicity in Sprague-Dawley male rats. Treatment of rats with SAME (100, 200mg/kg b.w.) effectively ameliorated the alterations induced with CCl_4 in lipid peroxidation, antioxidant defenses, biochemical markers, genotoxicity and renal lesions.

Sphaeranthus indicus L. Family: Asteraceae

Mathew *et al.* [626] evaluated the nephroprotective activity of the ethanol extract of entire plant of *Sphaeranthus indicus* cisplatin-induced nephrotoxicity. The ethanol extract significantly reduced the elevated serum creatinine and urea levels. Renal antioxidant defence systems, such as SOD, CAT, GPx activities and reduced GSH level that are depleted by cisplatin therapy were restored to normal by treatment with the extract. Cisplatin-induced lipid peroxidation was also found to be markedly reduced by treatment with the extract.

Stipa tenacissima L. Family: Poaceae

Inhibition of CaOx monohydrate crystal growth using aqueous extract of leaves of *Stipa tenacissima* was investigated by Beghalia *et al.* [61]. Activity was tested in bioassays. In the presence of plant extract, the length and the width of the crystals were reduced. It was found that extract of the plant inhibited potently the nucleation and growth phases. Inhibition of the crystal formation was 96.18% at 25% concentration, 84.12% at 50% concentration, 95.58% at 75% concentration and 95.58 at 100% concentration.

Strychnos potatorum L.f. Family: Loganiaceae

Varghese *et al.* [627] evaluated the protective activity of ethanolic extract of *Strychnos potatorum* seeds in rats in GM induced nephrotoxicity. The alcoholic extract of *S. potatorum* at a dose level of 200 mg/kg/body weight was found to normalize the raised blood urea, blood protein and serum creatinine. Investigation of the possible protective effect of *S. potatorum* revealed that 10 days administration of 200 mg/kg of alcoholic extract along with GM reduced the GM-induced renal injury.

Binu and Vijayakumari [628] investigated the antiurolithiatic acgtivity of *S. potatorum*. Mainly four parts of the plant were taken for the study, leaf, stem, bark and seed and they were extracted with petroleum ether, chloroform, methanol and water. The per cent inhibition of turbidity increased with concentration of extract and methanol extract of seed showed maximum dissolution of CaOx stones *in vitro*.

Swertia chirata Buch.-Ham. ex Wall. Family: Gentianaceae

Parmar *et al.* [629] evaluated the antiurolithiatic activity of *Swertia chirata* stems in rats. The ethylene glycol feeding resulted in an increase level of promoters with a decreased level of inhibitors as compared to normal control rats. All these conditions were significantly reversed with treatment of *S. chirata*.

Histopathological analysis also revealed deposition of CaOx crystals and disruption of tubular cells and juxtaglomerular cells. That deposition and disruption were also reduced in rats treated with *S. chirata*.

Syzygium cumini (L.) Skeels Family: Myrtaceae

Sreedevi *et al*. [630] assessed the protective activity of ethanol extract of fruits of *Syzygium cumini* on cisplatin-induced nephrotoxicity in albino rats. Animals which received ethanol extract of fruits of *S. cumini* significantly reversed the effects induced by cisplatin in dose dependent manner.

Sanjuna *et al*. [631] evaluated the *in vitro* antiurolithiatic activity of *S. cumini* leaves. Ethanolic extract showed their maximum efficiencies in the dissolution of CaOx crystals. Ethanolic extract of *S. cumini* leaves was found to be more effective in dissolution of CaOx than standard drug Neeri.

Tamarindus indica L. Family: Fabaceae

The effect of tartaric acid and tamarind on the growth of calcium hydrogen phosphate dehydrate crystals (CHPD) was investigated by Joseph *et al*. [632]. Chaudhary *et al*. [633] have conducted studies on the aqueous extracts of *Tamarindus indica* and *Terminalia arjuna* bark to establish a scientific basis for their antiurolithiatic property. Both the plants were found to retard the growth of COM crystals. However, tamarind fraction having molecular weight less than 10 kDa was found to be more effective. Inhibition of COM growth was also observed by purified fractions of both the plants. Out of these two plants, *Tamarindus indica* showed greater inhibition of COM crystal growth.

Aqueous extract of *Tamarindus indica* fruit pulp was evaluated by Kumar *et al*. [102] for its antiurolithiatic potential in albino Wistar rats. The administration of the drugs has resulted in reduction in the weight of stones compared to the control group, but neither was significantly reduced.

Ullah *et al*. [634] investigated the protective effects of hydroalcoholic extract of *T. indica* fruits against GM-induced renal toxicity. Animals treated by co-therapy with GM and *T. indica* had significantly improved renal structure and function. Co-therapy of *T. indica* for a period of three weeks successfully prevented functional and morphological derangements caused by GM as assessed by different renal function parameters and histological examinations.

The effect of ingestion of 3 and 10 g of tamarind pulp (*T. indica*) was studied in normal subjects and in stone formers. Tamarind intake at the dose of 10 g showed significant beneficial effect in inhibiting spontaneous crystallization in both normal subjects and in stone formers [635].

Tamarix gallica L. Family: Tamaricaceae

The inhibitor effect of acid fraction of the extract of *Tamarix gallica* on the crystallization of CaOx was investigated by Bensetal and Ouahrani [636]. The extract of *T. gallica* is very rich by acid compounds that are used as an inhibitor of nephrolithiasis (CaOx). Authors concluded that the extract of *T. gallica* acts at the stage of growth. The acid fraction of the extract of *T. gallica* gave an activity remarkable in the formation of urinary lithiasis (CaOx); this effectiveness is due to the presence of functions of acid.

Tamilnadia uliginosa (Retz.) Tirveng. & Sastre [Syn.: *Catunaregam ulginosa* (Retz.) Sivar.] Family: Rubiaceae

Sreedevi and Sravanthi [637] evaluated the protector activity of ethanolic extract of roots of *Tamilnadia uliginosa* (Syn.: *Catunaregam ulginosa*) (EECU) in cisplatin-induced nephrotoxicity in albino rats. EECU reversed the effects induced by cisplatin in a dose-dependent manner in both curative and prophylactic regimens. Histological studies substantiated the above results.

Taraxacum officinale (L.) Webber ex F.H.Wigg. Family: Asteraceae

Grases *et al.* [96] studied the effects of *Taraxacum officinale* to prevent and treat renal calculi formation in female Wistar rats. The infusion does not affect calciuria and citraturia values, they do not diminish calcinuria or increase the crystallization inhibitory capacity of the urine.

Taxillus tomentosus (Roth) van Tiegh. Family: Loranthaceae

Venkateswarlu *et al.* [638] investigated the potential of antiurolithiatic activity of ethanolic extract of *Taxillus tomentosus* plant (EETT). The EETT (200mg/kg BW and 400mg/kg BW) showed good antiurolithiatic activity when compared to the standard drug cystone (CST).

Tecoma stans (L.) Juss. ex Kunth Family: Bignoiaceae

The protector effect of ethyl acetate extract of dried flowers of *Tecoma stans* on GM-induced nephrotoxicity in albino rats was investigated by Raju *et al.* [639]. The ethyl acetate floral extract of *T. stans* significantly protected rat kidneys from GM-induced histopathological changes. GM-induced glomerular congestion, peritubular and blood vessel congestion, epithelial desquamation, accumulation of inflammatory cells and necrosis of the kidney cells were found to be reduced in the groups receiving the ethyl acetate floral extract of *T. stans* along with GM in a dose dependent manner. The floral extract also reduced the GM-induced increase in serum creatinine, serum uric acid, BUN and serum urea levels.

Kameshwaran *et al.* [640] evaluated the antiurolithiatic activity of aqueous and methanolic extracts of *T. stans* flowers in rats. Treatment with aqueous extract and methanolic extract of *T.stans* flowers significantly lowered the increased levels of oxalate, calcium and phosphate in urine and also significantly reduced their retention in kidney. The treatment with aqueous extract and alcoholic extract of *T. stans* flowers significantly lowered the elevated serum levels of BUN, creatinine and uric acid in both regimens. The histopathological study of the kidney also supported the above results. The results were comparable to that of standard drug (Cystone).

Tectona grandis L.f. Family: Lamiaceae

A study was undertaken by Patel *et al.* [641] to evaluate the *in vitro* antilithiatic activity on *Tectona grandis* seeds. Ethanolic extract of *T. grandis* was the most effective in inhibiting of calcium and phosphate precipitate *in vitro*.

Tephrosia purpurea (L.) Pers. Family: Fabaceae

Aqueous extract of the roots of *Tephrosia purpurea* was evaluated by Swathi *et al.* [642] for its antilithiatic activityin GM and ammonium oxalate models of urolithiasis. The aqueous extract of *T. purpurea* was found to be effective in reducing the formation of and dissolving existing CaOx and magnesium ammonium phosphate stones.

Jain *et al.* [643] evaluated the protective and curative effects of *T. purpurea* leaves against GM-induced acute nephrotoxicity in albino rats. In the preventive regimen, the extract showed significant reductions in the elevated blood urea and serum creatinine. Histopathological changes were in accordance with the biochemical findings. Also in the curative regimen, the blood urea and serum creatinine levels revealed significant curative effects. In *in vivo* antioxidant activity, the GSH level was significantly increased in the extract-treated groups, whereas MDA was reduced significantly.

Termnalia arjuna (Roxb. ex DC.) Wight & Arn. Family: Combretaceae

Manna *et al.* [644] evaluated the protective role of the water extract of the bark of *Termnalia arjuna* (TA) on CCl_4 induced oxidative stress and resultant dysfunction in the kidneys of mice. Aqueous extract of TA successfully prevented the alterations of the effects in the experimental animals.

Das *et al.* [645] evaluated the protective effect of aqueus bark extract of *T. arjuna* against dehydration induced oxidative stress and uremia in male Wister albino rats. The results suggest that dehydration induced oxidative stress and uremia in male rats may be protected by using *T. arjuna* bark extract.

The inhibitory potency of crude extracts or fractions of successive solvent extractions of *T. arjuna* bark was evaluated by Chaudhary *et al.* [646] on various stages of formation of calcium phosphate and on the growth of CaOx monohydrate crystals *in vitro*. *T. arjuna* bark has the potential to inhibit the formation of both calcium phosphate and CaOx crystals *in vitro*. Butanol fraction of *T. arjuna* extract was the most effective in inhibiting formation of calcium phosphate and CaOx crystals *in vitro*.

Venkateswarlu *et al.* [647] evaluated the nephroprotective effect of ethanolic extract of *T. arjuna* bark (EETAB) at the doses against Cisplatin induced nephrotoxicity in rats. Rats treated with EETAB significantly reduced the elevated levels of BUN, Cr, TP, MDA and significantly increased the levels of SOD, GSH, and CAT by restoring kidney architecture.

Mittal *et al.* [648] examined the antilithiatic potency of the aqueous extract (AE) of *T. arjuna*. *T. arjuna* extract exhibited a concentration dependent inhibition of nucleation and aggregation of CaOx crystals. The AE of *T. arjuna* bark also inhibited the growth of CaOx crystals. At the same time, the AE also modified the morphology of CaOx crystals from hexagonal to spherical shape with increasing concentrations of AE and reduced the dimensions such as area, perimeter, length and width of CaOx crystals in a dose dependent manner.

Mittal *et al.* [649] evaluated the antiurolithiatic properties of the Tris-Cl extract (TE) of *T. arjuna*. The antilithiatic activity of TE of *T. arjuna* was investigated on nucleation, aggregation, and growth of the CaOx crystals, as well as its protective potency was tested on oxalate-induced cell injury of NRK-52E renal epithelial cells. The TE of *T. arjuna* exhibited a concentration-dependent inhibition of nucleation and growth of CaOx crystals. When NRK-52E cells were injured by exposure to oxalate for 48 h, the TE prevented the cells from injury and CaOx crystal adherence resulting in increased cell viability in a dose-dependent manner.

Mittal *et al.* [650, 651] investigated the antiurolithiatic efficacy of aqueous extract of bark of *T. arjuna* on oxalate-induced injury to renal tubular epithelial cells. The results confirmed that oxalate injured MDCK cells were protected by *T. arjuna* extract. On treatment with a range concentrations, the cell viability increased in a concentration dependent manner. Moreover, the extract prevented the interaction of the CaOx crystals with the cell surface and reduced the number of apoptotic cells.

Terminalia bellirica Roxb. Family: Combretaceae

Upadhyay *et al.* [652] investigated the anti-urolithiatic effect of methanolic extract *Terminalia bellirica* (METB) fruits on ethylene glycol-induced renal stone in albino rats. MeTB significantly reduced the ethylene glycol induced disturbance in various physical and biochemical parameters in urine as well as in serum. MeTB prevented the depletion of GSH level and decrease in the level of SOD in ethylene glycol induced renal injury in rats.

Terminalia chebula Retz. Family: Combretaceae

Prasad *et al.* [653] reported the preventive effect of *Terminalia chebula* on nickel chloride ($NiCl_2$) induced renal oxidative stress, toxicity and cell proliferation response in male Wistar rats. Prophylactic treatment of rats with *T. chebula* daily for one week resulted in the diminution of $NiCl_2$ mediated damage as evident from the down regulation of GSH content, GST, GR, LPO, H_2O_2 generation, BUN, serum creatinine, DNA synthesis and ODC activity with concomitant restoration of GPx activity.

The antiurolithiatic property of aqueous extract of fruit of *T. chebula* in Wistar albino rats. The results indicate that ethylene glycol treatment decreases calcium level in urine and increased it in the kidney tissue homogenate, which were prevented in animal receiving simultaneous treatment of extract. Extract treatment decreased the elevated levels of oxalate and phosphate in urine as well as kidney tissue homogenate. The extract supplementation also prevented the elevation of serum levels creatinine, uric acid and BUN. Histopathological study revealed that extract reduced histological changes and retained the normal architecture of kidney tissue [654].

Tayal *et al.* [655] evaluated the antilithiatic properties of *T. chebula*. The antilithiatic activity of *T. chebula* was investigated on nucleation and growth of the CaOx crystals. The protective potency of the plant extract was also tested on oxalate induced cell injury of both NRK-52E and MDCK renal epithelial cells. The percentage inhibition of CaOx nucleation was found 95.84% at 25µg/mL of *T. chebula* aqueous extract which remained almost constant with the increasing concentration of the plant extract; however, plant extract inhibited CaOx crystal growth in a dose dependent pattern. When MDCK and NRK-52E cells were injured by exposure to oxalate for 48 hours, the aqueous extract prevented the injury in a dose-dependent manner. On treatment with the different concentrations of the plant extract, the cell viability increased and LDH release decreased in a concentration dependent manner

Terminalia muelleri Benth. Family: Combretaceae

Fahmy *et al.* [656] investigated the nephroprotective activity of polyphenol-rich fraction (TMEF) obtained from *Terminalia muelleri* against CCl_4-induced toxicity in mice. TMEF pretreatment significantly inhibited the CCl_4-induced renal MDA, creatinine, uric acid, urea and cholesterol. Furthermore, TMEF administration significantly increased GSH, SOD and protein levels at the tested doses of TMEF. Pretreatment with TMEF protected from ballooning degeneration, liver necrosis, renal inflammation, and degeneration of the kidney tubules.

Tetraclinis articulata (Vahl) Mast. Family: Cupressaceae

Beghalia *et al.* [193] investigated the effect of extracts of *T. articulata* on the CaOx crystals *in vitro*. With the addition of *T. articulata*, the best inhibitory concentrations 87.94% and 84.12% were encountered at the concentration of 100% and 50% respectively.

Thea sinensis L. [Syn.: *Camellia sinensis* (L.) Kuntze] Family: Theaceae

The effects of green tea (*Thea sinensis* Syn.: *Camellia sinensis*) tannin on nephrectomized rats were examined by Yokozawa *et al.* [657]. There were increases in BUN, serum creatinine, and urinary protein, and a decrease in creatinine clearance in the nephrectomized control rats, whereas better results for these parameters were obtained in rats given green tea tannin after nephrectomy, demonstrating a suppressed progression of the renal failure. When the renal parenchyma was partially resected, the remnant kidney showed a decrease in the activity of radical scavenger enzymes. Green tea tannin, however, was found to lighten the kidney under such oxidative stress. Mesangial proliferation and glomerular sclerotic lesions, which were conspicuous in the rats that were not given green tea tannin after nephrectomy, were also relieved.

A study was conducted by Yokozawa *et al.* [658] to clarify whether green tea tannin ameliorated cisplatin-induced renal injury in a renal epithelial cell line, swine-derived LLC-PK1 cells in culture. Green tea tannin was shown to suppress the cytotoxicity of cisplatin, the suppressive effect increasing with the dose of green tea tannin. The effect of cisplatin was then investigated in rats given green tea tannin for 40 days before cisplatin administration and in control rats given no green tea tannin. In control rats, blood, urinary and renal parameters and the activities of antioxidative enzymes in renal tissue deviated from the normal range, indicating dysfunction of the kidneys. In contrast, rats given green tea tannin showed decreased blood levels of urea nitrogen and creatinine, and decreased urinary levels of protein and glucose, reflecting less damage to the kidney. In this group, the activity of CAT in the renal tissue was increased, while the level of MDA was decreased, suggesting the involvement of radicals in the normalizing of kidney function. Based on the evidence available it appeared that green tea tannin eliminated oxidative stress and was beneficial to renal function.

El-Beshbishy [659] elucidated the antioxidant capacity of green tea extract (GTE) against Tamoxifen Citrate (TAM)-induced liver injury. The model of TAM-intoxication elicited significant declines in the antioxidant enzymes (GST, GPx, SOD and CAT) and reduced GSH concomitant with significant elevations in TBARS (thiobarbituric acid reactive substance) and liver transaminases; sGPT (serum glutamate pyruvate transaminase) and sGOT (serum glutamate oxaloacetate transaminase) levels. The oral administration of 1.5% GTE to TAM-intoxicated rats, produced significant increments in the antioxidant enzymes and reduced GSH concomitant with significant decrements in TBARS and liver transaminases levels.

Green tea extract was administered orally by Leena and Balaram [660] to rats to investigate its effect on cisplatin (3mg/kg) induced nephrotoxicity. Green tea extract restored the level of creatinine, urea, BUN and uric acid in serum of animals treated with cisplatin as compared to the animals treated with cisplatin alone. It was further found that administration of green tea extract restored the level of antioxidant enzymes such as, SOD, CAT and reduced GSH, and membrane bound enzymes like Na^+ K^+ ATPase, Ca^{2+} ATPase and Mg^{2+} ATPase and decreased lipid peroxidation (MDA) in kidney of animals which were altered after chronic treatment with cisplatin.

Jeong *et al*. [661] evaluated whether epigallocatechin gallate (EGCG), a main constituent of green tea polyphenols, could protect against cellular toxicity by oxalate and whether green tea supplementation attenuates the development of nephrolithiasis in an animal model and Cells of the NRK-52E line. The administration of EGCG inhibited free-radical production induced by oxalate. Green tea supplementation decreased the excretion of urinary oxalate and the activities of urinary gammaglutamyltranspeptidase and N-acetylglucosaminidase. The number of crystals within kidneys in treated group was significantly lower than in untreated group.

Khan *et al*. [662] evaluated the protective effect of green tea (GT) in GM-induced nephrotoxicity in male Wistar rats. GT given to GM rats reduced nephrotoxicity parameters, enhanced antioxidant defence and energy metabolism. The activity of BBM enzymes and transport of Pi declined by GM whereas GT enhanced BBM enzymes and Pi transport.

Khan *et al*. [663] has undertaken a study to see whether green tea (GT) can prevent cisplatin(CP)-induced nephrotoxic and other deleterious effects. GT consumption increased the activities of the enzymes of carbohydrate metabolism, brush border membrane, oxidative stress, and ^{32}Pi transport. GT ameliorated CP-induced nephrotoxic and other deleterious effects due to its intrinsic biochemical/antioxidant properties.

Abdel-Raheem *et al.* [664] investigated the possible protective effect of GTE against GM-induced nephrotoxicity. The simultaneous administration of GTE plus GM protected kidney tissues against nephrotoxic effect of GM as evidenced from amelioration of histopathological alterations and normalization of kidney biochemical parameters.

Ahn *et al.* [665] compared the effects of green tea polyphenol (GTP) pre-treatment with those of GTP post-treatment on cisplatin (CP)-induced nephrotoxicity in rat. Pretreatment with GTP resulted in markedly reduced elevation of serum creatinine and BUN amounts and changes of GGT and AP activity in kidney induced by CP. CP-induced histopathological changes, including tubular necrosis and dilation, were ameliorated in GTP pre-treated rats, compared to CP alone or GTP post-treated rats.

Thespesia populnea (L.) Sol. ex Correa Family: Malvaceae

Mika and Guruvayoorappan [666] investigated the effect of *Thespesia populnea* on Cisplatin induced Nephrotoxicity. Administration of cisplatin resulted in significant increase in the levels of serum urea creatinine, ALT, AST and bilirubin as compared to normal animals. On the other hand, introduction of *T. populnea* extract caused a significant reduction in the levels of serum markers namely urea, creatinine, ALT, AST and bilirubin. Increase in the levels of urea and creatinine in serum as well as ALT, AST and bilirubin is suggestive of both kidney and liver damage. *T. populnea* extract ameliorated cisplatin induced kidney and liver damage as indicated by reduction in the levels of serum urea, creatinine, AST, ALT and bilirubin.

Tinospora cordifolia (Willd.) Miers ex Hook. f. & Thoms. Family: Menispermaceae

The role of *Tinospora cordifolia* stem extract was investigated by Khanam *et al.* [667] for its curative effect in male wistar rats against the cisplatin-induced nephrotoxicity. Oral administration of plant extract cured the cisplatin induced kidney damage. Administration of cisplatin followed by alcoholic extract of *T. cordifolia* decreased the increased levels of serum creatinine, BUN and alkaline phosphatase in rats. These biochemical observations were supplemented by histopathological examination of kidney section.

Uppuluri *et al.* [668] investigated the protective role of the *Tinospora cordifolia* root ethanol extract against cisplatin induced nephrotoxicity in albino rats. In curative regimen, the extract significantly reduced the elevated serum creatinine and urea levels. Renal antioxidant defense systems, such as SOD, CAT, GPx activities and reduced GSH level, depleted by cisplatin therapy were restored to normal by treatment with the extract.

Sharma *et al.* [669] investigated the protector effect of aqueous extract of *T. cordifolia* against GM induced nephrotoxicity in albino rats. *T. cordifolia* pre-treated groups exhibited significant limitation in rise in levels of BUN and serum creatinine in a dose dependent manner. Histolopathological observations further corroborated the biochemical findings.

Trachyspermum ammi (L.) Sprague Family: Apiaceae

The antilithiatic activity of *Trachyspermum ammi* anticalcifying protein (TAP) was studied by Kaur *et al.* [670] in urolithiatic rat model. The antilithiatic potential of TAP was confirmed by its ability to maintain renal functioning, reduce renal injury and decrease crystal excretion in urine and retention in renal tissues.

Kaur *et al.* [671] examined the efficacy of *T. ammi* on CaOx crystallization *in vitro*. An anticalcifying protein from the seeds of *T. ammi* was purified by three step purification scheme based on its ability to inhibit CaOx crystallization *in vitro*. Amino acid analysis of *T. ammi* anticalcifying protein (TAP) showed abundant presence of acidic amino acids (Asp and Glu). Due to a significant similarity of TAP with unnamed protein product of *V. vinifera*, presence of two EF hand domains in TAP was anticipated, signifying its calcium binding properties which is a feature of most kidney stone inhibitory proteins.

Tragia involucrata L. Family: Euphorbiaceae

Palani *et al.* [672] investigated the protective and antioxidant activities of ethanol extract of *Tragia involucrata* (TI) on acetaminophen (APAP) induced toxicity in male albino rats. TI inhibited the hematological effects of APAP. TI significantly increased activities of renal SOD, CAT, GSH, and GPx and decreased MDA content of APAP-treated rats. Apart from these, histopathological changes also showed the protective nature of the TI extract against APAP induced necrotic damage of renal tissues.

Trema guineensis (Schum. & Thonn.) Ficalho Family: Ulmaceae

Cyril *et al.* [673] investigated the potential nephroprotective activity of aqueous and hydroethanolic extracts of *Trema guineensis* leaves in rat. *T.guineensis* aqueous and hydroethanolic extracts used to treat animals suffering from nephrotoxicity would have significantly reduced biochemical parameters considered as markers of nephrotoxicity. Moreover, the aqueous extract and vitamin E restored the toxic effect of GM into equal significance.

Trianthema portulacastrum L. Family: Aizoaceae

Balamurugan *et al.* [674] evaluated the protective effect of ethanolic extract of *Trianthema portulacastrum* leaves in GM-induced renal damage in rats. i.p administration of ethanolic extract of *T. portulacastrum* restored the levels of the biochemical factors determined significantly and exhibited a significant potential to scavenge free radicals with respect to control.

Sree lakshmi *et al.* [348] evaluated the effect of ethanolic extract of leaves of *T. portulacastrum* (EETP) on experimentally induced urolithiasis. Treatment with ethanolic extract of *T. portulacastrum* at both the doses (200 mg/kg and 400 mg/kg b.wt) showed a significant restoration of urinary and serum parameters on EG&AC induction. The extracts at both doses showed significant increase in antioxidant enzymes activity and decrease in MDA levels.

Tribulus terrestris L. Family: Zygophyllaceae

The ethanol extract of *Tribulus terrestris* (fruit) was evaluated by Anand *et al.* [675] for activity against artificially induced urolithiasis in albino rats. The extract exhibited dose-dependent antiurolithiatic activity and almost completely inhibited stone formation. Other biochemical parameters in urine and serum, and the histopathology of urinary bladder, which were altered during the process of stone formation, were also normalized by the plant extract in a dose-dependent manner.

An ethanolic extract of the fruits of *T. terrestris* showed significant dose dependent protection against uroliths induced by glass bead implantation in albino rats [676]. On subsequent fractionation of the ethanol extract, maximum activity was localised in the 10% aqueous methanol fraction. It provided significant protection against deposition of calculogenic material around the glass bead. It also protected leucocytosis and elevation in serum urea levels. Further, fractionation leads to decreased activity. This could be either due to loss of active compounds during fractionation, or the antiurolithiatic activity of *T. terrestris* being a combined effect of several constituents present in the methanolic fraction.

The effect of an aqueous extract of *T. terrestris* on the metabolism of oxalate in male rats fed sodium glycolate was investigated by Sangeeta *et al.* [677]. The supplementation of *T. terrestris* with sodium glycolate caused a reduction in liver GAO and GAD activities, whereas liver LDH activity remained unaltered. The isoenzyme pattern of kidney LDH revealed that normalization of kidney LDH by

T. terrestris feeding was mainly due to an increase in the LDH 5 fraction.

T. terrestris possess protective effect against the GM induced nephrotoxicity in both structural and functional terms [678]. Abdel-Kader *et al.* [679] evaluated the nephroprotective activities of the ethanolic plant extract and petroleum ether, dichloromethane and aqueous methanol fractions against CCl_4 induced toxicity in adult Wistar rats. Effect of the total 95% ethanol extract at 400 mg/kg on kidney was promising. The best effect was observed on the urea and creatinine levels. Both MDA and non-protein sulfhydryl groups in kidney tissues were improved to levels comparable with those obtained by silymarin.

Al-Ali *et al.* [680] studied the aqueous extract of the leaves and fruits of *T. terrestris* and the hair of *Z. mays*, to determine their diuretic activity of *T. terrestris*. The aqueous extract of *T. terrestris*, in oral dose of 5g/kg elicited a positive diuresis, which was slightly more than that of furosemide. *Z. mays* aqueous extract did not result in significant diuresis when given alone in oral dose of 5g/kg, while combination of *Z. mays* and *T. terrestris* extracts produced the same extent of diuresis as that produced by *T. terrestris* alone. Na(+), K(+) and Cl(+) concentrations in the urine had also much increased.

Joshi *et al.* [681] reported that herbal extracts of *T. terrestris* inhibit growth of CaOx monohydrate crystals *in vitro*. Aggarwal *et al.* [682] evaluated the antilithiatic properties of *T. terrestris*. *T. terrestris* extract exhibited a concentration dependent inhibition of nucleation and the growth of CaOx crystals. When NRK-52E cells were injured by exposure to oxalate for 72 h, *T. terrestris* extract prevented the injury in a dose-dependent manner. On treatment with the different concentrations of the plant, the cell viability increased and LDH release decreased in a concentration dependent manner. The data suggests that *T. terrestris* extract not only has a potential to inhibit nucleation and the growth of the CaOx crystals but also has a cytoprotective role.

Arasaratnam *et al.* [683] determined the effect of *T. terrestis* extract on urinary risk factors in normal subjects and urolithic patients. In urolithic patients the mean serum calcium level increased significantly and the mean urinary calcium level decreased significantly after treatment for one week with *T. terrestris* extract. The mean uric acid level of the urolithic patients decreased significantly in serum and urine after treatment with *T. terrestris* extract. The mean citrate, oxalate, proteins and glycosaminoglycan levels decreased significantly in urine samples of the urolithic patients after treatment with the extract.

Pachana *et al.* [684] studied the crystallization of CaOx by the precipitation of calcium chloride and sodium oxalate in the absence and presence of small caltrops (*T. terrestris*). The effects of small caltrops concentration on CaOx crystal forms and morphologies were investigated. The results showed that small caltrops affected the crystal morphologies that were mainly hexagonal, octahedral, and dendritic. Higher small caltrops concentration raised the formation of CaOx dihydrate (COD) crystals in an octahedral shape.

Kulkarni *et al.* [144] evaluated the nephroprotective and anti-nephro-toxic properties of roots of *T. trrestris* by using GM induced nephrotoxic model in Wistar strain albino rats. The drug has shown only nephroprotective activity.

Raoofi *et al.* [685] investigated the influence of hydroalcoholic extract of *T. terrestris* plant on cisplatin (CIS) induced renal tissue damage in male mice. The altered parameters reached to the normal range after administration of fruit extracts of *T.terrestris* for 4 days.

Meher *et al.* [249] investigated the renal protective effect of aqueous extract of *T. terrestris*. Aqueous extract of fruit showed protection to kidney against GM-induced renal injury in rats. The water extract of *T. terrestris* was cytoprotective towards NRF52E (normal rat kidney epithelial cells) [686] with prophylactic and curative effect *in vivo* [687, 688] confirming the protective effect on the renal epithelial cells by the aqueous extract. n-butanol extract of *T. terrestris* was the most potent fraction *in vitro*.

The preventive and curative urolithiatic efficacy in experimentally induced nephrolithiatic Wistar rats was evaluated by Kaushik *et al.* [689, 690] following oral administration of aqueous extract of *T. terrestris*. Treatment showed augmented renal function, restoration of normal renal architecture and increase in body weight. Microscopic analysis of urine revealed excretion of small sized urinary crystals, demonstrating that treatment potentially modulated the morphology of renal stones. Tissue enzymatic estimation affirmed the antioxidant efficacy of treatment with reduced free radical generation. Significant upregulation of p38MAPK at both the gene and protein level was noted in hyperoxaluric group and interestingly treatment reversed it.

Trichosanthes dioica Roxb. Family: Cucurbutaceae

Chaudhury and Paranjpe [691] reported nephroprotective effect of *Trichosanthes dioica*. Solomon *et al.* [692] evaluated the protective effect of *T. dioica* extract against GM-induced nephrotoxicity in rats. Kidney weight was determined and estimation of BUN, serum creatinine, uric acid, CAT, SOD, GPx, lipid peroxidation, urinary electrolytes was performed. Decrement in serum urea and creatinine along with reduction in uric acid was observed. Similarly, restoration of antioxidant enzymes and normalization of urinary electrolytes and kidney weight was observed.

Gupta *et al.* [693] evaluated the protective potential of *T. dioica* leaves extract (TLE) against GM induced nephrotoxicity and renal dysfunction. TLE 200 and 400 mg/kg treatment to GM treated rats recorded significant decrements in plasma and urine urea and creatinine, urinary Na+ and K+ level, renal lipid peroxidation along with significant increment in renal enzymatic and non-enzymatic antioxidants. Histological observations of kidney tissues too correlated with the biochemical observations.

Trigonella foenum-graecum L. Family: Fabaceae

Ahsan *et al.* [84] investigated the effect of *Trigonella foenum-graecum* seeds on experimentally-induced kidney stones. Daily oral treatment with *T. foenum-graecum* significantly decreased the quantity of CaOx deposited in the kidney.

Laroubi *et al.* [695] evaluated the protective effect of *T. foenum-graecum* (Tfg) on nephrolithiasic rats. The results showed that the amount of calcification in the kidneys and the total calcium amount of the renal tissue in rats treated with Tfg were significantly reduced compared with the untreated group.

The therapeutic efficacy of fenugreek seed extract with trigonelline as marker (SFSE-T) was evaluated in experimental urolithiasis in rats. Subacute oral treatment of SFSE-T (60 mg/kg) showed reversal of EG+AC induced changes in urine (decreased 24-h urine output, pH, excretion of creatinine, citrate, and chloride and increased uric acid and oxalate excretion) and serum (increased creatine, uric acid and BUN) parameters and decreased creatine clearance. Histopathology examination of the kidneys sections from SFSE-T (60 mg/kg) treated rats showed lowered number of crystals, cell damage and tubulointerstitial damage index as compared with EG+AC control rats [696].

Shekha *et al.* [697] investigated the effect of *T. foenum-graecum* on the prevention of renal calculi formation. Ethylene glycol group led to increases in kidney weight, MDA and platelet count, while cystone and fenugreek combat the effect of EG. Haematological examination showed that the hemoglobin and red blood cell count in rats treated EG were significantly lower than those in the controls while Fenugreek and Cystone decreased the EG effect.

The beneficial influence of dietary fenugreek seeds and onion (*Allium cepa*) on nephrotoxicity was evaluated by Pradeep and Srinivasan [698] in streptozotocin-induced diabetic rats. Dietary interventions were made with 10% fenugreek seeds or 3% onion (freeze-dried) or their combination for 6 weeks. Animals maintained on these dietary interventions countered nephromegaly, increase in creatinine clearance and oxidative stress in renal tissue. These dietary interventions significantly countered the increased renal cholesterol and triglycerides in diabetic condition. The up-regulation of the receptor for advanced glycation end products, inflammatory cytokines and oxidative stress markers in the renal tissue of diabetic rats was effectively countered. Renal 8-hydroxy-2-deoxyguanosine, its excretion, DNA fragmentation and mitochondrial DNA deletion were significantly annulled in diabetic rats by these dietary interventions. Generally, the beneficial effect was more in the combined intervention although not additive.

Pathan *et al.* [699] suggested that ethanolic extract of *Coleus barbatus* and *T. foenum-graecum* roots and their combination have positive effect on urolithiasis.

Hilmi *et al.* [700, 701] compared the ameliorative effect of silymarin with ethanol extract of *T. foenum-graecum* in an experimental model of GM- induced nephrotoxic rats. Biochemical indices like serum creatinine and serum urea levels were estimated to determine nephrotoxicity and amelioration of nephrotoxicity in all rat groups. Significant amelioration was observed in all the biochemical parameters in *T. foenum-graecum* and silymarin treated groups. The ameliorating effect of *T. foenum-graecum* is much more effective in comparison to that of silymarin in nephrotoxicity.

Uraria picta (Jacq.) DC. Family: Fabaceae

Kale *et al.* [702] evaluated the protective activity of water extract of *Uraria picta* on acetaminophen induced nephrotoxicity in Wistar albino rats. Treatment with the aqueous extract of *U. picta* significantly reduced the elevated levels of urine urea and BUN levels and also elevated levels of serum creatine and urine creatine compared to acetaminophen group.

Urtica dioica L. Family: Urticaceae

Methanolic extract of aerial parts of *Urtica dioica* was screened by Zhang *et al.* [703] for antiurolithiatic activity against ethylene glycol and ammonium chloride-induced CaOx renal stones in male rats. Treatment with the methanolic extract of *U. dioica* was found to decrease the elevated levels of urinary calcium, oxalate and creatinine, and significantly decrease the renal deposition of calcium and oxalate. Furthermore, renal histological observations revealed a significant reduction in CaOx crystal deposition in the test rats.

Vaccinium macrocarpon Aiton Family: Vacciniaceae

Influence of Cranberry juice on the urinary risk factors for CaOx renal calculi formation was investigated by McHarg *et al.* [704]. Urinary variables were assessed in a randomized cross-over trial in 20 South African men (students) with no previous history of kidney stones. The ingestion of cranberry juice significantly and uniquely altered three key urinary risk factors. Oxalate and phosphate excretion decreased while citrate excretion increased. In addition, there was a decrease in the relative supersaturation of CaOx, which tended to be significantly lower than that induced by water alone.

Kesseler *et al.* [562] evaluated the influence of cranberry (*Vaccinium macrocarpon*) juice on urinary stone risk factors. Investigations were carried out in 12 healthy male subjects aged 18-38 y. Cranberry juice decreased the urinary pH, whereas the excretion of oxalic acid and the relative supersaturation for uric acid were increased. Since cranberry juice acidifies urine it could be useful in the treatment of brushite and struvite stones as well as urinary tract infection.

Vaccinium myrtillus L. Family: Vacciniaceae

Pandir and Kara [705] investigated the effect of bilberry (*Vaccinium myrtillus*) on cisplatin-induced toxic effects in rat kidney. SOD, CAT, and GPx activities were decreased and MDA levels were increased in the cisplatin group compared to the cisplatin + bilberry group, and the differences were statistically significant. Kidney tissue damage was significantly higher in untreated group than in treated group.

Valeriana wallichii DC. Family: Valerianaceae

Ullah *et al.* [706] evaluated the nephroprotective effect of *Valeriana wallichii* against GM-induced nephrotoxicity. It was concluded from the findings that *V. wallichii* failed to deliver protective effects against GM-induced renal damage in spite of strong flavonoid contents and antioxidant properties.

Vepris heterophylla (Engl.) R. Let. Family: Rutaceae

Ntchapda *et al.* [707] assessed the diuretic properties of *Vepris heterophylla* leaves water extract. The findings indicated that the aqueous extract of *V. heterophylla* at doses ranging from 150 to 250 mg/kg caused a significant and dose-dependent increase of urinary water and electrolytes excretion in normal rats. The aqueous extract of the leaves of *V. heterophylla* accelerated the elimination of overloaded fluid. At the maximum of diuretic response, urinary osmolarity decreased significantly when compared with controls. Oral administration of aqueous extract at different doses produced a significant diuresis and slight increase in electrolytes excretion.

Verbena officinalis L. Family: Verbenaceae

Grases *et al.* [96] evaluated the effects of *Verbena officinalis* to prevent and treat renal calculi formation in female Wistar rats. The infusion does not affect calciuria and citraturia values, they do not diminish calcinuria or increase the crystallization inhibitory capacity of the urine. It can be concluded that beneficial effects caused by these herb infusions on urolithiasis can be attributed to some disinfectant action, and tentatively to the presence of saponins.

Vernonia amygdalina Delile Family: Asteraceae

Imafidon *et al.* [708] determined the effects of polyphenol-rich extract of the leaves of *Vernonia amygdalina* (PEVA) in rats with Cd-induced nephropathy. With marked improvements in renal histoarchitecture, PEVA treatment showed a duration and non dose-dependent ameliorative potential.

Komolafe *et al.* [205] evaluated the effect of *V. amygdalina* extract on the histomorphometry of the kidney in STZ induced diabetic rats. The histology and morphometric analysis revealed that the kidney in the group treated with *V. amygdalina* showed no significant increase in density compared to control.

Vernonia cinerea Less. Family: Asteraceae

Sreedevi *et al.* [709] examined the effect of petroleum ether, ethyl acetate and alcoholic extracts of aerial parts of *Vernonia cinerea* on cisplatin-induced nephrotoxicity in albino rats. Among the three extracts, alcoholic extract showed pronounced curative activity, ethyl acetate extract exhibited good prophylactic activity and petroleum ether extract showed moderate protection in both curative and prophylactic models against cisplatin-induced toxicity.

Hiremath and Jalalpure [710] evaluated the antiurolithiatic potential of whole plant hydro-alcoholic (30:70) extract of *V. cinerea*. Treatment with hydro-alcoholic extract of *V. cinerea* showed significant dose-dependent activity. A progressive increase in urine output, body weight, and decline in concentrations of stone-forming components such as calcium, oxalates, and phosphates was observed.

Viburnum opulus L. Family: Adoxaceae

Ilhan *et al.* [711] evaluated the antiurolithiatic effect of the various extracts prepared from the fruits of *Viburnum opulus*. Lyophilized juice of *V. opulus* (LJVO) and lyophilized commercial juice of *V. opulus* (LCJVO) exerted potential antiurolithiatic activity which was attributed to its diuretic effect along with the inhibitory action on the oxalate levels and free radical production.

Vigna mungo (L.) Hepper Family: Fabaceae

Nitin *et al.* [712] investigated the nephroprotective activity of aqueous extract of seeds of *Vigna mungo* (AEVM) against rifampicin-induced kidney damage in rats. Pretreatment with AEVM significantly prevented the physical, biochemical, and histological changes induced by rifampicin in the kidney.

Vitex negundo L. Family: Verbenaceae

Nephroprotective activity of extracts of *Vitex negundo* roots was investigated by Mishra *et al*. [111] against GM-induced acute nephrotoxicity in Wistar rats. The extracts of root significantly attenuated the nephrotoxicity by elevation of body weight, CAT, GPx and SOD or lowcring urine LDH and creatinine, serum urea; serum creatinine and LPO respectively.

Vitis vinifera L. Family: Vitaceae

The protection conferred by grape seed extract against GM-induced nephrotoxicity has been evaluated by El-Ashmawy *et al*. [713] in adult Swiss albino mice. Pretreatment with grape seed extract (7 days) and simultaneously (14 days) with GM significantly protected the kidney tissue by ameliorating its antioxidant activity.

Safa *et al*. [714] determined the protective effect of red grape seed extract (RGSE) on GM-induced nephrotoxicity in rats. On day 68, serum creatinine and BUN concentrations were highest in group 3, which was significantly higher than in group 1, while slightly higher than in group 2. Fractional excretion of sodium was not significantly different between the three groups. Histopathological evaluation showed that rats in group 3 had significantly higher degrees of severe acute tubular necrosis and interstitial mononuclear cell infiltration than the rats in groups 1 and 2.

Bhargavi *et al*. [715] investigated the protective activity of methanolic extract of seeds of *V. vinifera* (MEVV) against rifampicin induced and CCl_4 induced kidney damage in male albino Wistar rats. Pretreatment with MEVV and standard drug cystone significantly prevented the physical, biochemical and histological changes produced by rifampicin and carbon tetrachloride toxicity.

Withania coagulans (Stocks) Dunal Family: Solanaceae

Sharma *et al*. [716] explored the nephroprotective effect of *Withania coagulans* fruit extract and its modulatory effects against cisplatin-induced nephrotoxicity. Withaferin A was found 3.56 mg/g of *W. coagulans* fruit extract. It significantly prevented the rise in serum urea and creatinine level and also preserved rat kidneys from oxidative stress and free radical induced DNA damage. Histopathological study showed extract treatment eliminates tubular swelling, cellular necrosis, and protein cast deposition in cisplatin treated kidney tissue. It averted the decline in GSH content, activities of SOD and CAT. These parameters were restored to near normal levels by extract in a dose of 400 mg/kg, per oral.

Withania somnifera (L.) Dunal Family: Solanaceae

Panda *et al.* [717] evaluated the nephroprotective activity of *Withania somnifera* in cadmium-induced heptotoxicity in male mouse. A significant increase in the LPO in kiney tissues was found following the cadmium treatment. Both cadmium and *W. sonifera*-treated mice showed decrease in in LPO in the tissue homogenate when compared with that of mice treated with cadmium only. A significant decrease in SOD and CAT activities after cadmium administration and nearly normal values were obtained when *W. somnifera* was administered along with cadmium.

Jeyanthi and Subramanian [718] investigated the protective effect of *W. somnifera* on GN-induced nephrotoxicity. *W. somnifera* significantly reversed the changes as evidenced microscopically and there were no significant changes in the levels of sodium in the experimental animals compared to control.

Jeyanthi and Subramanian [719] investigated the protective effect of *Withania somnifera* root powder on GN induced nephrotoxicity in male Wistar rats. *W. somnifera* treatment altered the antioxidant status and significantly reversed the levels as seen microscopically. The results showed that the root powder of *W. somnifera* with the presence of natural antioxidants, bioflavanoids, and other bioactive compounds scavenged the free radicals generated by GN and ameliorated the severity of GN-induced nephrotoxicity by enhancing the antioxidant system and protecting the cellular integrity of kidney and liver tissues.

Sharma *et al.* [720] assessed the efficacy of *W. somnifera* in reducing lead-induced changes in mice kidney. The influences of lead were prevented partially by concurrent daily administration of WS root extract. Histological examination of kidney also revealed patho-physiological changes in lead nitrate exposed group and treatment with WS improved renal histopathology.

Shimmi *et al.* [721] evaluated the protector activity of *W. somnifera* root against GM-induced nephrotoxicity in male Wistar albnino rats. 92.3% of rats in *W. sominfera* pretreated and GM-treated group showed almost normal structure and 7.69% showed mild histological changes.

Kushwaha *et al.* [722] evaluated the curative activity of *W. somnifera* on GM-induced nephrotoxicity in rats. BUN and serum creatinine values were significantly low as compared to GT group in all test duration in phase-1. In phase two there was no significant difference of these markers in two groups.

Govindappa *et al.* [723] evaluated the *in vivo* nephroprotective and nephrocurative function of *W. somnifera* in GM-induced nephrotoxic Wistar rats. *W. somnifera* significantly restored the renal function on GM-induced nephrotoxicity. This phenomenon was accompanied with significantly reduced BUN, creatine, alkaline phosphatase, gamma-glutamyltransferase, albumin, total protein, calcium, potassium and kidney MDA concentrations. Additionally, *W. somnifera* significantly increased antioxidant activities of GSH and SOD to protect renal tissue damage from GM in wistar rats.

Zea mays L. Family: Poaceae

The effects on the CaOx urolithiasis urinary risk factors of *Zea mays (stigmata maydis)*, in herb infusion form, combined with different diets have been studied by Grases *et al.* [724] using male Wistar rats. From the reported study, the possible antilithiasic effects of *Z.mays* infusion can be exclusively assigned to some diuretic activity. Thus, no influence on important urinary risk factors such as citraturia, calciuria or urinary pH values was detected. It is interesting to emphasize that the diuretic effect of the herb infusion was clearly dependent on the diet and was maximum when the rats were fed with the standard one.

Rathod *et al.* [725] proved aqueous extracts of corn silk of *Z. mays* executed on generated CaOx crystals by homogenous precipitation method for *in-vitro* anti-lithiatic activity. The aqueous extract of corn silk of *Z. mays* has shown significant activity on comparison to the synthetic drug Spironolactone, furosemide and poly-herbal formulation Cystone. Corn silk was playing an important physical role in treatment by increasing the contraction of smooth muscles which led to increase the urinary output and increased the percentage the passage of urinary stones through the urinary tracts.

Antiurolithic activity of corn silk was also investigated by Talekar *et al.* [726] in animal models. The histopathological studies and X-rays showed significant data to confirm the efficacy of corn silk in urolithiasis.

Sabiu *et al.* [727] evaluated the protective effect of ethyl acetate fraction of *Z.mays*, *Stigma maydis* in acetaminophen-induced oxidative onslaughts in the kidneys of Wistar rats. The acetaminophen-mediated significant elevations in the serum concentrations of creatinine, urea, uric acid, sodium, potassium, and tissue levels of oxidized GSH, protein-oxidized products, lipid peroxidized products, and fragmented DNA were dose-dependently assuaged in the fraction-treated animals. The fraction also markedly improved creatinine clearance rate, GSH, and calcium concentrations as well as activities of SOD, CAT, GR, and GPx in the nephrotoxic rats. The observed effects compared favorably with that of vitamin C and are informative of the fraction's ability to prevent progression of renal pathological conditions and preserve kidney functions as evidently supported by the histological analysis..

Okokon *et al.* [728] evaluated the renoprotective potentials of *Z. mays* against alloxan-induced injuries in diabetic rats. The husk extract and fractions caused significant increases in the levels of oxidative stress markers (SOD, CAT, GPx, GSH) in the kidney and MDA level was decreased in the treated diabetic rats. The extract and fractions caused significant reduction of elevated serum levels of creatinine, urea and chloride in the diabetic rats. The extract/fractions caused increases in WBC, PCV, monocyte, neutrophil, platelet and eosinophil counts without affecting other parameters. Histology of kidney revealed absence or significant reductions in pathological features in the treated diabetic rats compared to untreated diabetic rats.

Okokon *et al.* [729] evaluated the nephroprotective property of cornhusk extract against gentimicin-induced kidney injuries to ascertain the folkloric claim of its usefulness in the treatment of poisoning. Administration of the husk extract (187-748 mg/kg) caused significant reduction of high levels of serum creatinine, urea and electrolytes concentrations (K+, Na+, Cl and HCO_3) caused by the toxicants. The effects were dose-dependent in most cases. The chemical pathological changes were consistent with histopathological observations suggesting marked nephroprotective potentials.

Zingiber officinale Roscoe Family: Zingiberaceae

The nephroprotective effects of ethanol extract of *Zingiber officinale* alone and in combination with vitamin E were evaluated by Ajith *et al.* [730] using induced nephrotoxicity in mice. The results of the study indicated that *Z. officinale* significantly and dose dependently protected the nephrotoxicity induced by cisplatin. The serum urea and creatinine levels in the cisplatin alone treated group were significantly elevated with respect to normal group of animals. The levels were reduced in the *Z. officinale* plus cisplatin, vitamin E plus cisplatin, and *Z. officinale* with vitamin E plus vitamin E treated groups. The activities of SOD, CAT GPx and level of GSH were elevated and level of MDA declined the *Z. officinale* plus cisplatin and *Z. officinale* with vitamin E plus cisplatin treated groups significantly. The protective effect of *Z. officinale* was found to be better than that of vitamin E. The results also demonstrated that the combination of *Z. officinale* with vitamin E showed better protection compared to their alone treated groups.

The nephroprotective effect of aqueous ethanol extract of *Z. officinale* was evaluated by Ajith *et al.* [731] against doxorubicin-induced acute renal damage in rat. Serum urea and creatinine levels were reduced in the *Z. officinale* plus DXN treated groups. The renal antioxidant enzymes activities such as SOD, CAT GPx, levels of GSH and GST activity were restored and that of MDA declined significantly in the *Z. officinale* plus DXN treated group. The nephroprotection is mediated by preventing the DXN-induced decline of renal antioxidant status, and also by increasing the activity of GST.

Uz *et al.* [732] analyzed the protective effect of dietary ginger (*Zingiber officinals*), on renal I/R injury in rats. Serum urea, creatinine, and cystatin C (CYC) levels were significantly elevated in the ischemia group, but these levels remained unchanged in the ginger + I/R group compared to the I/R group. Reduction of GPx and SOD enzyme activity was significantly improved by the treatment with ginger compared to I/R group. Administration of ginger resulted in significant reduction levels of tissue MDA, NO, protein carbonyl contents (PCC) in the ginger + I/R group compared with the I/R group. Ginger supplementation in the diet before I/R injury resulted in higher total antioxidant capacity (TAC) and lower total oxidant status (TOS) levels than I/R group. The ginger supplemented diet prior to I/R process demonstrated marked reduction of the histological features of renal injury.

Lakshmi and Sudhakar [733] evaluated the nephroprotective effect of ethyl acetate extract of rhizome of *Z.officinale* in Wistar rats. GM-induced glomerular congestion, peritubular and blood vessel congestion, epithelial desquamation, accumulation of inflammatory cells and necrosis of kidney cells were found to be reduced in the groups receiving the ethylacetate and dried fresh juice extract of *Z. officinale* along with GM. The extracts also normalized the GM-induced increase in serum-creatine, serum uric acid, BUN and serum urea levels. This is also evidenced by the histopathological studies.

Protective effect of ginger against alcohol-induced renal damage and antioxidant enzymes in male albino rats was investigated by Shanmugam *et al.* [734]. The altered parameters came to normalcy with treatment with ethanolic extract of ginger. The biochemical findings were supplemented by histopathological examination of the kidney. Severe congestion and degenerative changes in tubules in alcohol treated rats were restored by ginger extract treatment.

Ramudu *et al.* [735] evaluated the nephro-protective effect of ginger against chronic alcohol-induced oxidative stress and tissue damage. Ginger extract supplementation to the rats reversed the effects and attained the antioxidant status to normal levels. Furthermore, degenerative changes in renal cells with alcohol treatment were minimized to nearness in architecture by ginger supplementation.

Ramudu *et al.* [736] investigated the effect of ginger administration on altered blood glucose levels, intra- and extra-mitochondrial enzymes and tissue injuries in streptozotocin (STZ)-induced diabetic rats. Authors found highly elevated blood glucose levels in the diabetic group, and the glucose levels were significantly lowered by ginger administration. Activities of intra- and extra-mitochondrial enzymes were significantly decreased in the kidneys of the diabetic rats, while this was significantly reversed by 30 days of ginger treatment. They also observed consistent renal tissue damages in the diabetic rats; however, these injuries recovered in the ginger-treated diabetic rats as shown in histopathological studies.

Hamed *et al.* [737] evaluated the potential of successive ginger extracts (petroleum ether, chloroform, and ethanol) against nephrotoxicity induced by CCl_4 in rats. Treatment with ginger extracts resulted in markedly decreased levels of LPO, PGE(2), collagen and kidney function tests, while increased levels of GSH, SOD and serum protein were observed. Extracts of ginger, particularly the ethanol, resulted in an attractive candidate for the treatment of nephropathy induced by CCl_4 through scavenging free radicals, improved kidney functions, inhibition of inflammatory mediators, and normalizing the kidney histopathological architecture.

Nasri *et al.* [738] evaluated the curative and protective effects of *Z. officinale* (ginger) against GM tubular toxicity in rats. Ginger could prevent degeneration of the renal cells and reduce the severity of tubular damage caused by GM. However, it could not regenerate the GM degeneration. The results indicate that ginger is effective as a prophylaxis agent, but has not curative effect.

The potential protective effect of ginger *(Z. officinale)* rhizome extract on hyperglycemia-induced oxidative stress, inflammation and apoptosis was investigated by Al Hroob *et al.* [739]. Treatment with *Z. officinale* ameliorated hyperglycemia, hyperlipidemia and kidney function. In addition, *Z. officinale* minimized the histological alterations in the kidney of diabetic rats. *Z. officinale* extract significantly attenuated oxidative stress, inflammation and apoptosis, and enhanced antioxidant defenses in the diabetic kidney.

Zingiber zerumbet (L.) Roscoe ex Sm. Family: Zingiberaceae

The effects of ethyl acetate extract of *Zingiber zerumbet* rhizome on PCM-induced nephrotoxicity were examined by Hamid *et al.* [740]. Treatment with *Z. zerumbet* extract at doses of 200 and 400 mg/kg prevented the PCM-induced nephrotoxicity and oxidative impairments of the kidney, as evidenced by a significantly reduced level of plasma creatinine, plasma and renal MDA, plasma protein carbonyl, and renal advanced oxidation protein product (AOPP). Furthermore, both doses were also able to induce a significant increment of plasma and renal levels of GSH and plasma SOD activity. The nephroprotective effects of *Z. zerumbet* extract were confirmed by a reduced intensity of renal cellular damage, as evidenced by histological findings. Moreover, *Z. zerumbet* extract administered at 400 mg/kg was found to show greater protective effects than that at 200 mg/kg.

CONCLUSION

Medicinal plants are important sources of drugs for the treatment of several ailments. The consideration of scientists has been attracted to the utilization of medicinal plants for the treatment and management of different renal problems, including kidney stones. This chapter described more than 500 medicinal species with nephroprotective activities in detail. This is a single point of reference for all researchers. Drugs can be developed from this information for hepatoprotection and hepatocuring.

ABBREVIATIONS

ALT	Alanine amino transferase
AST	Aspartate amino transferase
ALP	Alkaline phosphatase
BUN	Blood Urea Nitrogen
CaOx	Calcium oxalate
CAT	Catalase
CCl$_4$	Carbon tetrachloride
DPPH2	2-diphenyl-1-picrylhydrazyl
EG	Ethylen glycol
GM	Gentamicin
GPx	Glutathione peroxidase
GR	Glutathione reductase
GSH	Glutathione
GST	Glutathione-S-transferase
LDH	Lactate dehydrogenase
MDA	Malondialdehyde
NO	Nitric oxide
SOD	Superoxide dismutase

REFERENCES

[1]   Javaid R, Aslam M, Nizami Q, Javaid R. Role of antioxidant herbal drugs in renal disorders: An overview. Free Radic Antioxid 2012; 2(1): 1-6.
[http://dx.doi.org/10.5530/ax.2012.2.2]

[2]   Lakshmi SM, Reddy TUK, Rani KSS. A review on medicinal plants for nephroprotctive activity. Asian J Pharm Clin Res 2012; 5(4): 8-14.

[3]   Dhole AR, Dhole VR, Magdum CS, Shreenivas M. Herbal therapy for urolithiasis: A brief review. Res J Pharmacol Pharmacodyn 2013; 5(1): 6-11.

[4]   Peesa JP. Nephroprotective potential of herbal medicines: A review. Asian J Pharm Tech 2013; 3(3): 115-8.

[5]   Ahmad QZ, Jahan N, Ahmad G. Tajuddin. An appraisal of nephroprotection and the scope of natural products in combating renal disorders. J Nephrol Ther 2014; 4: 170. [http://dx.doi.org/10.4172/2161-0959.1000170]

[6]   Sundararajan R, Bharampuram A, Koduru R. A review on phytoconstituents for nephroprotective activity. Pharmacophore 2014; 5(1): 160-82.

[7]   Janakiraman M, Jayaprakash K. Nephroprotective potential of medicinal plants: A review. Int J Sci Res 2015; 4(9): 543-7.

[8]   Sabiu S, O'Neill FH, Ashafa AOT. The purview of phytotherapy in the management of kidney disorders: a systematic review on Nigeria and South Africa. Afr J Tradit Complement Altern Med 2016; 13(5): 38-47. [PMID: 28487892]

[9]   Khajavi Rad A, Mohebbati R, Hosseinian S. Drug-induced nephrotoxicity and medicinal plants. Iran J Kidney Dis 2017; 11(3): 169-79. [PMID: 28575877]

[10]   Vaya RK, Sharma A, Singhvi IJ, Agarwal DK. Nephroprotective plants: A review. J Biosci Tech 2017; 8(1): 801-12.

[11]   Al-Snafi AE, Talab TA. A review of medicinal plants with nephroprotective effects. GSC Biol Pharmaceut Sci 2019; 8(1): 114-22. [http://dx.doi.org/10.30574/gscbps.2019.8.1.0108]

[12]   Das S, Vasudeva N, Sharma S. Kidney disorders and management through herbs: A review. J Phytopharmcol 2019; 8(1): 21-7. [http://dx.doi.org/10.31254/phyto.2019.8106]

[13]   Prasad KVSRG, Sujatha D, Bharathi K. Herbal drugs in urolithiasis-a review. Pharmacogn Rev 2007; 1(1): 175-8.

[14]   Butterweck V, Khan SR. Herbal medicines in the management of urolithiasis: alternative or complementary? Planta Med 2009; 75(10): 1095-103. [http://dx.doi.org/10.1055/s-0029-1185719] [PMID: 19444769]

[15]   Pareta SK, Patra KC, Mazumder PM, Sasmal D. Establishing the principle of herbal therapy for antiurolithiatic activity: A review. J Pharmacol & Toxicol 2011; 6(3): 321-32. [http://dx.doi.org/10.3923/jpt.2011.321.332]

[16]   Yadav RD, Jain SK. Herbal plants used in the treatment of urolithiasis a review. Int J Pharm Sci Res 2011; 2(6): 1412-20.

[17]   Joy JM, Prathyusha S, Mohanalakshmi S, Praveen Kumar AVS, Ashok Kumar CK. Potent herbal wealth with litholytic activity: A review. Innovative Drug Discovery 2012; 2(2): 66-75.

[18]   Nagal A, Singla RK. Herbal resources with antiurolithiatic effects: A review. Indo-Global J Pharmaceut Sci 2013; 3(1): 6-14.

[19]   Aggarwal A, Singla SK, Tandon C. Urolithiasis: phytotherapy as an adjunct therapy. Indian J Exp Biol 2014; 52(2): 103-11. [PMID: 24597142]

[20]   Rathod N, Chitme HR, Chandra R. *In vivo* and *in vitro* models for evaluating anti-urolithiasis activity

of herbal drugs. Intern J Pharmaceut Biosci 2014; 3(5): 309-29.

[21]   Al-Snafi AE. Medicinal plants with anti-urolithiatic effects (part 1). Int J Pharm 2015; 5(2): 98-103.

[22]   Al-Snafi AE. Arabian medicinal plants with antiurolithiatic and diuretic effects - plant based review (Part 1). IOSR J Pharm 2018; 8(6): 67-80.

[23]   Kasote DM, Jagtap SD, Thapa D, Khyade MS, Russell WR. Herbal remedies for urinary stones used in India and China: A review. J Ethnopharmacol 2017; 203: 55-68.
       [http://dx.doi.org/10.1016/j.jep.2017.03.038] [PMID: 28344029]

[24]   Makbul SAH, Kalam MA. Bioactive compounds from unani medicinal plants and their application in urolithiasis. 2019.

[25]   Zeng X, Xi Y, Jiang W. Protective roles of flavonoids and flavonoid-rich plant extracts against urolithiasis: a review. Crit Rev Food Sci Nutr 2018.
       [http://dx.doi.org/10.1080/10408398.2018.1439880] [PMID: 29432040]

[26]   Christina AJ, Muthumani P. Phytochemical investigation and anti lithiatic activity of *Abelmoschus moschatus* Medikus. Int J Pharm Pharm Sci 2013; 5(1): 108-13.

[27]   Djamhuri T, Khildah Y. Inhibitory activity of kidney stone formation (anti-nephrolithiasis) ethanol extract of red Gedi leaves (*Abelmoschus moschatus* Medik.) in male white rats. Galenika J Pharmacy 2015; 2(2): 32-9.

[28]   Lakshmi SM, Reddy TUK, Kumar CKA, Kumar DS, Prathysha S. Protective effect of *Abutilon indicum* L. (Malvaceae) against cisplatin induced nephrotoxicity in rats. Innovare J Life Sci 2013; 1(2): 35-9.

[29]   Reddy TU, Lakshmi SM, Kumar CKA, Prathyusha S, Kumar DS. Protective effect of *Abutilon indicum* L. (Malvaceae) against acetaminophen induced nephrotoxicity in rats. Innovare J Life Science 2013; 1(2): 40-3.

[30]   Shanmugapriya S, Anuradha R, Kiruthika R, Venkatalakshmi P, Velavan S. Formulation and evaluation of *Abutilon indicum* and *Boerhavia diffusa* for the determination of nephroprotective activities. J Sci Trans Environ Technov 2015; 9(2): 101-6.

[31]   Jesurun RSJ, Lavakumar S. Nephroprotective effect of ethanolic extract of *Abutilon indicum* root in gentamicin induced acute renal failure. Int J Basic Clin Pharmacol 2016; 5(3): 841-5.

[32]   Al-Majed AA, Mostafa AM, Al-Rikabi AC, Al-Shabanah OA. Protective effects of oral arabic gum administration on gentamicin-induced nephrotoxicity in rats. Pharmacol Res 2002; 46(5): 445-51.
       [http://dx.doi.org/10.1016/S1043661802001251] [PMID: 12419649]

[33]   Mahmoud MF, Diaai AA, Ahmed F. Evaluation of the efficacy of ginger, Arabic gum, and *Boswellia* in acute and chronic renal failure. Ren Fail 2012; 34(1): 73-82.
       [http://dx.doi.org/10.3109/0886022X.2011.623563] [PMID: 22017619]

[34]   Sathya M, Kokilavani R. Effect of ethanolic extract of *Acalypha indica* Linn. on ethylene glycol – induced kidney calculi in rats. Int J Pharm Pharm Sci 2012; 4 (Suppl.): 305-8.

[35]   Awari DM, Mute V, Babhale SP, Chaudhari SP. Antilithiatic effect of *Achyranthes aspera* leaves extract on ethylene glycol induced nephrolithiasis. J Pharma Res 2009; 2: 994-7.

[36]   Farook NAM, Rajesh SP, Nalini R. Inhibition of mineralization of urinary stone forming minerals by medicinal plants. E-J Chem 2009; 6(3): 938-42.
       [http://dx.doi.org/10.1155/2009/124168]

[37]   Aggarwal A, Tandon S, Singla SK, Tandon C. Reduction of oxalate induced renal tubular epithelial cell (NRK-52) injury and inhibition of calcium oxalate crystallization *in vitro* by aqueous extract of *Achyranthes aspera*. Int J Green Pharm 2010; 4: 159-64.
       [http://dx.doi.org/10.4103/0973-8258.69173]

[38]   Aggarwal A, Singla SK, Gandhi M, Tandon C. Preventive and curative effects of *Achyranthes aspera*

Linn. extract in experimentally induced nephrolithiasis. Indian J Exp Biol 2012; 50(3): 201-8. [PMID: 22439435]

[39]   Christi VE, Senthamarai R. A comparative study of antilithiatic effect of three traditional plants and their antioxidant activity. World J Pharmaceut Sci 2014; 2(10): 1290-9.

[40]   Pareta SK, Patra KC, Harwansh RK. *in-vitro* calcium oxalate crystallization inhibition by *Achyranthes indica* Linn. hydroalcoholic extract: An approach to antilithiasis. Int J Pharma Bio Sci 2011; 2(1): 432-7.

[41]   Prasad L, Khan TH, Jahangir T, Sultana S. *Acorus calamus* extracts and nickel chloride: prevention of oxidative damage and hyperproliferation response in rat kidney. Biol Trace Elem Res 2006; 113(1): 77-92.
[http://dx.doi.org/10.1385/BTER:113:1:77] [PMID: 17114817]

[42]   Palani S, Raja S, Kumar RP, Parameswaran P, Kumar BS. Therapeutic efficacy of *Acorus calamus* on acetaminophen induced nephrotoxicity and oxidative stress in male albino rats. Acta Pharmaceutica Sciencia 2010; 52: 89-100.

[43]   Sandeep D, Krishnan Nair CK. Amelioration of cisplatin-induced nephrotoxicity by extracts of *Hemidesmus indicus* and *Acorus calamus*. Pharm Biol 2010; 48(3): 290-5.
[http://dx.doi.org/10.3109/13880200903116048] [PMID: 20645815]

[44]   Ghelani H, Chapala M, Jadav P. Diuretic and antiurolithiatic activities of an ethanolic extract of *Acorus calamus* L. rhizome in experimental animal models. J Tradit Complement Med 2016; 6(4): 431-6.
[http://dx.doi.org/10.1016/j.jtcme.2015.12.004] [PMID: 27774431]

[45]   Ahmed A, Jahan N, Wadud A, Bilalm A, Hajera S. *in vitro* effect of hydro alcoholic extract of *Adiantum capillus-veneris* Linn. on calcium oxalate crystallization. Intern J Green Pharm 2013; 7(2): 106-10.
[http://dx.doi.org/10.4103/0973-8258.116385]

[46]   Ahmed A, Wadud A, Jahan N, Bilal A, Hajera S. Efficacy of *Adiantum capillus veneris* Linn in chemically induced urolithiasis in rats. J Ethnopharmacol 2013; 146(1): 411-6.
[http://dx.doi.org/10.1016/j.jep.2013.01.011] [PMID: 23333749]

[47]   Parameshwar P, Rao YN, Naik V, Reddy SH. Evaluation of antilithiatic activity of *Adonis aestivalis* Linn. in male Wister rats. Pharm Lett 2011; 3(2): 104-7.

[48]   Kore KJ, Shete RV, Jadhav PJ. RP-HPLC method os simultaneous nephroprotective role of *A. marmelos* extract. Int J Res Pharm Chem 2011; 1(3): 617-23.

[49]   Dwivedi J, Singh M, Sharma S, Sharma S. Antioxidant and nephroprotective potential of *Aegle marmelos* leaves extract. J Herbs Spices Med Plants 2017; 23(4): 363-77.
[http://dx.doi.org/10.1080/10496475.2017.1345029]

[50]   Movaliya V, Khamar D, Setty MM. Nephroprotective activity of aqueous extract of *Aerva javanica* roots in cisplatin induced renal toxicity in rats. Pharmacologyonline 2011; 1: 68-74.

[51]   Padala K, Ragini V. Anti urolithiatic activity of extracts of *Aerva javanica* in rats. Intern J Drug Dev & Res 2014; 6(4): 35-45.

[52]   Selvam R, Kalaiselvi P, Govindaraj A, Bala Murugan V, Sathish Kumar AS. Effect of *A. lanata* leaf extract and Vediuppu chunnam on the urinary risk factors of calcium oxalate urolithiasis during experimental hyperoxaluria. Pharmacol Res 2001; 43(1): 89-93.
[http://dx.doi.org/10.1006/phrs.2000.0745] [PMID: 11207071]

[53]   Shirwaikar A, Issac D, Malini S. Effect of *Aerva lanata* on cisplatin and gentamicin models of acute renal failure. J Ethnopharmacol 2004; 90(1): 81-6.
[http://dx.doi.org/10.1016/j.jep.2003.09.033] [PMID: 14698513]

[54]   Soundararajan P, Mahesh R, Ramesh T, Begum VH. Effect of *Aerva lanata* on calcium oxalate

urolithiasis in rats. Indian J Exp Biol 2006; 44(12): 981-6.
[PMID: 17176671]

[55]   Soumya PS, Poornima K, Ravikumar G, Kalaiselvi M, Gomathi D, Uma C. Nephroprotective effect of *Aerva lanata* against mercuric chloride induced renal injury in rats. J Pharm Res 2011; 4(8): 2474-6.

[56]   Nirmaladevi R, Chandrikka JU, Annadurai G, Kalpana S, Shrinidhi Raj T. Evaluation of *Aerva lanata* flower extract for its antilithiatic potential *in vitro* and *in vivo*. Intern J Pharm Pharmaceut Sci Res 2013; 3(2): 67-71.

[57]   Elmas O, Erbas O, Yigitturk G. The efficacy of *Aesculus hippocastanum* seeds on diabetic nephropathy in a streptozotocin-induced diabetic rat model. Biomed Pharmacother 2016; 83: 392-6.
[http://dx.doi.org/10.1016/j.biopha.2016.06.055] [PMID: 27424320]

[58]   Sumalatha G, Tanuja M, Babu Rao C, Revathi B, Varun D. Anti-urolithiatic and *in-vitro* antioxidant activity of leaves of *Ageratum conyzoides* in rat. World J Pharm Pharm Sci 2013; 2(2): 636-49.

[59]   Bhuvaneswari S, Vidya V, Thangathirupathi A. Antiurolithiatic activity of different extracts of *Ageratum conyzoides* (Linn.). J Pharmaceut Scientific Innovation 2015; 4(2): 140-3.
[http://dx.doi.org/10.7897/2277-4572.04231]

[60]   Giachetti D, Taddei E, Taddei I. Diuretic and uricosuric activity of *Agrimonia eupatoria* L. Boll Soc Ital Biol Sper 1986; 62(6): 705-11.
[PMID: 3790308]

[61]   Beghalia M, Ghalem S, Allali H, Belouatek A, Marouf A. Inhibition of calcium oxalate monohydrate crystal growth using Algerian medicinal plants. J Med Plants Res 2008; 2(3): 66-70.

[62]   Ahmadi M, Rad AK, Rajaei Z, Hadjzadeh MA, Mohammadian N, Tabasi NS. *Alcea rosea* root extract as a preventive and curative agent in ethylene glycol-induced urolithiasis in rats. Indian J Pharmacol 2012; 44(3): 304-7.
[http://dx.doi.org/10.4103/0253-7613.96298] [PMID: 22701236]

[63]   Suzuki K, Kawamara K, Tsugawa R. Formation and growth inhibition of calcium oxalate crystals by alismatis rhizome. Scanning Microsc 1999; 13(2-3): 183-9.

[64]   Azebaze AG, Ouahouo BM, Vardamides JC, *et al.* Antimicrobial and antileishmanial xanthones from the stem bark of *Allanblackia gabonensis* (Guttiferae). Nat Prod Res 2008; 22(4): 333-41.
[http://dx.doi.org/10.1080/14786410701855811] [PMID: 18322848]

[65]   Ige SF, Akhigbe RE, Adewale AA, *et al.* Effect of *Allium cepa* (Onion) extract on cadmium-induced nephrotoxicity in rats. Kidney Res J 2011; 1: 41-7.
[http://dx.doi.org/10.3923/krj.2011.41.47]

[66]   Kaur S, Tandon CD, Sharma R. Protective effects of garlic oil against propylene glycol induced toxicity on the kidney of young and aged mice. Med Sci Res 1996; 24(10): 683.

[67]   Maldonado PD, Barrera D, Medina-Campos ON, Hernández-Pando R, Ibarra-Rubio ME, Pedraza-Chaverrí J. Aged garlic extract attenuates gentamicin induced renal damage and oxidative stress in rats. Life Sci 2003; 73(20): 2543-56.
[http://dx.doi.org/10.1016/S0024-3205(03)00609-X] [PMID: 12967679]

[68]   Pedraza-Chaverrí J, Maldonado PD, Medina-Campos ON, *et al.* Garlic ameliorates gentamicin nephrotoxicity: relation to antioxidant enzymes. Free Radic Biol Med 2000; 29(7): 602-11.
[http://dx.doi.org/10.1016/S0891-5849(00)00354-3] [PMID: 11033412]

[69]   Abirami N, Jagadeeswari R. Amelioration of mercuric chloride induced nephrotoxicity and oxidative stress by garlic extract. Anc Sci Life 2006; 26(1-2): 73-7.
[PMID: 22557228]

[70]   Al-Qattan K, Thomson M, Ali M. Garlic (*Allium sativum*) and ginger (*Zingiber officinale*) attenuate structural nephropathy progression in streptozotocin-induced diabetic rats. Eur E J Clin Nutr Metab 2008; 3: e62-71.

[http://dx.doi.org/10.1016/j.eclnm.2007.12.001]

[71] Gulnaz H, Tahir M, Munir B, Sami W. Protective effects of garlic oil on acetaminophen induced nephrotoxicity in male albino rats. Biomed 2010; 26: 9-15.

[72] Savas M, Yeni E, Ciftci H, *et al*. The antioxidant role of oral administration of garlic oil on renal ischemia-reperfusion injury. Ren Fail 2010; 32(3): 362-7.
[http://dx.doi.org/10.3109/08860221003611711] [PMID: 20370453]

[73] Abdelaziz I, Kandeel M. The protective effects of *Nigella sativa* oil and *Allium sativum* extract on amikacin-induced nephrotoxicity. Int J Pharmacol 2011; 7: 697-703.
[http://dx.doi.org/10.3923/ijp.2011.697.703]

[74] Bagheri F, Gol A, Dabiri S, Javadi A. Preventive effect of garlic juice on renal reperfusion injury. Iran J Kidney Dis 2011; 5(3): 194-200.
[PMID: 21525580]

[75] Anusuya N, Devi DP, Dhinek A, Mythily S. Nephroprotcetive effect of ethanolic extract of garlic (*Allium sativum*) on cisplatin induced nephrotoxicity in male wistar rats. Asian J Pharm Clin Res 2013; 6: 97-100.

[76] Nasri H, Nematbakhsh M, Rafieian-Kopaei M. Ethanolic extract of garlic for attenuation of gentamicin-induced nephrotoxicity in Wistar rats. Iran J Kidney Dis 2013; 7(5): 376-82.
[PMID: 24072150]

[77] Rafieian-Kopaei M, Baradaran A, Merrikhi A, Nematbakhsh M, Madihi Y, Nasri H. Efficacy of co-administration of garlic extract and metformin for prevention of gentamicin-renal toxicity in wistar rats: A biochemical study. Int J Prev Med 2013; 4(3): 258-64.
[PMID: 23626881]

[78] Chatterjee P, Mukherjee A, Nandy S. Protective effects of the aqueous leaf extract of *Aloe barbadensis* on gentamicin and cisplatin-induced nephrotoxic rats. Asian Pac J Trop Biomed 2012; 9(1): S1754-63.
[http://dx.doi.org/10.1016/S2221-1691(12)60490-0]

[79] Kaushik P, Kaushik D, Yadav J, Pahwa P. Protective effect of *Alpinia galanga* in STZ induced diabetic nephropathy. Pak J Biol Sci 2013; 16(16): 804-11.
[http://dx.doi.org/10.3923/pjbs.2013.804.811] [PMID: 24498833]

[80] Talebi A, Karimi A, Ouguerram K, *et al*. Lack of nephroprotective efficacy of *Althaea officinalis* flower extract against gentamicin renal toxicity in male rats. Int J Prev Med 2014; 5(11): 1360-3.
[PMID: 25538830]

[81] Amuthan A, Chogtu B, Bairy KL, Sudhakar , Prakash M. Evaluation of diuretic activity of *Amaranthus spinosus* Linn. aqueous extract in Wistar rats. J Ethnopharmacol 2012; 140(2): 424-7.
[http://dx.doi.org/10.1016/j.jep.2012.01.049] [PMID: 22331031]

[82] Kengar S, Dattatray T, Jaywant J. Nephroprotective effect of *Amaranthus spinosus* root extract in carbon tetrachloride-induced histological toxicity in male albino rat. Int J Drug Dev Res 2017; 9(2): 5-7.

[83] Prasad KVSRG, Bharathi K, Srinivasan KK. Evaluation of *Ammannia baccifera* Linn. for antiurolithic activity in albino rats. Indian J Exp Biol 1994; 32(5): 311-3.
[PMID: 7927522]

[84] Ahsan SK, Tariq M, Ageel AM, al-Yahya MA, Shah AH. Effect of *Trigonella foenum-graecum* and *Ammi majus* on calcium oxalate urolithiasis in rats. J Ethnopharmacol 1989; 26(3): 249-54.
[http://dx.doi.org/10.1016/0378-8741(89)90097-4] [PMID: 2615405]

[85] Mutlag SH, Ismael DK, Al-Shawi NN. Study the possible hepatoprotective effect of different doses of *Ammi majus* seeds' extract against CCl_4 induced liver damage in rats. Pharm Glob 2011; 9: 1-5.
[IJCP].

[86] Khan ZA, Assiri AM, Al-Afghani HMA, Maghrabi TM. Inhibition of oxalate nephrolithiasis with

Ammi visnaga (AI-Khillah). Int Urol Nephrol 2001; 33(4): 605-8.
[http://dx.doi.org/10.1023/A:1020526517097] [PMID: 12452606]

[87]   Vanachayangkul P. 2008. *Ammi visnaga* L. for the prevention of Urolithiasis. Ph.D. theis.

[88]   Vanachayangkul P, Chow N, Khan SR, Butterweck V. Prevention of renal crystal deposition by an extract of *Ammi visnaga* L. and its constituents khellin and visnagin in hyperoxaluric rats. Urol Res 2011; 39(3): 189-95.
[http://dx.doi.org/10.1007/s00240-010-0333-y] [PMID: 21069311]

[89]   Muangman V, Viseshsindh V, Ratana-Olarn K, Buadilok S. The usage of *Andrographis paniculata* following extracorporeal shock wave lithotripsy (ESWL). J Med Assoc Thai 1995; 78(6): 310-3.
[PMID: 7561556]

[90]   Rao K. Anti-hyperglycemic and renal protective activities of *Andrographis paniculata* roots chloroform extract. Iran J Pharmacol Therap 2006; 5(1): 47-50.

[91]   Singh P, Srivastava MM, Khemani LD. Nephroprotective activities of root extracts of *Andrographis paniculata* (Burm. f.) Nees in gentamicin induced renal failure in rats: A time-dependent study. Arch Appl Sci Res 2009; 1(2): 67-73.

[92]   Singh P, Srivastava MM, Khemani LD. Renoprotective effects of *Andrographis paniculata* (Burm. f.) Nees in rats. Ups J Med Sci 2009; 114(3): 136-9.
[http://dx.doi.org/10.1080/03009730903174321] [PMID: 19736602]

[93]   Pratibhkumari PV, Prasad G. Efficacy of *Andrographis paniculata* on ethylene glycol induced nephrolithiasis in rats. J Pharm Sci. Innov (Camb, Mass) 2013; 2(3): 46-50.

[94]   Deshmukh AB, Patel JK. Aqueous extract of *Annona squamosa* (L.) ameliorates renal failure induced by 5/6 nephrectomy in rat. Indian J Pharmacol 2011; 43(6): 718-21.
[PMID: 22144782]

[95]   Al-Jawad FH, Al-Razzuqi RA, Al-Jeboori AA. *Apium graveolens* accentuates urinary Ca^{+2} excretions in experimental model of nephrocalcinosis. Intern J Green Pharm 2011; 5(2): 100-2.
[http://dx.doi.org/10.4103/0973-8258.85160]

[96]   Grases F, Melero G, Costa-Bauzá A, Prieto R, March JG. Urolithiasis and phytotherapy. Int Urol Nephrol 1994; 26(5): 507-11.
[http://dx.doi.org/10.1007/BF02767650] [PMID: 7860196]

[97]   Gürocak S, Küpeli B. Consumption of historical and current phytotherapeutic agents for urolithiasis: a critical review. J Urol 2006; 176(2): 450-5.
[http://dx.doi.org/10.1016/j.juro.2006.03.034] [PMID: 16813863]

[98]   Guinnin FDF, Sangaré MM, Atègbo JM, Sacramento IT, Issotina ZA, Klotoé JR, *et al.* Evaluation of hepatoprotective and nephroprotective activities of ethanolic extract leaves of *Aristolochia albida* Duch. against CCl_4-induced hepatic and renal dysfunction. J Pharm Biomed Sci 2017; 7(7): 264-9.

[99]   Arivazhagan SJJ, Vimaastalin R. Nephroprotective activity of *Aristolochia indica* leaf extract against gentamicin induced renal dysfunction. Intern J Res Biochem Biophys 2014; 4(2): 13-8.

[100] Bhattacharjee C, Dutta A. Nephroprotective activity of bark of *Artocarpus heterophyllus* Lam. Int J Biol Adv Res 2017; 8(6): 259-63.

[101] Christina AJM, Ashok K, Packialakshmi M, Tobin GC, Preethi J, Murugesh N. Antilithiatic effect of *Asparagus racemosus* Willd on ethylene glycol-induced lithiasis in male albino Wistar rats. Methods Find Exp Clin Pharmacol 2005; 27(9): 633-8.
[http://dx.doi.org/10.1358/mf.2005.27.9.939338] [PMID: 16357948]

[102] Kumar MCS, Udupa AL, Sammodavardhana K, Rathnakar UP, Udupa S, Prabhath KG. Antiurolithiatic activity of aqueous extracts of *Asparagus racemosus* Willd. and *Tamarindus indica* Linn. in rats. Pharmacologyonline 2009; 2: 625-30.

[103] Jagannath N, Chikkannasetty SS, Govindadas D, Devasankaraiah G. Study of antiurolithiatic activity

of *Asparagus racemosus* on albino rats. Indian J Pharmacol 2012; 44(5): 576-9.
[http://dx.doi.org/10.4103/0253-7613.100378] [PMID: 23112416]

[104] Li M, Wang W, Xue J, Gu Y, Lin S. Meta-analysis of the clinical value of *Astragalus membranaceus* in diabetic nephropathy. J Ethnopharmacol 2011; 133(2): 412-9.
[http://dx.doi.org/10.1016/j.jep.2010.10.012] [PMID: 20951192]

[105] Ezz-Din D, Gabry MS, Farrag ARH, Moneim AEA. Physiological and histological impact of *Azadirachta indica* (neem) leaves extract in a rat model of cisplatin-induced hepato and nephrotoxicity. J Med Plants Res 2011; 5(23): 5499-506.

[106] Hwisa NT, Assaleh FH, Sumalatha G, El Melad F, Babu Rao C, Prakash K. A Study on antiurolithiatic activity of *Melia Azadirachta* L. aqueous extract in rats. Am J Pharmacol Sci 2014; 2(1): 27-31.
[http://dx.doi.org/10.12691/ajps-2-1-6]

[107] Konda VR, Arunachalam R, Eerike M, *et al.* Nephroprotective effect of ethanolic extract of *Azima tetracantha* root in glycerol induced acute renal failure in Wistar albino rats. J Tradit Complement Med 2015; 6(4): 347-54.
[http://dx.doi.org/10.1016/j.jtcme.2015.05.001] [PMID: 27774418]

[108] Shahid M, Subhan F. Protective effect of *Bacopa monniera* methanol extract against carbon tetrachloride induced hepatotoxicity and nephrotoxicity. Pharmacol Online 2014; 2: 18-28.

[109] Patel VB, Patel DG, Makwana AG, Patel JM, Brahmbhatt MR. Comparative study of *Rivea hypocraterformis, Cynodon dactylon* and *Balanites aegyptiaca* using antilithiatic activity *in-vitro*. Int J Pharm Sci Res 2010; 1(12): 85-7.

[110] Atif M, Ahmed MI, Mahmood SB, Qurram MA. Evaluation of anti-urolithiatic activity of hydroalcoholic and aqueous leaf extract of *Barleria prionitis* in albino rats. Intern Res J Pharm 2014; 5(7): 587-92.
[http://dx.doi.org/10.7897/2230-8407.0507120]

[111] Mishra S, Pani SR, Sahoo S. Anti-nephrotoxic activity of some medicinal plants from tribal rich pockets of Odisha. Pharmacognosy Res 2014; 6(3): 210-7.
[http://dx.doi.org/10.4103/0974-8490.132598] [PMID: 25002801]

[112] Lakshmi BVS, Neelima N, Kasthuri N, Umarani V, Sudhakar M. Protective effect of *Bauhinia purpurea* on gentamicin-induced nephrotoxicity in rats. Indian J Pharm Sci 2009; 71(5): 551-4.
[http://dx.doi.org/10.4103/0250-474X.58196] [PMID: 20502576]

[113] Sivanagi Reddy T, Prasanna Shama K, Nirmala P, Shastry CS. Biochemical studies hepato and nephroprotective effect of Butterfly tree (*Bauhinia purpurea* Linn.) against acetaminophen induced toxicity. Int J Res Ayurveda Pharm 2012; 3(3): 455-60.

[114] Rana MA, Khan RA, Nasiruddin M, Khan AA. Amelioration of cisplatin-induced nephrotoxicity by ethanolic extract of *Bauhinia purpurea*: An *in vivo* study in rats. Saudi J Kidney Dis Transpl 2016; 27(1): 41-8.
[http://dx.doi.org/10.4103/1319-2442.174068] [PMID: 26787565]

[115] Pani SR, Mishra S, Sahoo S, Panda PK. Nephroprotective effect of *Bauhinia variegata* (Linn.) whole stem extract against cisplatin-induced nephropathy in rats. Indian J Pharmacol 2011; 43(2): 200-2.
[http://dx.doi.org/10.4103/0253-7613.77370] [PMID: 21572659]

[116] Rajani GP, Sharma V, Komala N. Effect of ethanolic and aqueous extracts of *Bauhinia variegata* Linn. on gentamicin-induced nephrotoxicity in rats. Indian J Pharmaceut Edu Res 2010; 45(2): 192-8.

[117] Sharma RK, Rajani G, Sharma V, Komala N. Effect of ethanolic and aqueous extracts of *Bauhinia variegata* Linn. on gentamicin-induced nephrotoxicity in rats. Indian J Pharm Educ Res 2011; 45: 192-8.

[118] Prusty KB, Harish B, Mamatha CH. Evaluation of nephro-protective activity of the methanolic extract of leaves of *Bauhinia variegata* Linn. (Family-*Caesalpiniaceae*). J Pharm Sci Technol 2012; 2: 16-9.

[119] Patel RK, Patel SB, Shah JG. Antiurolithiatic activity of ethanolic extract of seeds of *Benincasa hispida* (Thunb). Pharmacologyonline 2011; 3: 586-91.

[120] Varghese HS, Kotagiri S, Vrushabendra SBM, Archana SP, Raj GG. Nephroprotective activity of *Benincasa hispida* (Thunb.) Cogn. fruit extract against paracetamol induced nephrotoxicity in rats. Res J Pharm Biol Chem Sci 2013; 4(1): 322-32.

[121] Mingyu D, Mingzhang L, Quihong Y, Weiming U, Jianxing X, Weinming X. A study on *Benincasa hispida* contents effective for protection of kidney. Jiangsu J Agric Sci 1995; 11: 46-52.

[122] Sreedevi A, Barathi K, Prasad KVSRG. Effect of decotion of root bark of *Berberis aristata* against cisplatin induced nephrotoxicity in rats. Int J Pharm Pharm Sci 2009; 2(3): 51-6.

[123] Pervez S, Saeed M, Khan H, Shahid M, Ullah I. Nephro-protective effect of *Berberis baluchistanica* against gentamicin-induced nephrotoxicity in rabbit. Bangladesh J Pharmacol 2018; 13: 222-30.
[http://dx.doi.org/10.3329/bjp.v13i3.36621]

[124] Ashraf H, Heidari R, Nejati V, Ilkhanipoor M. Aqueous extract of *Berberis integerrima* root improves renal dysfunction in streptozotocin induced diabetic rats. Avicenna J Phytomed 2013; 3(1): 82-90.
[PMID: 25050261]

[125] Anwar R, Sultan R, Batool F. Ameliorating effect of *Berberis lycium* root bark extracts against cisplatin-induced nephro-pathy in rat. Bangladesh J Pharmacol 2018; 13: 248-54.
[http://dx.doi.org/10.3329/bjp.v13i3.36705]

[126] Bashir S, Gilani AH, Siddiqui AA, *et al*. *Berberis vulgaris* root bark extract prevents hyperoxaluria induced urolithiasis in rats. Phytother Res 2010; 24(8): 1250-5.
[http://dx.doi.org/10.1002/ptr.3196] [PMID: 20564494]

[127] Jyothilakshmi V, Thellamudhu G, Kumar A, Khurana A, Nayak D, Kalaiselvi P. Preliminary investigation on ultra high diluted *B. vulgaris* in experimental urolithiasis. Homeopathy 2013; 102(3): 172-8.
[http://dx.doi.org/10.1016/j.homp.2013.05.004] [PMID: 23870376]

[128] Byahatti VV, Pai KV, D'Souza MG. Effect of Phenolic Compounds from *Bergenia ciliata* (Haw.) Sternb.leaves on Experimental kidney stones. Anc Sci Life 2010; 30(1): 14-7.
[PMID: 22557418]

[129] Saha S, Verma RJ. *Bergenia ciliata* extract prevents ethylene glycol induced histopathological changes in the kidney. Acta Pol Pharm 2011; 68(5): 711-5.
[PMID: 21928716]

[130] Saha S, Verma RJ. Inhibition of calcium oxalate crystallisation *in vitro* by an extract of *Bergenia ciliata*. Arab J Urol 2013; 11(2): 187-92.
[http://dx.doi.org/10.1016/j.aju.2013.04.001] [PMID: 26558080]

[131] Joshi VS, Parekh BB, Joshi MJ, Vaidya AB. Herbal extract of *Tribulus terrestris* and *Bergenia ligulata* inhibit growth of calcium oxalate monohydrate crystals *in vitro*. J Cryst Growth 2005; 275: 1403-8.
[http://dx.doi.org/10.1016/j.jcrysgro.2004.11.240]

[132] Bashir S, Gilani AH. Antiurolithic effect of *Bergenia ligulata* rhizome: an explanation of the underlying mechanisms. J Ethnopharmacol 2009; 122(1): 106-16.
[http://dx.doi.org/10.1016/j.jep.2008.12.004] [PMID: 19118615]

[133] Harsoliya MS, Pathan JK, Khan N, Bhatl D, Patel VM. Effect of ethanolic extract of *Bergenia ligulata, Nigella sativa* and combination on calcium oxalate urolithiasis in rats. Int J Drug Formulat Res 2011; 2(2): 268-80.

[134] Saranya R, Geetha N. Inhibition of clacium oxalate crystallization *in vitro* by the extract of Beet root (*Beta vulgaris* L). Int J Pharm Pharm Sci 2014; 6(2): 361-5.

[135] Shah SK, Patel KM, Vaviya PM. Evaluation of antiurolithiatic activity of *Betula utilis* in rats using

ethylene glycol model. Asian J Pharm Res 2017; 7(2): 81-7.
[http://dx.doi.org/10.5958/2231-5691.2017.00014.4]

[136]   Pawar AT, Vyawahare NS. Anti-urolithiatic activity of standardized extract of *Biophytum sensitivum* against zinc disc implantation induced urolithiasis in rats. J Adv Pharm Technol Res 2015; 6(4): 176-82.
[http://dx.doi.org/10.4103/2231-4040.165017] [PMID: 26605159]

[137]   Chandavarkar S, Desai SNM, Gautam G. Nephroprotective activity of different extracts of *Biophytum sensitivum* (Linn.) DC. Int J Herb Med 2017; 5(1): 31-4.

[138]   Raut AA, Sunder S, Sarkar S, Pandita NS, Vaidya ADB. Preliminary study on crystal dissolution activity of *Rotula aquatica, Commiphora wightii* and *Boerhaavia diffusa* extracts. Fitoterapia 2008; 79(7-8): 544-7.
[http://dx.doi.org/10.1016/j.fitote.2008.06.001] [PMID: 18644427]

[139]   Chauhan CK, Joshi MJ, Vaidya ADB. Growth inhibition of struvite crystals in the presence of herbal extract *Boerhaavia diffusa* Linn. Am J Infect Dis 2009; 5(3): 170-9.
[http://dx.doi.org/10.3844/ajidsp.2009.170.179]

[140]   Indhumathi T, Shilpa K, Mohandass S. Evaluation of nephroprotective role of *Boerhavia diffusa* leaves against mercuric chloride induced toxicity in experimental rats. J Pharm Res 2011; 4(6): 1848-50.

[141]   Pareta SK, Patra KC, Mazumder PM, Sasmal D. Aqueous extract of *Boerhaavia diffusa* root ameliorates ethylene glycol-induced hyperoxaluric oxidative stress and renal injury in rat kidney. Pharm Biol 2011; 49(12): 1224-33.
[http://dx.doi.org/10.3109/13880209.2011.581671] [PMID: 21846174]

[142]   Yasir F, Waqar MA. Effect of indigenous plant extracts on calcium oxalate crystallization having a role in urolithiasis. Urol Res 2011; 39(5): 345-50.
[http://dx.doi.org/10.1007/s00240-011-0374-x] [PMID: 21643743]

[143]   Chitra V, Gowri K, Udayasri N. Antilithiatic activity of alcoholic extract of *Boerhaavia diffusa* roots on ethylene glycol induced lithiasis in rats. Int J Pharm Pharm Sci 2012; 4(2): 149-53.

[144]   Kulkarni YR, Apte BK, Kulkarni PH, Patil RR. Evaluation of nephroprotective and anti-nephro-toxic properties of Rakta Punarnava roots (*Boerhavia diffusa* L.) Gokshur fruits (*Tribulus terrestris* L.) in drug induced nephrotoxicity. Intern Res J Pharm 2012; 3(7): 329-34.

[145]   Srinivas S, Arun Kumar B. Effects of *Boerhavia diffusa* roots and *Drynaria quercifolia* rhizome extracts on urolithiatic rats. J Pharm Res 2012; 5(5): 2846-51.

[146]   Karwasra R, Kalra P, Nag TC, Gupta YK, Singh S, Panwar A. Safety assessment and attenuation of cisplatin induced nephrotoxicity by tuberous roots of *Boerhaavia diffusa*. Regul Toxicol Pharmacol 2016; 81: 341-52.
[http://dx.doi.org/10.1016/j.yrtph.2016.09.020] [PMID: 27667768]

[147]   Mosquera DMG, Ortega YH, Quero PC, Martínez RS, Pieters L. Antiurolithiatic activity of *Boldoa purpurascens* aqueous extract: An *in vitro* and *in vivo* study. J Ethnopharmacol 2020; 253: 112691.
[http://dx.doi.org/10.1016/j.jep.2020.112691] [PMID: 32092500]

[148]   Gadge NB, Jalalpure SS. Curative treatment with extracts of *Bombax ceiba* fruit reduces risk of calcium oxalate urolithiasis in rats. Pharm Biol 2012; 50(3): 310-7.
[http://dx.doi.org/10.3109/13880209.2011.604332] [PMID: 22321032]

[149]   Rajamurugan R, Suyavaran A, Selvaganabathy N, *et al. Brassica nigra* plays a remedy role in hepatic and renal damage. Pharm Biol 2012; 50(12): 1488-97.
[http://dx.doi.org/10.3109/13880209.2012.685129] [PMID: 22978659]

[150]   Naga Kishore R, Mangilai T, Anja Neyulu N, Abhinayani G, Sravya N. Investigation of anti urolithiatic activity of *Brassica oleracea gongylodes* and *Desmostachya bipinnata* in experimentally induced urolithiasis in animal models. Int J Pharm Pharm Sci 2014; 6(6): 602-4.

[151] Kim YH, Kim YW, Oh YJ, *et al.* Protective effect of the ethanol extract of the roots of *Brassica rapa* on cisplatin-induced nephrotoxicity in LLC-PK1 cells and rats. Biol Pharm Bull 2006; 29(12): 2436-41.
[http://dx.doi.org/10.1248/bpb.29.2436] [PMID: 17142978]

[152] Cordeiro M, Kaliwal B. Hepatoprotective and nephroprotective activity of bark extract of *Bridelia retusa* in CCl₄ treated female mice. Intern J Mol Biol 2011; 2(1)

[153] Harlalka GV, Patil CR, Patil MR. Protective effect of *Kalanchoe pinnata* Pers. (Crassulaceae) on gentamicin-induced nephrotoxicity in rats. Indian J Pharmacol 2007; 39(4): 201-5.
[http://dx.doi.org/10.4103/0253-7613.36540]

[154] Phatak RS, Hendre AS. *in-vitro* antiurolithiatic activity of *Kalanchoe pinnata* extract. Intern J Pharmacogn Phytocheml Res 2015; 7(2): 275-9.

[155] Gahlaut A, Pawar SD, Mandal TK, Dabur R. Evaluation of clinical efficacy of *Bryophyllum pinnatum* Salisb. for treatment of lithiasis. Int J Pharm Pharm Sci 2012; 4(4): 505-7.

[156] Shukla AB, Mandavia DR, Barvaliya MJ, Baxi SN, Tripathi CR. Evaluation of anti-urolithiatic effect of aqueous extract of *Bryophyllum pinnatum* (Lam.) leaves using ethylene glycol-induced renal calculi. Avicenna J Phytomed 2014; 4(3): 151-9.
[PMID: 25050313]

[157] Phatak RS, Subhash HA. *in-vitro* atiurolithiatic activity of *Kalanchoe pinnata* extract. Int J Pharmacogn Phytochem Res 2015; 7(2): 275-9.

[158] Yadav D, Sharma AK, Srivastava S, Tripathi YB. Nephroprotective potential of standardized herbals described in Ayurveda: A comparative study. J Chem Pharm Res 2016; 8(8): 419-27.

[159] Maheshwari C, Meenakshi K, Babu P, Narayana RV. Protective effet of *Butea monosperma* flowers against gentamicin induced renal toxicity. Res J Pharm Tech 2012; 4(12): 1898-900.

[160] Sonkar N, Ganeshpurkar A, Yadav P, Dubey S, Bansal D, Dubey N. An experimetal evaluation of nephroprotective potential of *Butea monosperma* extract in albino rats. Indian J Pharmacol 2014; 46(1): 109-12.
[http://dx.doi.org/10.4103/0253-7613.125190] [PMID: 24550595]

[161] Brijesh S, Lohit B, Sahil S, Madhususan S. Antinephritic potential of n-butanolic fraction of *Butea monsperma* (Lam.) flowers on doxorubin-induced nephritic syndrome in rats. Int J Res Ayurveda Pharm 2015; 6(4): 478-88.
[http://dx.doi.org/10.7897/2277-4343.06492]

[162] Sikandari S, Ahmed ML, Mathad P. Antilithiatic influence of *Butea monosperma* Lam and *Nigella sativa* Linn. on ethylene glycol induced nephrolithiasis in rats. Intern J Scientific & Res Publications 2015; 5(9): 1-9.

[163] Noorani A, Gupta K, Bhadada K, Kale MK. Protective effect of methanolic leaf extract of *Caesalpinia bonduc* L. on gentamicin - induced hepatotoxicity and nephrotoxicity in rats. Iranian J Pharmacol Therapeut 2011; 10: 21-5.

[164] Preethi KC, Kuttan R. Hepato and reno protective action of *Calendula officinalis* L. flower extract. Indian J Exp Biol 2009; 47(3): 163-8.
[PMID: 19405380]

[165] Verma PK, Raina R, Sultana M, Singh M, Kumar P. Total antioxidant and oxidant status of plasma and renal tissue of cisplatin-induced nephrotoxic rats: protection by floral extracts of *Calendula officinalis* Linn. Ren Fail 2016; 38(1): 142-50.
[http://dx.doi.org/10.3109/0886022X.2015.1103585] [PMID: 26513373]

[166] Dahiru D, Amos D, Sambo SH. Effect of ethanol extract of *Calotropis procera* root bark on carbon tetrachloride-induced hepatonephrotoxicity in female rats. Jordan J Biol Sci 2013; 6(3): 227-30.
[http://dx.doi.org/10.12816/0001538]

[167] Javed S, Khan JA, Khaliq T, Javed I, Abbas RZ. Experimental evaluation of nephroprotective potential of *Calotropis procera* (Ait.) flowers against gentamicin induced toxicity in albino rabbits. Pak Vet J 2015; 35(2): 222-6.

[168] Okwuosa CN, Achukwu PUA, Nwachukwu DC, Eze AA, Azubuike NC. Nephroprotective activity of stem bark extracts of *Canarium schweinfurthii* on acetaminophen-induced renal injuries in rats. Int J Med Health Dev 2009; 14(1): 234-41.

[169] Kalantar M, Goudarzi M, Khodayar MJ, Babaei J, Foruozandeh H, Bakhtiari N, *et al.* Protective effects of the hydrochloric extract of *Capparis spinosa* L. against cyclophosphamide induced nephrotoxicity in mice. Jundishapur J Nat Pharm Prod 2016; 11(4): e37240. [http://dx.doi.org/10.17795/jjnpp-37240]

[170] Tlili N, Feriani A, Saadoui E, Nasri N, Khaldi A. *Capparis spinosa* leaves extract: Source of bioantioxidants with nephroprotective and hepatoprotective effects. Biomed Pharmacother 2017; 87: 171-9. [http://dx.doi.org/10.1016/j.biopha.2016.12.052] [PMID: 28056421]

[171] Olagunjua JA, Adeneyeb AA, Fagbohunkac BS. Nephroprotective activities of the aqueous seed extract of *Carica papaya* Linn. in carbon tetrachloride induced renal injured Wistar rats: a dose- and time-dependent study. Biol Med (Aligarh) 2009; 1: 11-9.

[172] Nayeem K, Gupta D, Nayana H, Joshi RK. Anti-urolithiatic potential of the fruit extracts of *Carica papaya* on ethylene glycol induced urolithiatic rats. J Pharm Res 2010; 3(11): 2772-5.

[173] Debnath S, Babre N, Manjunath YS, Mallareddy V, Parameshwar P, Hariprasath K. Nephroprotective evaluation of ethanolic extract of the seeds of papaya and pumpkin fruit in cisplatin-induced nephrotoxicity. J Pharm Sci Technol 2010; 2(6): 241-6.

[174] Patil KS, Jagadish K, Preeti B. The effects of seed extract of *Carthamus tinctorious* on nephroprotective and diuretic activities in rats. J Trop Med 2009; 9(2): 354-8.

[175] Lin WC, Lai MT, Chen HY, *et al.* Protective effect of Flos carthami extract against ethylene glycol-induced urolithiasis in rats. Urol Res 2012; 40(6): 655-61. [http://dx.doi.org/10.1007/s00240-012-0472-4] [PMID: 22398437]

[176] Sadiq S, Nagi AH, Shahzad M, Zia A. The reno-protective effect of aqueous extract of *Carum carvi* (black zeera) seeds in streptozotocin induced diabetic nephropathy in rodents. Saudi J Kidney Dis Transpl 2010; 21(6): 1058-65. [PMID: 21060174]

[177] Abou El-Soud NH, El-Lithy NA, El-Saeed G, *et al.* Renoprotective effects of caraway (*Carum carvi* L.) essential oil in streptozotocin induced diabetic rats. J Appl Pharm Sci 2014; 4(2): 27-33.

[178] Swamiranga Reddy K, Hanumanna P. Venkata nagendra Prasad S, Surendra M, Swetha reddy K, Thanuja K. Anti-urolithiatic activity of *Carum copticum*. J Sci Res Pharm 2012; 1(2): 58-61.

[179] Annie S, Rajagopal PL, Malini S. Effect of *Cassia auriculata* Linn. root extract on cisplatin and gentamicin-induced renal injury. Phytomedicine 2005; 12(8): 555-60. [http://dx.doi.org/10.1016/j.phymed.2003.11.010] [PMID: 16121515]

[180] Ramesh C, Dharmendra KBK, John WE, Saleem BS, Girish K. Antiurolithiatic activity of wood bark extracts of *Cassia fistula* in rats. J Pharm Biomed Sci 2010; 2(2): 11-7.

[181] Gowrisri M, Kotagiri S, Vrushabendra Swamy BM, Archana Swamy P, Vishwanath KM. Anti-oxidant and nephroprotective activities of *Cassia occidentalis* leaf extract against gentamicin induced nephrotoxicity in rats. Res J Pharm Biol Chem Sci 2012; 3(3): 684-94.

[182] Ntchapda F, Barama J, Kemeta Azambou DR, Etet PFS, Dimo T. Diuretic and antioxidant activities of the aqueous extract of leaves of *Cassia occidentalis* (Linn.) in rats. Asian Pac J Trop Med 2015; 8(9): 685-93. [http://dx.doi.org/10.1016/j.apjtm.2015.07.030] [PMID: 26433651]

[183] El-Tantawy WH, Mohamed SAH, Abd Al Haleem EN. Evaluation of biochemical effects of *Casuarina equisetifolia* extract on gentamicin-induced nephrotoxicity and oxidative stress in rats. Phytochemical analysis. J Clin Biochem Nutr 2013; 53(3): 158-65.
[http://dx.doi.org/10.3164/jcbn.13-19] [PMID: 24249970]

[184] Ramesh C, Krishnadas N, Radhakrishnan R, Srinath R, Viswanatha GLS, Rajesh D, *et al*. Anti-urolithiatic activity of heart-wood extract of *Cedrus deodora* in rats. J Compl Int Med 2010; 7: 1-9.

[185] Choubey A, Choubey A, Jain P, Iyer D, Patil UK. Assessment of *Ceiba pentandra* on calcium oxalate urolithiasis in rats. Pharma Chem 2010; 2(6): 144-56.

[186] Joshi P, Patil S, Sambrekar SN. Evaluation of the antiurolithiatic activity of ethonolic extract of *Celosia argentea* (seeds) in rats. Universal J Pharmacy 2012; 1(1): 52-60.

[187] Kachchhi NR, Parmar RK, Tirgar PR, Desai TR, Bhalodia PN. Evaluation of the antiurolithiatic activity of methanolic extract of *Celosia argentea* roots in rats. Int J PhytoPharm 2012; 3(3): 249-55.

[188] Ashok P, Koti B, Viswanathswamy A. Effect of *Centratherum anthelminticum* on ethylene glycol induced urolithiasis in rats. RGUHS J Pharm Sci 2013; 3(1): 48-52.

[189] Galani VJ, Panchal RR. *in vitro* evaluation of *Centratherum anthelminticum* seeds for antinephrolithiatic activity. J Homeop Ayurv Med 2014; 3: 145-50.
[http://dx.doi.org/10.4172/2167-1206.1000145]

[190] Ahmed MM. Biochemical studies on nephroprotective effect of carob (*Ceratonia siliqua* L.) growing in Egypt. Nat Sci 2010; 8(3): 41-7.

[191] Khan MA, Pradhan D. Antiurolithiatic activity of *Ceropegia bulbosa* extract in rats. Pharm Sin 2012; 3(1): 148-52.

[192] Saleem U, Ali N, Ahmad B. Protective and curative effects of *Cestrum nocturnum* on rabbit kidney. Bangladesh J Pharmacol 2017; 12: 284-91.
[http://dx.doi.org/10.3329/bjp.v12i3.32410]

[193] Beghalia M, Ghalem S, Allali H, Belouatek A, Marouf A. Effect of herbal extracts of *Tetraclinis articulata* and *Chamaerops humilis* on calcium oxalate crystals *in vitro*. Gomal J Med Sci 2007; 5(2): 55-8.

[194] Sikarwar I, Dey YN, Wanjari MM, Sharma A, Gaidhani SN, Jadhav AD. *Chenopodium album* Linn. leaves prevent ethylene glycol-induced urolithiasis in rats. J Ethnopharmacol 2017; 195: 275-82.
[http://dx.doi.org/10.1016/j.jep.2016.11.031] [PMID: 27864113]

[195] Divya S, Banda T. Evaluation of anti-diuretic and anti-nephrolithiatic activities of ethanolic seeds extract of *Cicer arietinum* in experimental rats. Int J Pharmaceut Res Dev 2014; 5(12): 9-12.

[196] Biglarkhani M, Zargar MAA, Hashem-Dabagian F, Behbahani FA, Meyari A, Sadeghpour O. *Cicer arietinum* in the treatment of small renal stones: a doubl-blind, randomized and placebo-controlled trial. Res J Pharmacogn 2019; 6(1): 35-42.

[197] Noori S, Mahboob T. Role of electrolytes disturbances and Na(+)-K(+)-ATPase in cisplatin - induced renal toxicity and effects of ethanolic extract of *Cichorium intybus*. Pak J Pharm Sci 2012; 25(4): 857-62.
[PMID: 23010005]

[198] Ullah N, Khan MA, Khan T, Ahmad W. Protective effect of *Cinnamomum tamala* extract on gentamicin-induced nephritic damage in rabbits. Trop J Pharm Res 2013; 12(2): 215-9.

[199] Mishra A, Bhatti R, Singh A, Singh Ishar MP. Ameliorative effect of the cinnamon oil from *Cinnamomum zeylanicum* upon early stage diabetic nephropathy. Planta Med 2010; 76(5): 412-7.
[http://dx.doi.org/10.1055/s-0029-1186237] [PMID: 19876811]

[200] Ullah N, Khan M, Khan T, Ahmad W. Bioactive traditional plant *Cinnamomum zeylanicum* successfully combat against nephrotoxic effects of aminoglycosides. Bangladesh J Pharmacol 2013; 8:

15-21.
[http://dx.doi.org/10.3329/bjp.v8i1.12862]

[201] Reddy RCS, Swamy BMV, Swamy PA. Protective effect of *Cissampelos pareira* Linn. on paracetamol induced nephrotoxicity in male albino rats. Res J Pharm Biol Chem Sci 2012; 3(3): 695-705.

[202] Reddy DCS, Kumar GS, Swamy BV, Kumar KP. Protective effect of *Cissampelos pareira* Linn. extract on gentamicin-induced nephrotoxicity and oxidative damage in rats. Pharmacogn J 2014; 6: 59-67.
[http://dx.doi.org/10.5530/pj.2014.4.9]

[203] Sayana SB, Khanwelkar CC, Nimmagadda VR, Cavan VR. Antiurolithic activity of aqueous extract of roots of *Cissampelos pareira* in albino rats. Asian J Pharm Clin Res 2014; 7(3): 49-53.

[204] Amin HK. Effect of *Citrullus colocynthis* in ameliorating the oxidative stress and nephropathy in diabetic experimental rats. Intern J Pharmaceut Studies Res 2011; 2: 1-10.

[205] Komolafe OA, Ofusori DA, Adewole OS, Ajayi SA, Ijomone OM. Effects of four herbal plants on kidney histomorphology in STZ-induced diabetic Wistar rats. J Cytol Histol 2013; 5: 210.

[206] Ullah N, Khan MA, Asif AH, Khan T, Ahmad W. *Citrullus colocynthis* failed to combat against renal derangements, in spite of its strong antioxidant properties. Acta Pol Pharm 2013; 70(3): 533-8.
[PMID: 23757944]

[207] Ullah N, Khan MA, Khan T, Ahmad W. Nephroprotective potentials of *Citrus aurantium*: a prospective pharmacological study on experimental models. Pak J Pharm Sci 2014; 27(3): 505-10.
[PMID: 24811809]

[208] Joshi VS, Joshi MJ. Influence of inhibition of citric acid and lemon juice to the growth of calcium hydrogen phosphate dihydrate urinary crystals. Indian J Pure Appl Phy 2003; 41: 183-92.

[209] Touhami M, Laroubi A, Elhabazi K, *et al.* Lemon juice has protective activity in a rat urolithiasis model. BMC Urol 2007; 7: 18.
[http://dx.doi.org/10.1186/1471-2490-7-18] [PMID: 17919315]

[210] Kulaksizoğlu S, Sofikerim M, Cevik C. *in vitro* effect of lemon and orange juices on calcium oxalate crystallization. Int Urol Nephrol 2008; 40(3): 589-94.
[http://dx.doi.org/10.1007/s11255-007-9256-0] [PMID: 17721827]

[211] Chauhan CK, Joshi MJ. Growth inhibition of struvite crystals in the presence of juice of *Citrus medica* Linn. Urol Res 2008; 3695: 265-73.

[212] Shah AP, Patel SB, Patel KV, Gandhi TR. Effect of *Citrus medica* Linn. in urolithiasis induced by ethylene glycol model. Iranian J Phrmacol Therapeut 2014; 13: 35-9.

[213] Al-Yahya M, Mothana R, Al-Said M, Al-Dosari M, Al-Sohaibani M, Parvez MK, *et al.* Protective effect of *Citrus medica* 'otoroj' extract on gentamicin-induced nephrotoxicity and oxidative damage in rat kidney. Dig J Nanomater Biostruct 2015; 10: 19-29.

[214] Goldfarb DS, Asplin JR. Effect of grapefruit juice on urinary lithogenicity. J Urol 2001; 166(1): 263-7.
[http://dx.doi.org/10.1016/S0022-5347(05)66142-3] [PMID: 11435883]

[215] Trinchieri A, Lizzano R, Bernardini P, *et al.* Effect of acute load of grapefruit juice on urinary excretion of citrate and urinary risk factors for renal stone formation. Dig Liver Dis 2002; 34 (Suppl. 2): S160-3.
[http://dx.doi.org/10.1016/S1590-8658(02)80186-4] [PMID: 12408462]

[216] Hönow R, Laube N, Schneider A, Kessler T, Hesse A. Influence of grapefruit-, orange- and apple-juice consumption on urinary variables and risk of crystallization. Br J Nutr 2003; 90(2): 295-300.
[http://dx.doi.org/10.1079/BJN2003897] [PMID: 12908889]

[217] Poontawee W, Natakankitkul S, Wongmekiat O. Protective effect of *Cleistocalyx nervosum* var. *paniala* fruit extract against oxidative renal damage caused by cadmium. Molecules 2016; 21(2): 133.

[http://dx.doi.org/10.3390/molecules21020133] [PMID: 26805807]

[218] Upmanyu G, Tanu M, Gupta M, Gupta AK, Sushma A, Dhakar RC. Acute toxicity and diuretic studies of leaves of *Clerodendrum inerme*. J Pharm Res 2011; 4(5): 1431-2.

[219] Lu GW, Miura K, Yukimura T, Yamamoto K. Effects of extract from *Clerodendron trichotomum* on blood pressure and renal function in rats and dogs. J Ethnopharmacol 1994; 42(2): 77-82. [http://dx.doi.org/10.1016/0378-8741(94)90100-7] [PMID: 8072307]

[220] Piala JJ, Madissoo H, Rubin B. Diuretic activity of roots of *Clitoria ternatea* L. in dogs. Experientia 1962; 18(2): 89. [http://dx.doi.org/10.1007/BF02138275] [PMID: 14486285]

[221] Sarumathy K, Dhana M, Vijay T, Jayakanthi J. Evaluation of phytoconstituents, nephroprotective and antioxidant activities of *Clitoria ternatea*. J Appl Pharm Sci 2011; 1(5): 164-72.

[222] Devi KS, Damayanti M, Velmurugan D, Singh NR. Analysis of kidney stones by PXRD and evaluation of the antiurolithic potential of *Coix lacryma-jobi*. Int J Sci Res Publ 2015; 5: 1-5.

[223] Abou B, Felix YH, Edwige AKA, Nazaire DB. Evaluation of nephroprotective properties of aqueous and ethanolic extracts of *Gomphrena celosioides, Cola nitida* and *Entendrophragma angolense* against gentamicin induced renal dysfunction in the albino rats. Eur J Pharm Med Res 2016; 3(11): 62-9.

[224] Ghosh RB, Sur TK, Maity LN, Chakraborty SC. Antiurolithiatic activity of *Coleus aromaticus* benth in rats. Anc Sci Life 2000; 20(1-2): 44-7. [PMID: 22556997]

[225] Kpemissi M, Eklu-Gadegbeku K, Veerapur VP, *et al*. Nephroprotective activity of *Combretum micranthum* G. Don in cisplatin induced nephrotoxicity in rats: *in-vitro, in-vivo* and *in-silico* experiments. Biomed Pharmacother 2019a; 116: 108961. [http://dx.doi.org/10.1016/j.biopha.2019.108961] [PMID: 31146106]

[226] Kpemissi M, Eklu-Gadegbeku K, Veerapu VP, *et al*. Antioxidant and nephroprotection activities of Combretum micranthum: A phytochemical, in-vitro and exp-vivo studies. Helion 2019b' 5: e01365.

[227] Chauhan CK, Joshi MJ, Vaidya ADB. Growth inhibition of struvite crystals in the presence of herbal extract *Commiphora wightii*. J Mater Sci Mater Med 2009; 20 (Suppl. 1): S85-92. [http://dx.doi.org/10.1007/s10856-008-3489-z] [PMID: 18568390]

[228] Sharma V, Verma P. *Convolvulus arvensis* L. root extracts increase urine output and electrolytes in rats. Intern J Pharmaceut Res Dev 2011; 3(3): 193-7.

[229] Rajeshwari P, Rajeshwari G, Jabbirula SK, Vishnu VI. Evaluation of *in vitro* antiurolithiatic activity of *Convolvulus arvensis*. Int J Pharm Pharm Sci 2013; 5(3): 599-601.

[230] Brancalion AP, Oliveira RB, Sousa JP, *et al*. Effect of hydroalcoholic extract from *Copaifera langsdorffii* leaves on urolithiasis induced in rats. Urolithiasis 2012; 40(5): 475-81. [http://dx.doi.org/10.1007/s00240-011-0453-z] [PMID: 22237410]

[231] Aissaoui A, El-Hilaly J, Israili ZH, Lyoussi B. Acute diuretic effect of continuous intravenous infusion of an aqueous extract of *Coriandrum sativum* L. in anesthetized rats. J Ethnopharmacol 2008; 115(1): 89-95. [http://dx.doi.org/10.1016/j.jep.2007.09.007] [PMID: 17961943]

[232] Ezejiofor AN, Orish CN, Orisakwe OE. *Costus afer* ker gawl leaves against gentamicin-induced nephrotoxicity in rats. Iran J Kidney Dis 2014; 8(4): 310-3. [PMID: 25001137]

[233] de Cógáin MR, Linnes MP, Lee HJ, *et al*. Aqueous extract of *Costus arabicus* inhibits calcium oxalate crystal growth and adhesion to renal epithelial cells. Urolithiasis 2015; 43(2): 119-24. [http://dx.doi.org/10.1007/s00240-015-0749-5] [PMID: 25652357]

[234] Manjula K, Rajendran K, Eevera T, Kumaran S. Effect of *Costus igneus* stem extract on calcium oxalate urolithiasis in albino rats. Urol Res 2012; 40(5): 499-510.

[http://dx.doi.org/10.1007/s00240-012-0462-6] [PMID: 22298189]

[235] Mukadam M. Evaluation of anti–urolithiatic activity of *Costus igneus* and *Dolichos biflorus* Linn (horse gram) seeds. Glob J Res Anal 2019; 8(2): 49-51.

[236] Rajasekaran M. Nephroprotective effect of *Costus pictus* extract against doxorubicin-induced toxicity on Wistar rat. Bangladesh J Pharmacol 2019; 14(2): 93-100.
[http://dx.doi.org/10.3329/bjp.v14i2.39992]

[237] Araújo Viel T, Diogo Domingos C, da Silva Monteiro AP, Riggio Lima-Landman MT, Lapa AJ, Souccar C. Evaluation of the antiurolithiatic activity of the extract of *Costus spiralis* Roscoe in rats. J Ethnopharmacol 1999; 66(2): 193-8.
[http://dx.doi.org/10.1016/S0378-8741(98)00171-8] [PMID: 10433477]

[238] Gupta P, Patel N, Bhatt L, Zambare GN, Bodhankar SL, Jain BB, *et al.* Anti-urolithiatic effect of petroleum ether extract stem bark of *Crataeva adansonii* in rats. Pharm Biol 2006; 44(3): 160-5.
[http://dx.doi.org/10.1080/13880200600686400]

[239] Mekap SK, Mishra S, Sahoo S, Panda PK. Anturolithiatic activity of *Crataeva magna* Lour. bark. Indian J Nat Prod Resour 2011; 2(1): 28-33.

[240] Kumar P, Deshpande PJ, Singh LM. Clinical study with *Crataeva nurvala* in urinary tract infection. J Scientific Research in Plant Medicine 1982; 2(3): 75-9.

[241] Prabhakar YS, Kumar DS. The Varuna tree, *Crataeva nurvala*, a promising plant in the treatment of urinary stones-A review. Fitoterapia 1990; 61(2): 99-111.

[242] Varalakshmi P, Shamila Y, Latha E. Effect of *Crataeva nurvala* in experimental urolithiasis. J Ethnopharmacol 1990; 28(3): 313-21.
[http://dx.doi.org/10.1016/0378-8741(90)90082-5] [PMID: 2335959]

[243] Varalakshmi P, Latha E, Shamila Y, Jayanthi S. Effect of *Crataeva nurvala* on the biochemistry of the small intestinal tract of normal and stone-forming rats. J Ethnopharmacol 1991; 31(1): 67-73.
[http://dx.doi.org/10.1016/0378-8741(91)90145-4] [PMID: 1827653]

[244] Singh PP, Hussain F, Ghosh R, Ahmed A, Gupta RC. Effect of simultaneous sodium oxalate and methionine feeding with and without varuna (*Crataeva nurvala* Hook. & Forst) therapy on urolithiogenesis in guinea pigs. Indian J Clin Biochem 1992; 7: 23-6.
[http://dx.doi.org/10.1007/BF02867698]

[245] Shirwaikar A, Setty M, Bommu P. Effect of lupeol isolated from *Crataeva nurvala* Buch.-Ham. stem bark extract against free radical induced nephrotoxicity in rats. Indian J Exp Biol 2004; 42(7): 686-90.
[PMID: 15339033]

[246] Shirwaikar A, Manjunath SM, Bommu P, Krishnand B. Ethanolic extract of *Crataeva nurvala* stem bark reverses cisplatin-induced nephrotoxicity. Indian J Exp Biol 2004; 42(7): 559-64.
[PMID: 15339033]

[247] Agarwal S, Gupta Sj, Saxena AK, Gupta N, Agarwal S. Urolithiatic property of Varuna (*Crataeva nurvala*): An experimental study. Ayu 201; 31(3): 361-6.

[248] Shelkea TT, Bhaskarb VH, Adkara PP, Jhaa U, Oswala RJ. Nephroprotective activity of ethanolic extract of stem barks of *Crataeva nurvula* Buch Hum. Int J Pharm Sci Res 2011; 2(10): 2712.

[249] Meher SK, Chaudhuri SB, Marjit B, Mukherjee PK, Ram AK, Munshi S, *et al.* Nephroprotective action of *T. terrestris* Linn. and *Crataeva nurvala* Buchman in Albino rats. Indian J Pharmacol 2001; 33: 124-45.

[250] Bienvenu KF, Cyril DG, Florian YB, Felix YH, Timothée OA. Evaluation of nephroprotective properties of aqueous and hydroethanolic extracts of *Crinum scillifolium* against gentamicin induced renal dysfunction in the albino rats. J Adv Med Med Res 2019; 30(1): 1-10.
[http://dx.doi.org/10.9734/jammr/2019/v30i130160]

[251] Hosseinzadeh H, Sadeghnia HR, Ziaee T, Danaee A. Protective effect of aqueous saffron extract

(*Crocus sativus* L.) and crocin, its active constituent, on renal ischemia-reperfusion-induced oxidative damage in rats. J Pharm Pharm Sci 2005; 8(3): 387-93.
[PMID: 16401388]

[252]   Ajami M, Eghtesadi S, Pazoki-Toroudi H, Habibey R, Ebrahimi SA. Effect of *Crocus sativus* on gentamicin induced nephrotoxicity. Biol Res 2010; 43(1): 83-90.
[http://dx.doi.org/10.4067/S0716-97602010000100010] [PMID: 21157635]

[253]   Bandegi AR, Rashidy-Pour A, Vafaei AA, Ghadrdoost B. Protective effects of *Crocus sativus* L extract and crocin against chronic-stress induced oxidative damage of brain, liver and kidneys in rats. Adv Pharm Bull 2014; 4 (Suppl. 2): 493-9.
[PMID: 25671180]

[254]   el Daly ES. Protective effect of cysteine and vitamin E, *Crocus sativus* and *Nigella sativa* extracts on cisplatin-induced toxicity in rats. J Pharm Belg 1998; 53(2): 87-93.
[PMID: 9609969]

[255]   Okokon JE, Nwafor PA, Noah K. Nephroprotective effect of *Croton zambesicus* root extract against gentimicin-induced kidney injury. Asian Pac J Trop Med 2011; 4(12): 969-72.
[http://dx.doi.org/10.1016/S1995-7645(11)60228-9] [PMID: 22118033]

[256]   Pethakar SR, Hurkadale PJ, Hiremath RD. Evaluation of antiurolithiatic potentials of hydro-alcoholic extract of *Cucumis sativus* L. Indian J Pharmaceut Education Res 2017; 51: S607-13.
[http://dx.doi.org/10.5530/ijper.51.4s.89]

[257]   Balakrishnan A, Kokilavani R, Gurusamy K, Teepa KSA, Sathya M. Effect of ethanolic fruit extract of *Cucumis trigonus* Roxb. on antioxidants and lipid peroxidation in urolithiasis induced wistar albino rats. Anc Sci Life 2011; 31(1): 10-6.
[PMID: 22736884]

[258]   Abdel-Hady H, El-Sayed MM, Abdel-Hady AA, Hashah MM, Abdel-Hady AM, Aoushousha T, *et al.* Nephroprotective activityof methanolic extract of *Lantana camara* and squash (*Cucurbita pepo*) on cisplatin-induced nephrotxicity in rts and identification of certan chemical constituents of *Lantana camara* by HPLC-ESI-MS. Pharmacogn J 2018; 10(1): 136-47.
[http://dx.doi.org/10.5530/pj.2018.1.24]

[259]   Shehzad A, Saleem U, Shah MA. Vargas-de la Cruz, Khan AH, Ahmad B. Antiurolithiatic evaluation of *Cucurbita pepo* seds extract against sodium oxalate-induced renal calculi. Pharmacogn Mag 2020; 16: S174-80.
[http://dx.doi.org/10.4103/pm.pm_166_19]

[260]   Mahesh CM, Gowda KP, Gupta AK. Protective action of *Cuminum cyminum* against gentamicin induced nephrotoxicity. Pak J Pharm Sci 2010; 3(4): 753-7.

[261]   Jayasuda A. Anti-urolithiatic and antioxidant activity of fruit extract of *Cuminum cyminum* linn in rats. MPharm Dissertation, Rajv Gandhi University of Health Sciences, Bangalore 2011.

[262]   Kumar A, Singh JK, Ali M, *et al.* Evaluation of *Cuminum cyminum* and *Coriandrum sativum* on profenofos induced nephrotoxicity in Swiss albino mice. Elixir Applied Botany 2011; 39: 4771-3.

[263]   Kumar R, Ali M, Kumar A. Nephroprotective effect of *Cuminum cyminum* on chloropyrifos induced kidney of mice. Adv J Pharm Life sci Res, 2014; 2(4): 46-53.

[264]   Elhabib EM, Homeida MMA, Adam SEI. Effect of combined paracetamol and *Cuminum cyminum* or *Nigella sativa* used in Wistar Rats. J Pharmacol Toxicol 2007; 2: 653-9.
[http://dx.doi.org/10.3923/jpt.2007.653.659]

[265]   Venu A, Sandhyarani G, Purnachander M. Effect of fruit of *Cuminum cyminum* on ethylene glycol (eg) induced urolithiasis in rats. European J Biomed Pharmaceut Sci 2017; 4(8): 338-51.

[266]   Khorsandi L, Orazizadeh M. Protective effect of *Curcuma longa* extract on acetaminophen induced nephrotoxicity in mice. Daru 2008; 16: 155-9.

[267] Thuawaini MM, Kadhem HS, Al-Dierawi KH. Nephroprotective activity of *Matricaria chamomile* and *Curcuma longa* aqueous extracts on tetracycline – induced nephro-toxicity in albino rats. Int J Pharm Ther 2016; 7: 161-7.

[268] Thuawaini MM, Al-Farhan MBG, Abbas KF. Hepatoprotective and nephroprotecitve effects of aqueous extract of turmeric (*Curcuma longa*) in rifampicin and isoniazid-induced hepatotoxicity and nephrotoxicity in rats. Asian J Pharm Clin Res 2019; 12(3): 293-8.
[http://dx.doi.org/10.22159/ajpcr.2019.v12i3.30419]

[269] Pathak NN, Rajurkar SR, Tarekh S, Badgire VV. Nephroprotective efects of carvedilol and *Curcuma longa* against cisplatin-induced nephrotoxicity in rats. Asian J Med Sci 2014; 5(2): 91-8.
[http://dx.doi.org/10.3126/ajms.v5i2.5483]

[270] Ademiluyi AO, Oboh G, Ogunsuyi OB, Akinyemi AJ. Attenuation of gentamycin-induced nephrotoxicity in rats by dietary inclusion of ginger (*Zingiber officinale*) and turmeric (*Curcuma longa*) rhizomes. Nutr Health 2012; 21(4): 209-18.
[http://dx.doi.org/10.1177/0260106013506668] [PMID: 24197862]

[271] Rosita Y. Marianne. Nephroprotective activity of ethanol extract of *Curcuma mangga* Val. in paracetamol-induced male mice. Asian J Pharm Clin Res 2018; 11(13): 126-8.
[http://dx.doi.org/10.22159/ajpcr.2018.v11s1.26585]

[272] Murthy RLN, Nataraj H, Ramachandra Setty S. Nephroprotective activity of *Cyanotis fasciculata* against cisplatin induced nephroprotoxicity. Int Res J Pharm 2011; 2(9): 137-42.

[273] Christina AJ, Packia Lakshmi M, Nagarajan M, Kurian S. Modulatory effect of *Cyclea peltata* Lam. on stone formation induced by ethylene glycol treatment in rats. Methods Find Exp Clin Pharmacol 2002; 24(2): 77-9.
[http://dx.doi.org/10.1358/mf.2002.24.2.677130] [PMID: 12040886]

[274] Vijayan FP, Rani VK, Vineesh VR, Sudha KS, Michael MM, Padikkala J. Protective effect of *Cyclea peltata* Lam on cisplatin-induced nephrotoxicity and oxidative damage. J Basic Clin Physiol Pharmacol 2007; 18(2): 101-14.
[http://dx.doi.org/10.1515/JBCPP.2007.18.2.101] [PMID: 17715566]

[275] Ullah N, Khan MA, Khan T, Ahmad W. *Cymbopogon citratus* protects against the renal injury induced by toxic doses of aminoglycosides in rabbits. Indian J Pharm Sci 2013; 75(2): 241-6.
[PMID: 24019578]

[276] Al Haznawi AM, Attar AS, Abdulshakoor AA, Ramadan MA. Inhibition of calcium oxalate nephrotoxicity with *Cymbopogon schenanthus* (Al-Ethkher). M.Sc. thesis, Faculty of Applied Medical Sciences, Saudi Arabia. 2007.

[277] Atmani F, Sadki C, Aziz M, Mimouni M, Hacht B. *Cynodon dactylon* extract as a preventive and curative agent in experimentally induced nephrolithiasis. Urol Res 2009; 37(2): 75-82.
[http://dx.doi.org/10.1007/s00240-009-0174-8] [PMID: 19183977]

[278] Mousa-Al-Reza H, Rad AK, Rajaei Z, Sadeghian MH, Hashemi N, Keshavarzi Z. Preventive effect of *Cynodon dactylon* against ethylene glycol-induced nephrolithiasis in male rats. Avicenna J Phytomed 2011; 1(1): 14-23.

[279] Khajavi Rad A, Hadjzadeh MAR, Rajaei Z, Mohammadian N, Valiollahi S, Sonei M. The beneficial effect of *Cynodon dactylon* fractions on ethylene glycol-induced kidney calculi in rats. Urol J 2011; 8(3): 179-84.
[PMID: 21910095]

[280] Pinakin DJ, Sohin KZ, Jaydip VG, Manish AR. Evaluation of antiurolithalic activity of *Cyperus rotundus* Linn. rhizomes in rats. Inventi Rapid. Ethnopharmacology 2013; 2013(3): 1-6.

[281] Narware SK, Maithili V, Senthilkumar KL. Protective effect of *Dalbergia sisso* bark on hepatotoxicityand nephrotoxicity in albino rat. IOSR J Pharm 2012; 2(3): 410-28.

[282] Mital PR, Laxman PJ, Rameshvar PK. Protective effect of *Daucus carota* root extract against ischemia reperfusion injury in rats. Pharmacology 2011; 1: 432-9.

[283] Afzal M, Kazmi I, Kaur R, Ahmad A, Pravez M, Anwar F. Comparison of protective and curative potential of *Daucus carota* root extract on renal ischemia reperfusion injury in rats. Pharm Biol 2013; 51(7): 856-62.
[http://dx.doi.org/10.3109/13880209.2013.767840] [PMID: 23627465]

[284] Sodimbaku V, Pujari L, Mullangi R, Marri S. Carrot (*Daucus carota* L.): Nephroprotective against gentamicin-induced nephrotoxicity in rats. Indian J Pharmacol 2016; 48(2): 122-7.
[http://dx.doi.org/10.4103/0253-7613.178822] [PMID: 27127313]

[285] Pullaiah CP, Kedam T, Nelson VK, Kumar GVN, Reddy GD. Supplementation of *Daucus carota* L. extract prevents urolithiasis in experimental rats. Indian J Nat Prod Resour 2018; 9(3): 253-60.

[286] Kim E-S, Lee J-S, Akram M, *et al.* Protective activity of *Dendropanax morbifera* against cisplatin-induced acute kidney injury. Kidney Blood Press Res 2015; 40(1): 1-12.
[http://dx.doi.org/10.1159/000368466] [PMID: 25661683]

[287] Hirayama H, Wang Z, Nishi K, *et al.* Effect of *Desmodium styracifolium*-triterpenoid on calcium oxalate renal stones. Br J Urol 1993; 71(2): 143-7.
[http://dx.doi.org/10.1111/j.1464-410X.1993.tb15906.x] [PMID: 8461944]

[288] Xiang S, Zhou J, Li J, *et al.* Antilithic effects of extracts from different polarity fractions of *Desmodium styracifolium* on experimentally induced urolithiasis in rats. Urolithiasis 2015; 43(5): 433-9.
[http://dx.doi.org/10.1007/s00240-015-0795-z] [PMID: 26123751]

[289] Zhou J, Jin J, Li X, *et al.* Total flavonoids of *Desmodium styracifolium* attenuates the formation of hydroxy-L-proline-induced calcium oxalate urolithiasis in rats. Urolithiasis 2018; 46(3): 231-41.
[http://dx.doi.org/10.1007/s00240-017-0985-y] [PMID: 28567512]

[290] Jayakumari S, Anbu J. Ravi chandran V. Antiurolithiatic activity of *Dichrostachys cinerea* L. Wight & Arn. root extract. J Pharm Res 2011; 4(4): 1206-8.

[291] Sreedevi A, Bharathi K, Prasad KVSRG. Effect of alcoholic extract of root of *Dichrostachys cinerea* Wight & Arn. against cisplatin-induced nephrotoxicity in rats. Nat Prod Radiance 2009; 8(1): 12-8.

[292] Khan MR, Rizvi W, Khan GN, Khan RA, Shaheen S. Carbon tetrachloride-induced nephrotoxicity in rats: protective role of *Digera muricata*. J Ethnopharmacol 2009; 122(1): 91-9.
[http://dx.doi.org/10.1016/j.jep.2008.12.006] [PMID: 19118616]

[293] Moghaddam AH, Nabavi SM, Nabavi SF, Bigdellou R, Mohammadzadeh S, Ebrahimzadeh MA. Antioxidant, antihemolytic and nephroprotective activity of aqueous extract of *Diospyros lotus* seeds. Acta Pol Pharm 2012; 69(4): 687-92.
[PMID: 22876611]

[294] Peshin A, Singla SK. Anticalcifying properties of *Dolichos biflorus* (horse gram) seeds. Indian J Exp Biol 1994; 32(12): 889-91.
[PMID: 7896323]

[295] Garimella TS, Jolly CI, Narayanan S. *in vitro* studies on antilithiatic activity of seeds of *Dolichos biflorus* Linn. and rhizomes of *Bergenia ligulata* Wall. Phytother Res 2001; 15(4): 351-5.
[http://dx.doi.org/10.1002/ptr.833] [PMID: 11406861]

[296] Bijarnia RK, Kaur T, Singla SK, Tandon C. A novel calcium oxalate crystal growth inhibitory protein from the seeds of *Dolichos biflorus* (L.). Protein J 2009; 28(3-4): 161-8.
[http://dx.doi.org/10.1007/s10930-009-9179-y] [PMID: 19488841]

[297] Atodariya U, Roshni B, Siddhi U, Umesh U. Antiurolithiatic activity of *Dolichos biflorus* seeds. J Pharmacogn Phytochem 2013; 2(2): 209-21.

[298] Saha S, Verma RJ. Antinephrolithiatic and antioxidative efficacy of *Dolichos biflorus* seeds in a

lithiasic rat model. Pharm Biol 2015; 53(1): 16-30.
[http://dx.doi.org/10.3109/13880209.2014.909501] [PMID: 25243879]

[299] Deoda RS, Pandya H, Patel M, Yadav KN, Kadam PV, Patil MJ. Antilithiatic activity of leaves, bulb and stem of *Nymphea odorata* and *Dolichos lablab* beans. Res J Pharm Biol Chem Sci 2012; 3(1): 814-9.

[300] Long M, Qiu D, Li F, Johnson F, Luft B. Flavonoid of Drynaria fortunei protects against acute renal failure. Phytother Res 2005; 19(5): 422-7.
[http://dx.doi.org/10.1002/ptr.1606] [PMID: 16106396]

[301] Mustea I, Postesu D, Tamas M, Rasnita TD. Experimental evaluation of protective activity of *Echinacea pallida* against cisplatin toxicity. Phytother Res 1997; 11(3): 263-5.
[http://dx.doi.org/10.1002/(SICI)1099-1573(199705)11:3<263::AID-PTR77>3.0.CO;2-0]

[302] Portella VG, Cosenza GP, Diniz LRL, *et al.* Nephroprotective effect of *Echinodorus macrophyllus* Micheli on gentamicin induced nephrotoxicity in rats. Nephron Extra 2012; 2(1): 177-83.
[http://dx.doi.org/10.1159/000339181] [PMID: 22811691]

[303] Dungca NTP. Protective effect of the methanolic leaf extract of *Eclipta alba* (L.) Hassk. (Asteraceae) against gentamicin-induced nephrotoxicity in Sprague Dawley rats. J Ethnopharmacol 2016; 184: 18-21.
[http://dx.doi.org/10.1016/j.jep.2016.03.002] [PMID: 26945981]

[304] Ahmad F, Al-Subaie AM, Al-Ohalai AI, Mohammed AS. Phytochemical and nephroprotective activity of *Eclipta prostrata* against gentamicin-induced nephrotoxicity in Wistar rats. Int J Pharma Res Health Sci 2018; 6: 2559-64.

[305] Kakalij RM, Alla CP, Kshirsagar RP, Kumar BH, Mutha SS, Diwan PV. Ameliorative effect of *Elaeocarpus ganitrus* on gentamicin-induced nephrotoxicity in rats. Indian J Pharmacol 2014; 46(3): 298-302.
[http://dx.doi.org/10.4103/0253-7613.132163] [PMID: 24987177]

[306] Sahoo HB, Swain SR, Nandy S, Sagar R, Bhaiji A. Nephroprotective activity of ethanolic extract of *Elephantophus scaber* leaves on albino rats. Int Res J Pharm 2012; 3(5): 246-50.

[307] Kumari S, Dutta A, Farooqui S, *et al.* Nephrotoxicity induced by pan masala in Swiss mice and its protection by *Elettaria cardamomum* (L.) Maton. Int J Pharm Biol Sci 2013; 3(1): 231-8.

[308] Sanjuna C, Prasad M, Anjali M, *et al.* Evaluation of *in vitro* anti-urolithiatic activity of *Elettaria cardamomum*. World J Gastroenterol Hepatol Endosc 2019d; 1(1) WJGHE-1-111

[309] Bahuguna YM, Rawat MSM, Juyal V, Gnanarajan G. Antilithiatic effect of grains of *Eleusine coracana*. Saudi Pharm J 2009; 17(2): 182-8.

[310] Grases F, Ramis M, Costa-Bauzá A, March JG. Effect of *Herniaria hirsuta* and *Agropyron repens* on calcium oxalate urolithiasis risk in rats. J Ethnopharmacol 1995; 45(3): 211-4.
[http://dx.doi.org/10.1016/0378-8741(94)01218-O] [PMID: 7623486]

[311] Bhatt NM, Chauhan K, Gupta S, *et al.* Protective effect of *Enicostemma littorale* Blume methanolic extract on gentamicin-induced nephrotoxicity in rats. Am J Infect Dis 2011; 7: 83-90.
[http://dx.doi.org/10.3844/ajidsp.2011.83.90]

[312] Carneiro DM, Freire RC, Honório TC, *et al.* Randomized, double-blind clinical trial to assess the acute diuretic effect of *Equisetum arvense* (field horsetail) in healthy volunteers. Evid Based Complement Alternat Med 2014; 2014: 760683.
[http://dx.doi.org/10.1155/2014/760683] [PMID: 24723963]

[313] Sarwar Alam M, Kaur G, Jabbar Z, Javed K, Athar M. *Eruca sativa* seeds possess antioxidant activity and exert a protective effect on mercuric chloride induced renal toxicity. Food Chem Toxicol 2007; 45(6): 910-20.
[http://dx.doi.org/10.1016/j.fct.2006.11.013] [PMID: 17207565]

[314] Feyissa T, Asres K, Engidawork E. Renoprotective effects of the crude extract and solvent fractions of the leaves of *Euclea divinorum* Hierns against gentamicin-induced nephrotoxicity in rats. J Ethnopharmacol 2013; 145(3): 758-66.
[http://dx.doi.org/10.1016/j.jep.2012.12.006] [PMID: 23228914]

[315] Suganya S, Ragavendran P, Rajalakshmymenon B, Rathi MA, Thirumoorthi L, Meenakshi P, *et al.* Potential effect of *Euphorbia hirta* against nitrobenzene-induced nephrotoxicity. Pharmacol Online 2010; 2: 963-70.

[316] Suganya S, Sophia D, Raj CA, *et al.* Amelioration of nitrobenzene-induced nephrotoxicity by the ethanol extract of the herb *Euphorbia hirta.* Pharmacognosy Res 2011; 3(3): 201-7.
[http://dx.doi.org/10.4103/0974-8490.85009] [PMID: 22022170]

[317] Johnson PB, Abdurahman EM, Tiam EA, Abdu-Aguye I, Hussaini IM. *Euphorbia hirta* leaf extracts increase urine output and electrolytes in rats. J Ethnopharmacol 1999; 65(1): 63-9.
[http://dx.doi.org/10.1016/S0378-8741(98)00143-3] [PMID: 10350369]

[318] Pracheta P, Sharma V, Singh L, *et al.* Chemopreventive effect of hydroethanolic extract of *Euphorbia neriifolia* leaves against DENA-induced renal carcinogenesis in mice. Asian Pac J Cancer Prev 2011; 12(3): 677-83.
[PMID: 21627363]

[319] Chinnappan SM, George A, Thaggikuppe P, Choudhary YK, Choudhary VK, Ramani Y, *et al.* Nephroprotective effect of herbal extract *Eurycoma longifolia* on paracetamol-induced nephrotoxicity in rats. Evid Based Complement Alternat Med 2019; 2019: 1-6.
[http://dx.doi.org/10.1155/2019/4916519]

[320] Sharma S, Modi A, Narayan G, Hemalatha S. Protective effect of *Exacum lawii* on cisplatin-induced oxidative renal damage in rats. Pharmacogn Mag 2018; 13 (Suppl. 4): S807-16.
[PMID: 29491637]

[321] Perez RMG, Vargas RS, Perez SG, Zavala MS. Anti-urolithiatic activity of *Eysenhardtia polystachya* aqueous extract on rats. Phytother Res 1998; 12: 144-5.
[http://dx.doi.org/10.1002/(SICI)1099-1573(199803)12:2<144::AID-PTR202>3.0.CO;2-H]

[322] Kore K, Shete R, Kale B, Borade A. Protective role of hydroalcoholic extract of *Ficus carica* in gentamicin induced nephrotoxicity in rats. Int J Pharm Life Sci 2011; 2: 978-82.

[323] Irene II, Iheanacho UA. Acute effect of administration of ethanol extracts of *Ficus exasperata* Vahl on kidney function in albino rats. J Med Plants Res 2007; 1: 27-9.

[324] Swathi N, Sreedevi A, Bharathi K. Evaluation of nephroprotective activity of fruits of *Ficus hispida* on cisplatin-induced nephrotoxicity. Pharmacogn J 2011; 3: 62-8.
[http://dx.doi.org/10.5530/pj.2011.22.12]

[325] Khan N, Sultana S. Chemomodulatory effect of *Ficus racemosa* extract against chemically induced renal carcinogenesis and oxidative damage response in Wistar rats. Life Sci 2005; 77(11): 1194-210.
[http://dx.doi.org/10.1016/j.lfs.2004.12.041] [PMID: 15885707]

[326] Gowda KPS, Swamy BMV. Histopathological and nephroprotective study of aqueous stem bark extract of *Ficus racemosa* in drug induced nephrotoxic rats. IOSR J Pharm 2012; 2(2): 265-70.
[http://dx.doi.org/10.9790/3013-0220265270]

[327] Yadav YC, Srivastava DN. Nephroprotective and curative effects of *Ficus religiosa* latex extract against cisplatin-induced acute renal failure. Pharm Biol 2013; 51(11): 1480-5.
[http://dx.doi.org/10.3109/13880209.2013.793718] [PMID: 23870082]

[328] Hashmi N, Muhammad F, Javed I, *et al.* Nephroprotective effects of *Ficus religiosa* Linn. (peepal plant) stem bark against isoniazid and rifampicin-induced nephrotoxicity in albino rabbits. Pak Vet J 2013; 33: 330-4.

[329] Musabayane CT, Gondwe M, Kamadyaapa DR, Chuturgoon AA, Ojewole JAO. Effects of *Ficus*

thonningii (Blume) [Morarceae] stem-bark ethanolic extract on blood glucose, cardiovascular and kidney functions of rats, and on kidney cell lines of the proximal (LLC-PK1) and distal tubules (MDBK). Ren Fail 2007; 29(4): 389-97.
[http://dx.doi.org/10.1080/08860220701260735] [PMID: 17497459]

[330] Tanira MOM, Shah AH, Mohsin A, Ageel AM, Qureshi S. Pharmacological and toxicological investigations on *Foeniculum vulgare* dried fruit extract in experimental animals. Phytother Res 1996; 10: 33-6.
[http://dx.doi.org/10.1002/(SICI)1099-1573(199602)10:1<33::AID-PTR769>3.0.CO;2-L]

[331] Shaheen U, Manzoor Z, Khaliq T, Kanwal T, Muhammad F, Hassan IJ, *et al.* Evaluation of nephroprotective effects of *Foeniculum vulgare* Mill, *Solanum nigrum* Linn. and their mixture against gentamicin-induced nephrotoxicity in albino rats. Int J Pharm Sci Rev Res 2014; 25: 1-9.

[332] Jemal A. Evaluation of diuretic activity of aqueous and 80% methanol extracts of *Foeniculum vulgare* Mill (Apiaceae) leaf in rats. M.Sc. thesis, Addis Ababa University. 2015.

[333] Sadrefozalayi S, Farokhi F. Effect of the aqueous extract of *Foeniculum vulgare* (fennel) on the kidney in experimental PCOS female rats. Avicenna J Phytomed 2014; 4(2): 110-7.
[PMID: 25050308]

[334] Mazaheri S, Nematbakhsh M, Bahadorani M, *et al.* Effects of fennel essential oil on cisplatin-induced nephrotoxicity in ovariectomized rats. Toxicol Int 2013; 20(2): 138-45.
[http://dx.doi.org/10.4103/0971-6580.117256] [PMID: 24082507]

[335] Komolafe IJ, Akinlalu AO, Ogunsusi MO, Oluboade O. Protective effects of extract and fraction of root- bark of *Garcinia kola* (Heckel) on the renal biochemical parameters of gentamicin-induced nephrotoxic rats. Afr J Biochem Res 2016; 10(5): 30-7.
[http://dx.doi.org/10.5897/AJBR2016.0890]

[336] Inselmann G, Blöhmer A, Kottny W, Nellessen U, Hänel H, Heidemann HT. Modification of cisplatin-induced renal *p*-aminohippurate uptake alteration and lipid peroxidation by thiols, *Ginkgo biloba* extract, deferoxamine and torbafylline. Nephron J 1995; 70(4): 425-9.
[http://dx.doi.org/10.1159/000188640] [PMID: 7477647]

[337] Naidu MUR, Shifow AA, Kumar KV, Ratnakar KS. *Ginkgo biloba* extract ameliorates gentamicin-induced nephrotoxicity in rats. Phytomedicine 2000; 7(3): 191-7.
[http://dx.doi.org/10.1016/S0944-7113(00)80003-3] [PMID: 11185729]

[338] Okuyan B, Izzettin FV, Bingöl-Ozakpinar Ö, Turan P, Ozdemir ZN, Sancar M, *et al.* The effects of *Ginkgo biloba* on nephrotoxicity induced by cisplatin-based chemotherapy protocols in rats. IUFS J Biol 2012; 71: 103-11.

[339] Song J, Liu D, Feng L, Zhang Z, Jia X, Xiao W. Protective effect of standardized extract of *Ginkgo biloba* against Cisplatin-induced nephrotoxicity. Evid Based Complement Alternat Med 2013; 2013: 846126.
[http://dx.doi.org/10.1155/2013/846126] [PMID: 24371467]

[340] Liang Q, Li X, Zhou W, *et al.* An explanation of the underlying mechanisms for the *in vitro* and *in vivo* antiurolithic activity of *Glechoma longituba*. Oxid Med Cell Longev 2016; 2016(1): 3134919.
[http://dx.doi.org/10.1155/2016/3134919] [PMID: 27840669]

[341] Vijaya T, Nallani Rama RV. Antiurolithiatic activity of methanolic extract of dried leaves of *Glochidion velutinum* using ethylene glycol induced rats. Int J Biol Pharm Res 2013; 4(12): 878-84.

[342] El-Sayed NH, Awaad AS, Mabry TJ. Phytochemical studies and effect on urine volume of *Glossostemon bruguieri* Desf. constituents. Indian J Exp Biol 2004; 42(2): 186-9.
[PMID: 15282952]

[343] Ekor M, Farombi EO, Emerole GO. Modulation of gentamicin-induced renal dysfunction and injury by the phenolic extract of soybean (*Glycine max*). Fundam Clin Pharmacol 2006; 20(3): 263-71.
[http://dx.doi.org/10.1111/j.1472-8206.2006.00407.x] [PMID: 16671961]

[344] Ekor M, Emerole GO, Farombi EO. Phenolic extract of soybean (*Glycine max*) attenuates cisplatin-induced nephrotoxicity in rats. Food Chem Toxicol 2010; 48(4): 1005-12.
[http://dx.doi.org/10.1016/j.fct.2009.12.027] [PMID: 20109512]

[345] Ramasamy A, Jothivel N, Das S, *et al.* Evaluation of the protective role of *Glycine max* seed extract (soybean oil) in drug-induced nephrotoxicity in experimental rats. J Diet Suppl 2018; 15(5): 583-95.
[http://dx.doi.org/10.1080/19390211.2017.1358792] [PMID: 28956655]

[346] Narasimha DK, Reddy KR, Jayaveera KN, Bharathi T, Vrushabendra S, Rajkumar BM. Study on the diuretic activity of *Gossypium herbaceum* Linn leaves extract in albino rats. Pharmacologyonline 2008; 1: 78-81.

[347] Babu PV, Krishna MV, Ashwini T, Raju MG. Antilithiatic activity of *Grewia asiatica* in male rats. Int J Pharm Sci Res 2017; 8(3): 1326-35.

[348] Sree Lakshmi K, Prabhakaran V, Mallikarjuna G, Gowthami A. Antilithiatic activity of *Trianthema portulacastrum* L. and *Gymnema sylvestre* R.Br. against ethylene glycol induced urolithiasis. Int J Pharm Sci Rev Res 2014; 25(1): 16-22.

[349] Adeneye A, Olagunju J, Benebo AS, Elias SO, Adisa AO, Idowu BO, *et al.* Nephroprotective effects of the aqueous root extract of *Harungana madagascariensis* L. in acute and repeated dose acetaminophen renal injured rats. Int J Appl Res Nat Prod 2008; 1(1): 6-14.

[350] Tailor CS, Goyal A. Isolation of phyto constituents and *in vitro* anti lithiatic by titrimetric method, antioxidant activity by 1, 1-Diphenyl-2-Picryl hydrazyl scavenging assay method of alcoholic roots and rhizomes extract of *Hedychium coronarium* J.Koenig plant species. Asian J Pharm Clin Res 2015; 8(4): 225-9.

[351] Khan NI, Shenge JS, Naikwade NS. Antilithiatic effect of *Helianthus annuus* Linn. leaf extract in ethylene glycol and ammonium chloride induced nephrolithiasis. Int J Pharm Pharm Sci 2010; 2(4): 180-4.

[352] Musabayane CT, Munjeri O, Mdege ND. Effects of *Helichrysum ceres* extracts on renal function and blood pressure in the rat. Ren Fail 2003; 25(1): 5-14.
[http://dx.doi.org/10.1081/JDI-120017438] [PMID: 12617328]

[353] Onaran M, Orhan N, Farahvash A, *et al.* Successful treatment of sodium oxalate induced urolithiasis with *Helichrysum* flowers. J Ethnopharmacol 2016; 186: 322-8.
[http://dx.doi.org/10.1016/j.jep.2016.04.003] [PMID: 27085940]

[354] Bayir Y, Halici Z, Keles MS, *et al.* Helichrysum plicatum DC. subsp. plicatum extract as a preventive agent in experimentally induced urolithiasis model. J Ethnopharmacol 2011; 138(2): 408-14.
[http://dx.doi.org/10.1016/j.jep.2011.09.026] [PMID: 21963562]

[355] Sharma SK, Goyal N. Protective effect of *Heliotropium eichwaldi* against cisplatin-induced nephrotoxicity in mice. J Chin Integr Med 2012; 10(5): 555-60.
[http://dx.doi.org/10.3736/jcim20120511] [PMID: 22587978]

[356] Kotnis MS, Patel P, Menon SN, Sane RT. Renoprotective effect of *Hemidesmus indicus*, a herbal drug used in gentamicin-induced renal toxicity. Nephrology (Carlton) 2004; 9(3): 142-52.
[http://dx.doi.org/10.1111/j.1440-1797.2004.00247.x] [PMID: 15189175]

[357] Kaur A, Singh S, Shirwaikar A, Manjunath Setty M. Effect of ethanolic extract of *Hemidesmus indicus* roots on cisplatin induced nephrotoxicity in rats. J Pharm Res 2011; 4(8): 2523-5.

[358] Atmani F, Khan SR. Effects of an extract from *Herniaria hirsuta* on calcium oxalate crystallization *in vitro*. BJU Int 2000; 85(6): 621-5.
[http://dx.doi.org/10.1046/j.1464-410x.2000.00485.x] [PMID: 10759652]

[359] Atmani F, Farell G, Lieske JC. Extract from *Herniaria hirsuta* coats calcium oxalate monohydrate crystals and blocks their adhesion to renal epithelial cells. J Urol 2004; 172(4 Pt 1): 1510-4.
[http://dx.doi.org/10.1097/01.ju.0000131004.03795.c5] [PMID: 15371881]

[360] Atmani F, Slimani Y, Mimouni M, Aziz M, Hacht B, Ziyyat A. Effect of aqueous extract from *Herniaria hirsuta* L. on experimentally nephrolithiasic rats. J Ethnopharmacol 2004; 95(1): 87-93. b
[http://dx.doi.org/10.1016/j.jep.2004.06.028] [PMID: 15374612]

[361] Atmani F, Slimani Y, Mimouni M, Hacht B. Prophylaxis of calcium oxalate stones by *Herniaria hirsuta* on experimentally induced nephrolithiasis in rats. BJU Int 2003; 92(1): 137-40.
[http://dx.doi.org/10.1046/j.1464-410X.2003.04289.x] [PMID: 12823398]

[362] Atmani F, Yamina S, Nait MA, Mohammed B, Abdlekrim R. *in vitro* and *in vivo* antilithiatic effect of saponin rich fraction isolated from *Herniaria hirsuta*. J Bras Nefrol 2006; 28: 199-203.

[363] Meiouet F, El Kabbaj S, Daudon M. [*in vitro* study of the litholytic effects of herbal extracts on cystine urinary calculi]. Prog Urol 2011; 21(1): 40-7.
[http://dx.doi.org/10.1016/j.purol.2010.05.009] [PMID: 21193144]

[364] Reddy YR, Sujatha C, Raghavendra HG. Nephroprotective effect of *Hibiscus platanifolius* in gentamicin induced nephrotoxicity in rats. Creative J Pharmaceut Res 2016; 2(2): 26-33.

[365] Nirmaladevi R, Kalpana S, Kavitha D, Padma PR. Evaluation of antilithiatic potential of *Hibiscus rosa-sinensis* Linn, *in vitro*. J Pharm Res 2012; 5(8): 4353-6.

[366] Jena M, Mishra S, Mishra SS. Effect of aqueous extract of *Hibiscus rosa-sinensis* Linn on urinary volume and electrolyte extraction in albino rats. Int J Pharm Bio Sci 2013; 4(3): 304-9.

[367] Kirdpon S, Nakorn SN, Kirdpon W. Changes in urinary chemical composition in healthy volunteers after consuming roselle (*Hibiscus sabdariffa* Linn.) juice. J Med Assoc Thai 1994; 77(6): 314-21.
[PMID: 7869018]

[368] Prasongwatana V, Woottisin S, Sriboonlue P, Kukongviriyapan V. Uricosuric effect of Roselle (*Hibiscus sabdariffa*) in normal and renal-stone former subjects. J Ethnopharmacol 2008; 117(3): 491-5.
[http://dx.doi.org/10.1016/j.jep.2008.02.036] [PMID: 18423919]

[369] Woottisin S, Hossain RZ, Yachantha C, Sriboonlue P, Ogawa Y, Saito S. Effects of *Orthosiphon grandiflorus, Hibiscus sabdariffa* and *Phyllanthus amarus* extracts on risk factors for urinary calcium oxalate stones in rats. J Urol 2011; 185(1): 323-8.
[http://dx.doi.org/10.1016/j.juro.2010.09.003] [PMID: 21075390]

[370] Betanabhatala KS, Christina AJM, Sundar BS, Selvakumar S, Saravanan KS. Antilithiatic activity of *Hibiscus sabdariffa* Linn. on ethylene glycol induced lithiasis in rats. Nat Prod Radiance 2009; 8: 43-7.

[371] Kunworarath N, Muangnil P, Itharat A, Hiranyachattada S. Acute and subchronic treatment of *Hibiscus sabdariffa* Linn. extract on renal function and lipid peroxidation in cisplatin-induced acute renal failure rats. J Physiol Biomed Sci 2014; 27(1): 5-12.

[372] Jiménez-Ferrer E, Alarcón-Alonso J, Aguilar-Rojas A, *et al.* Diuretic effect of compounds from *Hibiscus sabdariffa* by modulation of the aldosterone activity. Planta Med 2012; 78(18): 1893-8.
[http://dx.doi.org/10.1055/s-0032-1327864] [PMID: 23150077]

[373] Khan A, Khan SR, Gilani AH. Studies on the *in vitro* and in *vivo* antiurolithic activity of *Holarrhena antidysenterica*. Urol Res 2012; 40(6): 671-81.
[http://dx.doi.org/10.1007/s00240-012-0483-1] [PMID: 22622371]

[374] Prasad KVSRG, Abraham R, Bharathi K, Srinivasan KK. Evaluation of *Homonia riparia* Lour. for antiurolithiatic activity in albino rats. Pharm Biol 1997; 35(4): 278-83.

[375] Shah JG, Patel BG, Patel SB, Patel RK. Antiurolithiatic and antioxidant activity of *Hordeum vulgare* seeds on ethylene glycol-induced urolithiasis in rats. Indian J Pharmacol 2012; 44(6): 672-7.
[http://dx.doi.org/10.4103/0253-7613.103237] [PMID: 23248392]

[376] Kang C, Lee H, Hah DY, *et al.* Protective effects of *Houttuynia cordata* Thunb. on gentamicin induced oxidative stress and nephrotoxicity in rats. Toxicol Res 2013; 29(1): 61-7.

[http://dx.doi.org/10.5487/TR.2013.29.1.061] [PMID: 24278630]

[377] Bibu KJ, Joy AD, Mercey KA. Therapeutic effect of ethanolic extract of *Hygrophila spinosa* T. Anders on gentamicin-induced nephrotoxicity in rats. Indian J Exp Biol 2010; 48(9): 911-7. [PMID: 21506499]

[378] Sathish R, Natarajan K, Nikhad MM. Effect of *Hygrophila spinosa* T. Anders. on ethylene glycol induced urolithiasis in rats. Asian J Pharm Clin Res 2010; 3(4): 61-3.

[379] Ingale KG, Thakurdesai PA, Vyawahare NS. Effect of *Hygrophila spinosa* in ethylene glycol induced nephrolithiasis in rats. Indian J Pharmacol 2012; 44(5): 639-42. [http://dx.doi.org/10.4103/0253-7613.100402] [PMID: 23112429]

[380] Ingale KG, Thakurdesai PA, Vyawahare NS. Protective effect of *Hygrophila spinosa* against cisplatin induced nephrotoxicity in rats. Indian J Pharmacol 2013; 45(3): 232-6. [http://dx.doi.org/10.4103/0253-7613.111909] [PMID: 23833364]

[381] Khalili M, Jalali MR, Mirzaei-Azandaryani M. Effect of hydroalcoholic extract of *Hypericum perforatum* L. leaves on ethylene glycol-induced kidney calculi in rats. Urol J 2012; 9(2): 472-9. [PMID: 22641490]

[382] Agarwal K, Varma R. Inhibition of calcium oxlate crystallization *in vitro* by various extracts of *Hyptis suaveolens* (L.) Poit. Int Res J Pharmacy 2012; 3(3): 261-4.

[383] Anbu J, Suman S, Swaroop Kumar K, Satheesh Kumar R, Nithya S, Kannadhasan R. Antiurolithiatic activity of ethyl acetate root extract of *Ichnocarpus frutescens* using ethylene glycol induced method in rats. J Pharma Sci Res 2011; 3(4): 1182-9.

[384] Priyadarsini G, Kumar A, Anbu J, Ashwini A, Ayyasamy S. Nephroprotective activity of decoction of *Indigofera tinctoria* (avurikudineer) against cisplatin induced nephropathy in rats. Int J Life Sci Pharma Res 2012; 2(4): 56-62.

[385] Sharmin R, Hossain ABMI, Rahman S, Momtaz A, Sharmin K. Mosaddek ASM. Study on the effect of ethanol extract of *Ipomoea aquatica* (Kalmi Shak) leaves on gentamicin induced nephrotoxic rats. ARC J Dental Sci 2016; 1(3): 9-14.

[386] Sathish R, Jeyabalan G. Study of *in vitro* antilithiatic effect of *Ipomoea batatas* (L) leaves and tuberous roots. Asian J Pharm Clin Res 2018; 11(2): 427-31. [http://dx.doi.org/10.22159/ajpcr.2018.v11i2.23319]

[387] Kalaiselvan A, Anand T, Soundarajan M. Reno productive activity of *Ipomoea digitata* in gentamicin induced kidney dysfunction. J Ecobiotech 2010; 2(2): 57-62.

[388] Das M, Malipeddi H. Antiurolithiatic activity of ethanol leaf extract of *Ipomoea eriocarpa* against ethylene glycol-induced urolithiasis in male Wistar rats. Indian J Pharmacol 2016; 48(3): 270-4. [http://dx.doi.org/10.4103/0253-7613.182886] [PMID: 27298496]

[389] Hamsa TP, Kuttan G. Protective role of *Ipomoea obscura* (L.) on cyclophosphamide-induced uro- and nephrotoxicities by modulating antioxidant status and pro-inflammatory cytokine levels. Inflame 2011; 19(3): 155-67. [http://dx.doi.org/10.1007/s10787-010-0055-3] [PMID: 20878549]

[390] Bag A, Mumtaz S. Hepatoprotective and nephroprotective activity of hydroalcoholic extract of *Ipomoea staphylina* leaves. Bangladesh J Pharmacol 2013; 8: 263-8. [http://dx.doi.org/10.3329/bjp.v8i3.14845]

[391] Bahuguna Y, Rawat MSM, Juyal V, Gupta V. Antilithiatic effect of *Jasminum auriculatum* Vahl. Int J Green Pharm 2009; 3(2): 155-8. [http://dx.doi.org/10.4103/0973-8258.54910]

[392] Haque R, Bin-Hafeez B, Parvez S, *et al.* Aqueous extract of walnut (*Juglans regia* L.) protects mice against cyclophosphamide-induced biochemical toxicity. Hum Exp Toxicol 2003; 22(9): 473-80. [http://dx.doi.org/10.1191/0960327103ht388oa] [PMID: 14580007]

[393] Stanic G, Samarzija I, Blazevic N. Time-dependent diuretic response in rats treated with juniper berry preparations. Phytother Res 1998; 12: 494-7.
[http://dx.doi.org/10.1002/(SICI)1099-1573(199811)12:7<494::AID-PTR340>3.0.CO;2-N]

[394] Lasheras B. Etude pharmacologique preliminaire de *Prunus spinosa* L. *Amelanchier ovalis* Medikus, *Juniperus communis* L. et *Urtica dioica* L. Plant Med Phytother 1986; 20: 219-26.

[395] Kumar A, Kumari NS, D'Souza P, Bhargavan D. Evaluation of renal protective activity of *Adhatoda zeylanica* (Medic) leaves extract in wistar rats. Nitte Univ J Health Sci 2013; 3(4): 55-66.
[http://dx.doi.org/10.1055/s-0040-1703701]

[396] Torki A, Hosseinabadi T, Fasihzadeh S, Sadeghimanesh A, Wibowo JP, Lorigooini Z. Solubility of calcum oxalate and calcium phosphate crystallization in the presence of crude extract and fractions from *Kelussia odoratissima* Mozaff. Phcog Res 2018; 10: 379-84.
[http://dx.doi.org/10.4103/pr.pr_68_18]

[397] El Badwi S, Bakhiet A, Gadir EA. Haemato-biochemical effects of aqueous extract of *Khaya senegalensis* stem bark on gentamicin-induced nephrotoxicity in Wistar rats. J Biol Sci 2012; 12: 361-6.
[http://dx.doi.org/10.3923/jbs.2012.361.366]

[398] Azu OO, Duru FIO, Osinubi AA, Noronha CC, Elesha SO, Okanlawon AO. Protective agent, *Kigelia africana* fruit extract against cisplatin induced kidney oxidant injury in Sprague dawley rats. Asian J Pharm Clin Res 2010; 3(2): 84-8.

[399] Kumar R, Kumar T, Kamboj V, Harish C. Pharmacological evalution of ethanolic extract of *Kigelia pinnata* fruit against ethylene glycol induced urolithiasis in rats. Asian J Plant Sci Res 2012; 2(1): 63-72.

[400] Mahurkar N, Mumtaz M, Ifthekar S. Protective effect of aqueous and methanolic extracts of *Lagenaria siceraria* seeds in gentamicin induced nephrotoxicity. Int J Res Ayurveda Pharm 2012; 3(3): 443-6.

[401] Takawale RV, Mali VR, Kapase CU, Bodhankar SL. Effect of *Lagenaria siceraria* fruit powder on sodium oxalate induced urolithiasis in Wistar rats. J Ayurveda Integr Med 2012; 3(2): 75-9.
[http://dx.doi.org/10.4103/0975-9476.96522] [PMID: 22707863]

[402] Prasad M, Sanjuna C, Anjali M, Sandhya N, Srikanth M, Himabindu J, *et al.* Evaluation of *in vitro* anti urolithiatic activity of *Lagenaria siceraria.* World J Gastroenterol Hepatol Endosc 2019; 1(1) WJGHE-1-107

[403] Mayee R, Thosar A. Evaluation of *Lantana camara* Linn. (Verbenaceae) for antiurolithiatic and antioxidant activities in rats. Int J Pharmaceut Clini Res 2011; 3(6): 10-4.

[404] Chatterjee P, Nandy S, Dwivedi A. Nephroprotective effect of methanolic extract of *Lantana camara* L. against acetaminophen and cisplatin-induced kidney injury. American J Pharm Tech Res 2012; 2(2): 487-501.

[405] Khalid S, Khan H, Anwar AA, Abrar S. Nephroprotective effect of ethanolic extract of *Lantana camara* Linn. flower on acute dose of cisplatin induced renal injured rats. RGUHS J Pharm Sci 2012; 2(2): 68-77.

[406] Vyas N, Argal A. Nephroprotective activity of ethanolic extract of roots and oleanolic acid isolated from roots of *Lantana camara.* Intern J Pharmacol & Clinical Sci 2012; 1(2): 54-60.

[407] Khan RA, Khan MR, Sahreen S. Evaluation of *Launaea procumbens* use in renal disorders: a rat model. J Ethnopharmacol 2010; 128(2): 452-61.
[http://dx.doi.org/10.1016/j.jep.2010.01.026] [PMID: 20096342]

[408] Makasana A, Ranpariya V, Desai D, Mendpara J, Parekh V. Evaluation for the anti-urolithiatic activity of *Launaea procumbens* against ethylene glycol-induced renal calculi in rats. Toxicol Rep 2014; 1: 46-52.

[http://dx.doi.org/10.1016/j.toxrep.2014.03.006] [PMID: 28962225]

[409] Bansode PA, Raichure GR, Lendave MA, Kolekar DM, Awtade KV, Kedar PR, *et al.* Urolithiatic activity of *Launaea procumbens* against calcium oxalate and calcium phosphate stones. European J Biomed & Pharmaceut Sci 2015; 2(2): 260-8.

[410] Adejuwon AS, Femi-Akinsotu O, Omirinde JO, Owolabi OR, Afodun AM. *Launaea taraxacifolia* ameliorates cisplatin-induced hepato-renal injury. European J Med Plants 2014; 4(5): 528-41.
[http://dx.doi.org/10.9734/EJMP/2014/7314]

[411] Sanjuna C, Anjali M, Prasad M, Sandhya N, Himabindhu J, Ramanjaneyulu K. Evaluation of *in vitro* antiurolithiatic activity of *Laurus nobilis* leaves. World J Gastroenterol Hepatol Endosc 2019; 1(1) WJGHE-1-106.

[412] Sreedevi A, Kokila J, Saisruthi K. Evaluation of leaves of *Lawsonia inermis* for nephroprotective activity. Int J Sci Res Rev 2019; 8(2): 2641-51.

[413] Nizami AN, Rahman MA, Ahmed NU, Islam MS. Whole *Leea macrophylla* ethanolic extract normalizes kidney deposits and recovers renal impairments in an ethylene glycol-induced urolithiasis model of rats. Asian Pac J Trop Med 2012; 5(7): 533-8.
[http://dx.doi.org/10.1016/S1995-7645(12)60094-7] [PMID: 22647815]

[414] Sreedevi A, Saisruthi K. Attenuation of cisplatin-induced nephrotoxicity by ethanol extract of seeds of *Lens culinaris* Medic. Anc Sci Life 2017; 37(2): 74-80.

[415] Shinde N, Jagtap A, Undale V, Kakade S, Kotwal S, Patil R. Protective effect of *Lepidium sativum* against doxorubicin-induced nephrotoxicity in rats. Res J Pharm Biol Chem Sci 2010; 1(3): 42-9.

[416] Yadav YC, Srivastava DN, Seth AK, Saini V. Nephroprotective and curative activity of *Lepidium sativum* L. seeds in albino rats using cisplatin induced acute renal failure. Pharma Chem 2010; 2(4): 57-64.

[417] Yadav YC, Srivastav DN, Seth AK, Saini V, Yadav KS. Nephropharmacological activity of ethanolic extract *Lepidium sativum* L. seeds in albino rats using cisplatin induced acute renal failure. Int J Pharm Sci Rev Res 2010; 4(3): 64-8.

[418] Balgoon MJ. Assessment of the protective effect of *Lepidium sativum* against aluminum-induced liver and kidney effects in albino rat. BioMed Res Int 2019; 2019: 4516730.
[http://dx.doi.org/10.1155/2019/4516730] [PMID: 31396529]

[419] Cho HJ, Bae WJ, Kim SJ, *et al.* The inhibitory effect of an ethanol extract of the spores of *Lygodium japonicum* on ethylene glycol-induced kidney calculi in rats. Urolithiasis 2014; 42(4): 309-15.
[http://dx.doi.org/10.1007/s00240-014-0674-z] [PMID: 24972555]

[420] Wu G, Cai Y, Wei H, *et al.* Nephroprotective activity of *Macrothelypteris oligophlebia* rhizomes ethanol extract. Pharm Biol 2012; 50(6): 773-7.
[http://dx.doi.org/10.3109/13880209.2011.632776] [PMID: 22077104]

[421] Chaitanya DAK, Kumar MS, Reddy AM, Mukherjee NSV, Sumanth NH, Ramesh R. Antiurolithiatic activity of *Macrotyloma uniflorum* seed extract of ethylene glycol induced urolithiasis in albino rats. J Innovative Trends in Pharmaceut Sci 2010; 1(5): 216-26.

[422] Palani S, Raja S, Karthi S, Archana S, Senthil Kumar B. *In-vivo* analysis of nephro & hepato protective effects and anti-oxidant activity of *Madhuca longifolia* against acetaminophen-induced toxicity & oxidative stress. J Pharm Res 2010; 3(1): 9-16.

[423] Sushma M, Prasad KVSRG, Jhansi Laxmi Bai D, Vijay R, Rao VUM. Prophylactic and curative effect of ethanolic extract of *Bassia malabarica* bark against cisplatin induced nephrotoxicity. Asian J Pharm Clin Res 2014; 7(4): 143-6.

[424] Sushma M, Sujatha D, Prasad KVSRG. Evaluation of protective effect of *Bassia malabarica* leaves against cisplatin induced nephrotoxicity and doxorubicin-induced cardiotoxicity in rats. Asian J Pharm Clin Res 2018; 11(6): 462-7.

[http://dx.doi.org/10.22159/ajpcr.2018.v11i6.26401]

[425] Palani S, Raja S, Santhosh Kalash R, Senthil Kumar B. Evaluation of nephroprotective and antioxidant activity of *Mahonia leschenaultia* Takeda on acetaminophen-induced toxicity in rat. Toxicol Enviroment Cem 2010; 92(4): 789-99.

[426] Patel TB, Dharmesh K. Golwala, Santosh KV. Antiurolithiatic activity of alcoholic leaf extract of *Mallotus philippensis* Lam. against ethylene glycol induced urolithiasis in rats. Aegaeum Journal 2020; 8(4): 759-65.

[427] Gazwi HSS, Mahnoud ME. Nephroprotective Effect of *Malva sylvestris* extract against CCl₄ induced nephrotoxicity in albino rats. J. Food and Dairy Sci. 3rd Mansoura International Food Congress (MIFC). 37-43.

[428] Rad AK, Ghazi L, Boroushaki MT, Khooei A, Keshavarzi Z, Hosseinian S, *et al.* Effect of commercial (vimang) and hydroalcoholic extract of *Mangifera indica* (Mango) on gentamicin-induced nephrotoxicity in rat. Avicenna J Phytomed 2011; 1(2): 98-105.

[429] Sanjuna C, Prasad M, Anjali M, Sandhya N, Manasa Y, Srikanth M, *et al.* Evaluation of *in vitro* antiurolithiatic activity of *Manilkara zapota* seeds. World J Gastroenterol Hepatol Endosc 2019; 1(1) WJGHE-1-108

[430] Salama RH, Abd-El-Hameed NA, Abd-El-Ghaffar S, Mohammed ZT, Ghandour NM. Nephroprotective effect of *Nigella sativa* and *Matricaria chamomilla* in cisplatin induced renal injury. Int J Clin Med 2011; 2: 185-95.
[http://dx.doi.org/10.4236/ijcm.2011.23031]

[431] Thuwaini MM, Kadhem HS, Al-Dierawi KH. Nephroprotective activity of *Matricaria chamomile* and *Curcuma longa* aqueous extracts on tetracycline-induced nephro-toxicity in albino rats. Int J Pharm Ther 2016; 7: 161-7.

[432] Christina AJ, Haja Najumadeen N, Vimal Kumar S, Manikandan N, Tobin GC, Venkataraman S, *et al.* Antilithiatic effect of *Melia azedarach* on ethylene glycol-induced nephrolithiasis in rats. Pharm Biol 2006; 44(6): 480-5.
[http://dx.doi.org/10.1080/13880200600812634]

[433] Bahuguna YM, Patil KS, Jalalpure SS. Phytochemical and pharmacological investigation of *Melia azedarach* leaves for antiurolithiatic activity. J Trop Med Plants 2008; 9: 344-52.

[434] Dharmalingam SR, Madhappan R, Chidambaram K, Ramamurthy S, Gopal K, Swetha P, *et al.* Anti-urolithiatic activity of *Melia azedarach* Linn. leaf extract in ethylene glycol-induced urolithiasis in male albino rats. Trop J Pharm Res 2014; 13(3): 391-7.
[http://dx.doi.org/10.4314/tjpr.v13i3.12]

[435] Singh RK, Gautam RK, Karchul MS. Evaluation of nephroprotective activity of *Mentha arvensis* in cisplatin induced nephrotoxicity. Asian J Pharm Clin Res 2014; 7: 188-91.

[436] Ullah N, Khan MA, Khan T, Asif AH, Ahmad W. Mentha piperita in nephrotoxicity--a possible intervention to ameliorate renal derangements associated with gentamicin. Indian J Pharmacol 2014; 46(2): 166-70.
[http://dx.doi.org/10.4103/0253-7613.129309] [PMID: 24741187]

[437] Akdogan M, Kilinç I, Oncu M, Karaoz E, Delibas N. Investigation of biochemical and histopathological effects of *Mentha piperita* L. and *Mentha spicata* L. on kidney tissue in rats. Hum Exp Toxicol 2003; 22(4): 213-9.
[http://dx.doi.org/10.1191/0960327103ht332oa] [PMID: 12755472]

[438] Manasa Reddy J, Prathyusha K, Himabindhu J, Ramanjaneyulu K. Evaluation of *in vitro* antiurolithiatic activity of *Mentha piperita.* J Pharmaceut Sci Med 2018; 3(8): 22-8.

[439] Satyavati D, Tripathy S, Srinivas K. Nephroprotective effect of ethanolic extract of flowers of *Michelia champaca* against cisplatin-induced nephropathy in rats. World J Pharm Pharm Sci 2013; 2(6): 6352-65.

[440] Joyamma V, Rao SG, Hrishikeshavan HJ, Aroor AR, Kulkarni DR. Biochemical mechanisms and effects of *Mimosa pudica* (Linn) on experimental urolithiasis in rats. Indian J Exp Biol 1990; 28(3): 237-40.
[PMID: 2365419]

[441] Ashok P, Koti BC, Vishwanathswamy AHM. Antiurolithiatic and antioxidant activity of *Mimusops elengi* on ethylene glycol-induced urolithiasis in rats. Indian J Pharmacol 2010; 42(6): 380-3.
[http://dx.doi.org/10.4103/0253-7613.71925] [PMID: 21189910]

[442] Jain A, Singhai AK. Nephroprotective activity of *Momordica dioica* Roxb. in cisplatin-induced nephrotoxicity. Nat Prod Res 2010; 24(9): 846-54.
[http://dx.doi.org/10.1080/14786410903132589] [PMID: 20461630]

[443] Jain A, Singhai AK. Effect of *Momordica dioica* Roxb on gentamicin model of acute renal failure. Nat Prod Res 2010; 24(15): 1379-89.
[http://dx.doi.org/10.1080/14786410802267569] [PMID: 19241280]

[444] Palani S, Raja S, Kumar RP, Selvaraj R, Kumar BS. Evaluation of phytoconstituents and anti-nephrotoxic and antioxidant activities of *Monochoria vaginalis*. Pak J Pharm Sci 2011; 24(3): 293-301.
[PMID: 21715262]

[445] Jan S, Khan MR. Protective effects of *Monotheca buxifolia* fruit on renal toxicity induced by CCl_4 in rats. BMC Complement Altern Med 2016; 16(1): 289.
[http://dx.doi.org/10.1186/s12906-016-1256-0] [PMID: 27530158]

[446] Verma NK, Patel SS, Saleem TM, Christiana AJM, Chidambaranathan N. Modulatory effect of noni-herbal formulation against ethylene glycol-induced nephrolithiasis in albino rats. J Pharm Sci Res 2009; 1: 83-9.

[447] Shenoy JP, Pai PG, Shoeb A, Gokul P, Kulkarni A, Kotian MS. An evaluation of diuretic activity of *Morinda citrifolia* (Linn.) (Noni) fruit juice in normal rats. Int J Pharm Pharm Sci 2011; 3(2): 119-21.

[448] Bhavani R. Effect of Noni (*Morinda citrifolia*) extract on treatment of ethylene glycol and ammonium chloride induced kidney disease. Int J Pharm Sci Res 2014; 5(6): 249-56.

[449] Karamcheti SA, Satyavati D, Siva Subramanian N, Pradeep HA. Pradeep kumar C, Deepika Sri Prashanthi G. Chemoprotective effect of ethanolic extract of *Morinda citrifolia* against cisplatin induced nephrotoxicity. Pharma Innov 2014; 3(1): 84-91.

[450] Karadi RV, Gadge NB, Alagawadi KR, Savadi RV. Effect of *Moringa oleifera* Lam. root-wood on ethylene glycol induced urolithiasis in rats. J Ethnopharmacol 2006; 105(1-2): 306-11.
[http://dx.doi.org/10.1016/j.jep.2005.11.004] [PMID: 16386862]

[451] Fahad J. Antiurolithiatic activity of aqueous extract of bark of *Moringa oleifera* (Lam.) in rats. Health 2010; 2(4): 352-5.
[http://dx.doi.org/10.4236/health.2010.24053]

[452] Sachan D. Effect of the ethanolic extract of *Moringa oleifera* Linn. plant on ethylene glycol induced lithiatic albino rats. Intern J Toxicological and Pharmacological Res 2012; 4(3): 26-8.

[453] Lakshmana G, Rajeshkumar D, Ashok Reddy P, *et al.* Determination of nephroprotective activity of ethanolic leaf extracts of *Moringa pterygosperma* on paracetamol-induced nephrotoxic rats. Int J Allied Med Sci Clin Res 2013; 1: 51-61.

[454] Ouédraogo M, Lamien-Sanou A, Ramdé N, *et al.* Protective effect of *Moringa oleifera* leaves against gentamicin-induced nephrotoxicity in rabbits. Exp Toxicol Pathol 2013; 65(3): 335-9.
[http://dx.doi.org/10.1016/j.etp.2011.11.006] [PMID: 22197459]

[455] Nafiu AO, Akomolafe RO, Alabi QK, Idowu CO, Odujoko OO. Effect of fatty acids from ethanol extract of *Moringa oleifera* seeds on kidney function impairment and oxidative stress induced by gentamicin in rats. Biomed Pharmacother 2019; 117: 109154.

[http://dx.doi.org/10.1016/j.biopha.2019.109154] [PMID: 31387184]

[456] Nematbakhsh M, Hajhashemi V, Ghannadi A, Talebi A, Nikahd M. Protective effects of the *Morus alba* L. leaf extracts on cisplatin-induced nephrotoxicity in rat. Res Pharm Sci 2013; 8(2): 71-7.
[PMID: 24019816]

[457] Maya S, Pramod C. Evaluation of antinephrolithiatic activity of ethanolic leaf extract of *Morus alba* L. in animal models. Int Res J Pharm 2014; 5(5): 427-33.
[http://dx.doi.org/10.7897/2230-8407.050588]

[458] Ullah N, Khan MA, Khan S, Ahmad H, Asif AH, Khan T. Nephro-protective potential of *Morus alba*, a prospective experimental study on animal models. Pharm Biol 2016; 54(3): 530-5.
[http://dx.doi.org/10.3109/13880209.2015.1052149] [PMID: 26067678]

[459] Hashim MI, Askar SJ. Ameliorating effects of *Morus alba* leaves extract on nephrotoxicity - induced by gentamicin in male rats. Indian J Nat Sci 2019; 9(52): 16626-37.

[460] Modi KP, Patel NM, Goyal RK. Protective effects of aqueous extract of *Mucuna pruriens* Linn. (DC.) seed against gentamicin induced oxidative stress and nephrotoxicity in rats. Iranian J Pharmacol Therapeut 2008; 7(2): 131-5.

[461] Mahipal P, Pawar RS. Nephroprotective effect of *Murraya koenigii* on cyclophosphamide induced nephrotoxicity in rats. Asian Pac J Trop Med 2017; 10(8): 808-12.
[http://dx.doi.org/10.1016/j.apjtm.2017.08.005] [PMID: 28942830]

[462] Prasad KVSRG, Bharathi K, Srinivasan KK. Evaluation of Musa (*paradisiaca* Linn. cultivar)--"Puttubale" stem juice for antilithiatic activity in albino rats. Indian J Physiol Pharmacol 1993; 37(4): 337-41.
[PMID: 8112813]

[463] Poonguzhali PK, Chegu H. The influence of banana stem extract on urinary risk factors for stones in normal and hyperoxaluric rats. Br J Urol 1994; 74(1): 23-5.
[http://dx.doi.org/10.1111/j.1464-410X.1994.tb16539.x] [PMID: 8044524]

[464] Jha U, Shelka TT, Oswal RS, Adkar PP, Navgire VN. Pharmacological screening of *Musa paradisica* Linn. against ethylene glycol induced renal calculi. Int J Res Ayurveda Pharm 2011; 2(3): 995-8.

[465] Prasobh GR, Revikumar KG. Effect of Musa tablet on ethylene glycol-induced urolithiasis in rats. Intern J Pharma Biosci 2012; pp. 1251-4.

[466] Kalpana S, Nirmaladevi R, Rai TS, Karthika P. Inhibition of calcium oxalate crystallization *in vitro* by extract of banana cultivar monthan. Int J Pharm Pharm Sci 2013; 4: 649-53.

[467] Thirumala K, Janarthan M, Firasat Ali M. Evalution of anti-urolithiatic activity of aqueous extract of stem core of *Musa paradisiaca* against ethylene glycol and ammonium chloride induced urolithiasis on Wistar rats. Indian J Res Pharm Biotech 2013; 1(6): 866-8.

[468] Panigrahi PN, Dey S, Sahoo M, Dan A. Antiurolithiatic and antioxidant efficacy of *Musa paradisiaca* pseudostem on ethylene glycol-induced nephrolithiasis in rat. Indian J Pharmacol 2017; 49(1): 77-83.
[PMID: 28458427]

[469] Nivetha J, Prasanna G. Nephroprotective effect of *Myristica fragrans* against gentamicin-induced toxicity in albino rats. Int J Adv Pharm Sci 2014; 5: 2039-45.

[470] Prathibhakumari PV, Prasad G. Anti-urolithiatic potential of aqueous fruit extract of *Neolamarckia cadamba* on Wistar albino rats. J Pharm Res 2012; 5(6): 3134-8.

[471] Ali BH. The effect of *Nigella sativa* oil on gentamicin nephrotoxicity in rats. Am J Chin Med 2004; 32(1): 49-55.
[http://dx.doi.org/10.1142/S0192415X04001710] [PMID: 15154284]

[472] Hadjzadeh MA, Khoei A, Hadjzadeh Z, Parizady M. Ethanolic extract of *nigella sativa* L seeds on ethylene glycol-induced kidney calculi in rats. Urol J 2007; 4(2): 86-90.
[PMID: 17701927]

[473] Bayrak O, Bavbek N, Karatas OF, *et al. Nigella sativa* protects against ischaemia/reperfusion injury in rat kidneys. Nephrol Dial Transplant 2008; 23(7): 2206-12.
[http://dx.doi.org/10.1093/ndt/gfm953] [PMID: 18211980]

[474] Begum NA, Dewan ZF, Nahar N, Mamun MR. Effect of n-Hexane extract of *Nigella sativa* on gentamicin induced nephrotoxicity in rats. Bangladesh J Pharmacol 2006; 1: 16-20.

[475] Yildiz F, Coban S, Terzi A, *et al.* Protective effects of *Nigella sativa* against ischemia-reperfusion injury of kidneys. Ren Fail 2010; 32(1): 126-31.
[http://dx.doi.org/10.3109/08860220903367577] [PMID: 20113278]

[476] Yaman I, Balikci E. Protective effects of *nigella sativa* against gentamicin-induced nephrotoxicity in rats. Exp Toxicol Pathol 2010; 62(2): 183-90.
[http://dx.doi.org/10.1016/j.etp.2009.03.006] [PMID: 19398313]

[477] Hadjzadeh MA, Keshavarzi Z, Tabatabaee Yazdi SA, Ghasem Shirazi M, Rajaei Z, Khajavi Rad A. Effect of alcoholic extract of *Nigella sativa* on cisplatin-induced toxicity in rat. Iran J Kidney Dis 2012; 6(2): 99-104.
[PMID: 22388606]

[478] Saleem U, Ahmad B, Rehman K, Mahmood S, Alam M, Erum A. Nephro-protective effect of vitamin C and *Nigella sativa* oil on gentamicin associated nephrotoxicity in rabbits. Pak J Pharm Sci 2012; 25(4): 727-30.
[PMID: 23009987]

[479] Benhelima A, Kaid-Omar Z, Hemida H, Benmahdi T, Addou A. Nephroprotective and diuretic effect of *Nigella sativa* l seeds oil on lithiasic wistar rats. Afr J Tradit Complement Altern Med 2016; 13(6): 204-14.
[http://dx.doi.org/10.21010/ajtcam.v13i6.30] [PMID: 28480381]

[480] Hosseinian S, Khajavi Rad A, Hadjzadeh MA, Mohamadian Roshan N, Havakhah S, Shafiee S. The protective effect of *Nigella sativa* against cisplatin-induced nephrotoxicity in rats. Avicenna J Phytomed 2016; 6(1): 44-54.
[PMID: 27247921]

[481] Canayakin D, Bayir Y, Kilic Baygutalp N, *et al.* Paracetamol-induced nephrotoxicity and oxidative stress in rats: the protective role of *Nigella sativa*. Pharm Biol 2016; 54(10): 2082-91.
[http://dx.doi.org/10.3109/13880209.2016.1145701] [PMID: 26956915]

[482] Hosseinian S, Hadjzadeh MA, Roshan NM, *et al.* Renoprotective effect of *Nigella sativa* against cisplatin-induced nephrotoxicity and oxidative stress in rat. Saudi J Kidney Dis Transpl 2018; 29(1): 19-29.
[http://dx.doi.org/10.4103/1319-2442.225208] [PMID: 29456204]

[483] Goswami P, Srivastava R. Protective effect of root extract of *Nothosaerva brachiata* Wight in ethylene glycol induced urolithiatic rats. Intern Res J Pharm 2015; 6(12): 808-12.
[http://dx.doi.org/10.7897/2230-8407.0612157]

[484] Shelke TT, Bhaskar VH, Jha U, Adkar PP, Oswal RJ. Effect of ethanolic extract of *Nymphaea alba* Linn. on urolithiatic rats. Intern J Pharmaceut Clinical Res 2011; 3(3): 55-7.

[485] Zaveri M, Desai N, Movaliya V. Effect of *Ocimum basilicum* on cisplatin models of acute renal failure. Adv Res Pharm Biol 2011; 1(2): 91-100.

[486] Sakr AS, Al-Amoudi WM. Effect of leave extract of *Ocimum basilicum* on deltamethrin induced nephrotoxicity and oxidative stress in albino rats. J Appl Pharm Sci 2012; 2(5): 22-7.
[http://dx.doi.org/10.7324/JAPS.2012.2507]

[487] Arhoghro EM, Anosike EO, Uwakwe AA. *Ocimum gratissimum* aqueous extract enhances recovery in cisplatin induced nephrotoxicity in albino Wistar rats. Indian J Drugs Dis 2012; 1(5): 129-42.

[488] Agarwal K, Varma R. *Ocimum gratissimum* L.: A medicinal plant with promising anti-urolithiatic

activity. Indian J Pharmaceut Sci Drug Res 2014; 6(1): 78-81.

[489] Ogundipe DJ, Akomolafe RO, Sanusi AA, Imafidon CE, Olukiran OS, Oladele AA. *Ocimum gratissimum* ameliorates gentamicin-induced kidney injury but decreases creatinine clearance following sub-chronic administration in rats. J Evid Based Complementary Altern Med 2017; 22(4): 592-602.
[http://dx.doi.org/10.1177/2156587217691891] [PMID: 29228801]

[490] Tavafi M, Ahmadvand H, Toolabi P. Inhibitory effect of olive leaf extract on gentamicin-induced nephrotoxicity in rats. Iran J Kidney Dis 2012; 6(1): 25-32.
[PMID: 22218116]

[491] Al-Sowayan NS, Mousa HM. Ameliorative effect of olive leaf extract on carbon tetrachloride-induced nephrotoxicity in rats. Life Sci J 2014; 11(5): 238-42.

[492] Alenzi M, Rahiman S, Tantry BA. Antiurolithic effect of olive oil in a mouse model of ethylene glycol-induced urolithiasis. Investig Clin Urol 2017; 58(3): 210-6.
[http://dx.doi.org/10.4111/icu.2017.58.3.210] [PMID: 28480348]

[493] Bwititi PT, Machakaire T, Nhachi CB, Musabayane CT. Effects of *Opuntia megacantha* leaves extract on renal electrolyte and fluid handling in streptozotocin (STZ)-diabetic rats. Ren Fail 2001; 23(2): 149-58.
[http://dx.doi.org/10.1081/JDI-100103487] [PMID: 11417947]

[494] Khan A, Bashir S, Khan SR, Gilani AH. Antiurolithic activity of *Origanum vulgare* is mediated through multiple pathways. BMC Complement Altern Med 2011; 11: 96.
[http://dx.doi.org/10.1186/1472-6882-11-96] [PMID: 22004514]

[495] Premgamone A, Sriboonlue P, Disatapornjaroen W, Maskasem S, Sinsupan N, Apinives C. A long-term study on the efficacy of a herbal plant, Orthosiphon grandiflorus, and sodium potassium citrate in renal calculi treatment. Southeast Asian J Trop Med Public Health 2001; 32(3): 654-60.
[PMID: 11944733]

[496] Kannappan N, Madhukar A. Mariymmal, Sindhura PU, Mannavalan R. Evaluation of nephroprotective activity of *Orthosiphon stamineus* Benth. extract using rat model. Int J Pharm Tech Res 2010; 2(3): 209-15.

[497] Maheswari C. Mariammal, Venkatnarayan R. Renal protective activity of *Orthosiphon stamineus* leaf extract against cisplatin induced renal toxicity. Int J Pharm Tech 2011; 3(1): 1584-92.

[498] Ramesh K, Manohar S, Rajeshkumar S. Nephroprotective activity of ethanolic extract of *Orthosiphon stamineus* leaves on ethylene glycol induced urolithiasis in albino rats. J Pharm Tech Res 2014; 6: 403-8.

[499] Ohkawa T, Ebisuno S, Kitagawa M, Morimoto S, Miyazaki Y, Yasukawa S. Rice bran treatment for patients with hypercalciuric stones: experimental and clinical studies. J Urol 1984; 132(6): 1140-5.
[http://dx.doi.org/10.1016/S0022-5347(17)50065-8] [PMID: 6094846]

[500] Ebisuno S, Morimoto S, Yoshida T, Fukatani T, Yasukawa S, Ohkawa T. Rice-bran treatment for calcium stone formers with idiopathic hypercalciuria. Br J Urol 1986; 58(6): 592-5.
[http://dx.doi.org/10.1111/j.1464-410X.1986.tb05892.x] [PMID: 3801813]

[501] Ebisuno S, Morimoto S, Yasukawa S, Ohkawa T. Results of long-term rice bran treatment on stone recurrence in hypercalciuric patients. Br J Urol 1991; 67(3): 237-40.
[http://dx.doi.org/10.1111/j.1464-410X.1991.tb15125.x] [PMID: 1902388]

[502] Li X, Wang W, Su Y, Yue Z, Bao J. Inhibitory effect of an aqueous extract of *Radix Paeoniae Alba* on calcium oxalate nephrolithiasis in a rat model. Ren Fail 2017; 39(1): 120-9.
[http://dx.doi.org/10.1080/0886022X.2016.1254658] [PMID: 28085537]

[503] Qi Z-L, Wang Z, Li W, *et al.* Nephroprotective effects of anthocyanin from the fruits of *Panax ginseng* (GFA) on cisplatin-induced acute kidney injury in mice: GFA alleviates cisplatin-induced nephrotoxicity. Phytother Res 2017; 31(9): 1400-9.

[http://dx.doi.org/10.1002/ptr.5867] [PMID: 28731262]

[504]   Ma Z-N, Liu Z, Wang Z, *et al*. Supplementation of American ginseng berry extract mitigated cisplatin-evoked nephrotoxicity by suppressing ROS-mediated activation of MAPK and NF-κB signaling pathways. Food Chem Toxicol 2017; 110: 62-73.
[http://dx.doi.org/10.1016/j.fct.2017.10.006] [PMID: 29024717]

[505]   Bouanani S, Henchiri C, Migianu-Griffoni E, Aouf N, Lecouvey M. Pharmacological and toxicological effects of *Paronychia argentea* in experimental calcium oxalate nephrolithiasis in rats. J Ethnopharmacol 2010; 129(1): 38-45.
[http://dx.doi.org/10.1016/j.jep.2010.01.056] [PMID: 20138208]

[506]   Shelke TT, Kothai R, Adkar PP, *et al*. Nephroprotective activity of ethanolic extract of dried fruits of *Pedalium murex* Linn. J Cell and Tissue Res 2009; 9(1): 1687-90.

[507]   Teepa KSA, Kokilavani R, Balakrishnan A, Gurusamy K. Effect of ethanolic fruit extract of *Pedalium murex* Linn. in ethylene glycol induced urolithiasis in male Wistar albino rats. Anc Sci Life 2010; 29(4): 29-34.
[PMID: 22557365]

[508]   Vyas B, Vyas R, Joshi S, Santani D. Antiurolithiatic activity of whole-plant hydroalcoholic extract of *Pergularia daemia* in rats. J Young Pharm 2011; 3(1): 36-40.
[http://dx.doi.org/10.4103/0975-1483.76417] [PMID: 21607052]

[509]   Alyami FA, Rabah DM. Effect of drinking parsley leaf tea on urinary composition and urinary stones' risk factors. Saudi J Kidney Dis Transpl 2011; 22(3): 511-4.
[PMID: 21566309]

[510]   Jassim AM. Protective effect of *Petroselinum crispum* (parsley) extract on histopathological changes in liver, kidney and pancreas induced by sodium valproate- in male rats. Kufa J Veter Med Sci 2013; 4(1): 20-7.

[511]   Gumaih H, Al-Yousofy F, Ibrahim H, Ali S, Alasbahy A. Evaluation of ethanolic seed extract of parsley on ethylene glycol induced calcium oxalate, experimental model. Int J Sci Res 2015; 6: 1683-8.

[512]   Al-Yousofy F, Gumaih H, Ibrahim H, Alasbahy A. Parsley! Mechanism as antiurolithiasis remedy. Am J Clin Exp Urol 2017; 5(3): 55-62.
[PMID: 29181438]

[513]   Jafar S, Mehri L, Hadi B, Jamshid M. The antiurolithiasic and hepatocurative activities of aqueous extracts of *Petroselinum sativum* on ethylene glycol-induced kidney calculi in rats. Acade J 2012; 7: 1577-83.

[514]   Aslam M, Dayal R, Javed K, Parray SA, Jetley S, Samim M. Nephroprotective effects of methanolic extract of *Peucedanum grande* against acute renal failure induced by potassium dichromate in rat. Int J Pharm Sci Drug Res 2013; 5(2): 45-9.

[515]   Kumar BN, Wadud A, Jahan N, *et al*. Antilithiatic effect of *Peucedanum grande* C. B. Clarke in chemically induced urolithiasis in rats. J Ethnopharmacol 2016; 194: 1122-9.
[http://dx.doi.org/10.1016/j.jep.2016.10.081] [PMID: 27825989]

[516]   Chaware V. Protective effect of the aqueous extract of *Phaseolus radiatus* seeds on gentamicin induced nephrotoxicity in rats. Int J Pharma Bio Sci 2012; 3: 73-5.

[517]   Sree Lakshmi N, Sujatha D, Bharathi K, Prasad KVSRG. Antiurolithiatic activity of *Phaeolus vulgaris* seeds against ethylene glycol-induced renal clculi in Wistar rats. Int J Green Pharm 2017; 11(4): 281-9.

[518]   Vinciya T. Evaluaton of antiurolithiatic activity of ethanolic and aqueous extract of *Phaseolus vulgaris* Linn. seeds. MPharm dissertation, The Tamil Nadu Dr MGRMedical University, Chennai, India

[519]   Das P, Kumar K, Nambiraj A, *et al*. Potential therapeutic activity of *Phlogacanthus thyrsiformis*

Hardow (Mabb) flower extract and its biofabricated silver nanoparticles against chemically induced urolithiasis in male Wistar rats. Int J Biol Macromol 2017; 103: 621-9.
[http://dx.doi.org/10.1016/j.ijbiomac.2017.05.096] [PMID: 28528955]

[520] Al-Qarawi AA, Abdel-Rahman H, Mousa HM, Ail BH, El-Mougy SA. Nephroprotective action of *Phoenix dactylifera* in gentamicin-induced nephrotoxicity. Pharm Biol 2008; 46: 227-30.
[http://dx.doi.org/10.1080/13880200701739322]

[521] Ali SA, Abdelaziz DH. The protective effect of date seeds on nephrotoxicity induced by carbon tetrachloride in rats. Int J Pharm Sci Rev Res 2014; 26(12): 62-8.

[522] Al-Gamli AH, Salama AAA, Elhassen SM, Osman ZM, El-Eraky W, Hassan A. Evaluation of anti urolithiatic activity of *Phoenix dactylefera* seeds extract in ethylene glycol induced urolithiasis in rats. Int J Pharm Pharm Res 2017; 9(2): 7-20.

[523] Sujatha D, Ranganayakulu D, Bharathi K, Prasad KVSR. Effect of ethanolic extract of *Phyla nodiflora* (Linn.) Greenes against calculi producing diet induced urolithiasis. Indian J Nat Prod Resour 2010; 1(3): 314-21.

[524] Adeneye AA, Benebo AS. Protective effect of the aqueous leaf and seed extract of *Phyllanthus amarus* on gentamicin and acetaminophen-induced nephrotoxic rats. J Ethnopharmacol 2008; 118(2): 318-23.
[http://dx.doi.org/10.1016/j.jep.2008.04.025] [PMID: 18554830]

[525] Obianime AW, Uche FI. The Phytochemical screening and the effects of methanolic extract of *Phyllanthus amarus* leaf on the biochemical parameters of Male guinea pigs. J Appl Sci Environ Manag 2008; 12(4): 73-7.

[526] Bakhtiary SA, Iqbal MM, Ibrahim M. Hepatoprotective and nephroprotective activity of *Phyllanthus amarus* Schum & Thonn. seed extract. Ann Phytomed 2012; 1(2): 97-104.

[527] Singh S, Swarn L, Kavindra NT. Protective role of *Phyllanthus fraternus* against cyclophosphamide induced nephrotoxicity in mice. J Sci Res 2014; 58: 75-85.

[528] Chandrasekar MJN, Bommu P, Nanjan M, Suresh B. Chemoprotective effect of *Phyllanthus maderaspatensis* in modulating cisplatin-induced nephrotoxicity and genotoxicity. Pharm Biol 2006; 44: 100-6.
[http://dx.doi.org/10.1080/13880200600592046]

[529] Boim MA, Heilberg IP, Schor N. *Phyllanthus niruri* as a promising alternative treatment for nephrolithiasis. Int Braz J Urol 2010; 36(6): 657-64.
[http://dx.doi.org/10.1590/S1677-55382010000600002] [PMID: 21176271]

[530] Melo EMA, Coelho STNS, Santos DR, Ajxzen H, Schor N. Urolitiase experimental: *Phyllanthus niruri.* AIDS Res Hum Retroviruses 1992; 8: 1937.

[531] Campos AH, Schor N. *Phyllanthus niruri* inhibits calcium oxalate endocytosis by renal tubular cells: its role in urolithiasis. Nephron J 1999; 81(4): 393-7.
[http://dx.doi.org/10.1159/000045322] [PMID: 10095174]

[532] Freitas AM, Schor N, Boim MA. The effect of *Phyllanthus niruri* on urinary inhibitors of calcium oxalate crystallization and other factors associated with renal stone formation. BJU Int 2002; 89(9): 829-34.
[http://dx.doi.org/10.1046/j.1464-410X.2002.02794.x] [PMID: 12010223]

[533] Barros ME, Schor N, Boim MA. Effects of an aqueous extract from *Phyllantus niruri* on calcium oxalate crystallization *in vitro.* Urol Res 2003; 30(6): 374-9.
[http://dx.doi.org/10.1007/s00240-002-0285-y] [PMID: 12599017]

[534] Nishiura JL, Campos AH, Boim MA, Heilberg IP, Schor N. *Phyllanthus niruri* normalizes elevated urinary calcium levels in calcium stone forming (CSF) patients. Urol Res 2004; 32(5): 362-6.
[http://dx.doi.org/10.1007/s00240-004-0432-8] [PMID: 15221244]

[535] Barros ME, Lima R, Mercuri LP, Matos JR, Schor N, Boim MA. Effect of extract of *Phyllanthus niruri* on crystal deposition in experimental urolithiasis. Urol Res 2006; 34(6): 351-7. [http://dx.doi.org/10.1007/s00240-006-0065-1] [PMID: 16896689]

[536] Gaddam SR, Lalitha PR, Gaddam RR, Dyaga VC. Evaluation of nephroprotective activity of the methanolic extract of *Phyllanthus niruri* (Family Euphorbiaceae). Int J Pharm Phytopharmacol Res 2015; 4(5): 276-80.

[537] Sabatullah A, Aslam M, Javed K, Siddiqui WA. Nephroprotective activity of hydroalcoholic extract of *Physalis alkekengi* (Solanaceae) fruit against cisplatin induced nephrotoxicity in rats. Planta Med 2010; 76(5): 101-6.

[538] Aslam M, Siddiqui WA. Sabahatullah, Javed K, Khan AH. Nephroprotective activity of hydroalcoholic extract of *Physalis alkekengi* (Solanaceae) fruit against cisplatin induced nephrotoxicity in rats. World J Pharm Res 2015; 4(9): 2059-70.

[539] Abdel-Moneim AE, El-Deib KM. The possible protective effects of *Physalis peruviana* on carbon tetrachloride-induced nephrotoxicity in male albino rats. Life Sci J 2012; 9: 1038-52.

[540] Yamgar S, Sali L, Salkar R, Jain NK, Gadgoli CH. Studies on nephroprotective and nephrocurative activity of ethanolic extract of *Picrorhiza kurroa* Royle and arogyawardhinibati in rats. Intern J Pharm & Technol 2010; 2(3): 472-89.

[541] Changizi-Ashtiyani S, Seddigh A, Najafi H, *et al.* *Pimpinella anisum* L. ethanolic extract ameliorates the gentamicin- induced nephrotoxicity in rats. Nephrology (Carlton) 2017; 22(2): 133-8. [http://dx.doi.org/10.1111/nep.12953] [PMID: 27860049]

[542] Aiswarya N, Rashmi RR, Preethi JS, *et al.* Nephroprotective effect of aqueous extract of *Pimpinella anisum* in gentamicin induced nephrotoxicity in Wistar Rats. Pharmacogn J 2018; 10(3): 403-7. [http://dx.doi.org/10.5530/pj.2018.3.66]

[543] Palani S, Raja S, Kumar RP, Jayakumar S, Kumar BS. Therapeutic efficacy of *Pimpinella tirupatiensis* (Apiaceae) on acetaminophen induced nephrotoxicity and oxidative stress in male albino rats. Int J Pharm Tech Res 2009; 1(3): 925-34.

[544] Hosseinzadeh H, Khooei AR, Khashayarmanesh Z, Motamed-Shariaty V. Antiurolithiatic activity of *Pinus eldarica* medw: fruits aqueous extract in rats. Urol J 2010; 7(4): 232-7. [PMID: 21170851]

[545] Ahmad QZ, Ahmad G. Tajuddin, Jafri MA. The study of Kabab chini (*Piper cubeba*) for nephroprotective effect in cisplatin induced nephrotoxicity. Unani Medicus 2010; 1(1): 85-91.

[546] Ahmad QZ, Jahan N, Ahmad G. Nephroprotective effect of Kabab chini (*Piper cubeba*) in gentamycin-induced nephrotoxicity. Saudi J Kidney Dis Transpl 2012; 23(4): 773-81. [http://dx.doi.org/10.4103/1319-2442.98159] [PMID: 22805390]

[547] Bano H, Jahan N, Makbul SAA, Kumar BN, Husain S, Sayed A. Effect of *Piper cubeba* L. fruit on ethylene glycol and ammonium chloride induced urolithiasis in male Sprague Dawley rats. Integr Med Res 2018; 7(4): 358-65. [http://dx.doi.org/10.1016/j.imr.2018.06.005] [PMID: 30591890]

[548] Heidarian E, Jafari-Dehkordi E, Valipour P, Ghatreh-Samani K, Ashrafi-Eshkaftaki L. Nephroprotective and anti-inflammatory effects of *Pistacia atlantica* leaf hydroethanolic extract against gentamicin-induced nephrotoxicity in rats. J Diet Suppl 2017; 14(5): 489-502. [http://dx.doi.org/10.1080/19390211.2016.1267062] [PMID: 28121473]

[549] Ghaedi T, Mirzaei A, Laameerad B. Protective effect of *Pistacia khinjuk* on gentamicin-induced nephrotoxicity in rats. World J Pharm Pharm Sci 2014; 3: 919-26.

[550] Ehsani V, Amirteimoury M, Taghipour Z, *et al.* Protective effect of hydroalcoholic extract of *Pistacia vera* against gentamicin-induced nephrotoxicity in rats. Ren Fail 2017; 39(1): 519-25. [http://dx.doi.org/10.1080/0886022X.2017.1326384] [PMID: 28558475]

[551] Aziz SA, See TL, Khuay LY, Osman K, Abu Bakar MA. *in vitro* effects of *plantago major* extract on urolithiasis. Malays J Med Sci 2005; 12(2): 22-6.
[PMID: 22605954]

[552] Sharifa AA, Jamaludin J, Kiong LS, Chea LA, Osman K. Antiurolithiatic terpenoid compound from *Plantago major* Linn. (Ekar Anjing). Sains Malays 2012; 41(1): 33-9.

[553] Jose MA. Ibrahim, Janardhan S. Modulatory effect of *Plectranthus amboinicus* Lour on ethylene glycol induced nephrolithiasis in rats. Indian J Pharmacol 2005; 37: 43-5.
[http://dx.doi.org/10.4103/0253-7613.13857]

[554] Palani S, Raja S, Naresh R, Kumar BS. Evaluation of nephroprotective, diuretic, and antioxidant activities of *Plectranthus amboinicus* on acetaminophen-induced nephrotoxic rats. Toxicol Mech Methods 2010; 20(4): 213-21.
[http://dx.doi.org/10.3109/15376511003736787] [PMID: 20367443]

[555] Radha B, Janarthan M, Durraivel S. Protective role of methanolic extract of *Polygonum glabrum* Willd. against cisplatin and gentamicin induced nephrotoxicity in albino rats. Indian J Res Pharm Biotech 2013; 1(6): 846-9.

[556] Shirwaikar A, Malini S, Kumari SC. Protective effect of *Pongamia pinnata* flowers against cisplatin and gentamicin induced nephrotoxicity in rats. Indian J Exp Biol 2003; 41(1): 58-62.
[PMID: 15267137]

[557] Karimi G, Khoei A, Omidi A, *et al.* Protective effect of aqueous and ethanolic extracts of *Portulaca oleracea* against cisplatin induced nephrotoxicity. Iran J Basic Med Sci 2010; 13: 31-5.

[558] Hozayen W, Bastawy M, Elshafeey H. Effects of aqueous purslane (*Portulaca oleracea*) extract and fish oil on gentamicin nephrotoxicity in albino rats. Nat Sci 2011; 9(2): 47-62.

[559] Kishore DV, Moosavi F, Varma RK. Effect of ethanolic extract of *Portulaca oleracea* on ethylene glycol and ammonium induced urolithiasis. Intern J Pharm Pharmaceutl Sci 2012; 5(2): 134-40.

[560] Gutierrez RM, Gomez YG, Ramirez EB. Nephroprotective activity of *Prosthechea michuacana* against cisplatin-induced acute renal failure in rats. J Med Food 2010; 13(4): 911-6.
[http://dx.doi.org/10.1089/jmf.2009.0175] [PMID: 20673060]

[561] Azaryan E, Malekaneh M, Shemshadi Nejad M, Haghighi F. Therapeutic effects of aqueous extracts of *Cerasus avium* stem on ethylene glycol- induced kidney calculi in rats. Urol J 2017; 14(4): 4024-9.
[PMID: 28670670]

[562] Kessler T, Jansen B, Hesse A. Effect of blackcurrant-, cranberry- and plum juice consumption on risk factors associated with kidney stone formation. Eur J Clin Nutr 2002; 56(10): 1020-3.
[http://dx.doi.org/10.1038/sj.ejcn.1601442] [PMID: 12373623]

[563] Ojewale OA, Adekoya OA, Faduyile FA, Yemitan OK, Odukanmi OA. Nephroprotective activities of ethanolic roots extract of *Pseudocedrela kotschyi* against oxidative stress and nephrotoxicity in alloxan-induced diabetic albino rats. Br J Pharmacol Toxicol 2014; 5(1): 26-34.
[http://dx.doi.org/10.19026/bjpt.5.5413]

[564] Adesia A. 2013.

[565] Mohan M, Shashank B, Vishnu Priya A. Protective effect of *Psidium guajava* L. leaves ethanolic extract on doxorubicin-induced nephrotoxicity in rats. Indian J Nat Prod Resour 2014; 5: 129-33.

[566] Saputri FC, Anjani FD, Mun'im A. Nephroprotective effect of *Pterocarpus indicus* Willd. leaves. J Young Pharm 2017; 9(1) (Suppl.): s43-5.
[http://dx.doi.org/10.5530/jyp.2017.1s.11]

[567] Tugcu V, Kemahli E, Ozbek E, *et al.* Protective effect of a potent antioxidant, pomegranate juice, in the kidey of rats with nephrolithiasis induced by ethylene glycol. J Endourol 2008; 22(12): 2723-31.
[http://dx.doi.org/10.1089/end.2008.0357] [PMID: 19025399]

[568] Ahmed MM, Ali SE. Protective effect of pomegranate peel ethanol extract against ferric nitrilotriacetate induced renal oxidative damage in rats. J Cell Mol Biol 2010; 7,8(2,1): 35-43.

[569] Boroushaki MT, Asadpour E, Sadeghnia HR, Dolati K. Effect of pomegranate seed oil against gentamicin -induced nephrotoxicity in rat. J Food Sci Technol 2014; 51(11): 3510-4.
[http://dx.doi.org/10.1007/s13197-012-0881-y] [PMID: 26396355]

[570] Singh AP, Singh AJ, Singh N. Pharmacological investigations of *Punica granatum* in glycerol-induced acute renal failure in rats. Indian J Pharmacol 2011; 43(5): 551-6.
[http://dx.doi.org/10.4103/0253-7613.84971] [PMID: 22021999]

[571] Ali NAM, Saeed SZ. Nephro-protective effect of *Punica granatum* in gentamicin-induced nephrotoxicity in rats. Med J Babylon 2012; 9: 220-8.

[572] Boroushaki MT, Sadeghnia HR, Banihasan M. Protective effect of pomegranate seed oil on hexacholorobutadiene –induced nephrotoxicity in rat. J Ren Fail 2010; 32: 612-7.
[http://dx.doi.org/10.3109/08860221003778056]

[573] Rathod NR, Biswas D, Chitme HR, Ratna S, Muchandi IS, Chandra R. Anti-urolithiatic effects of *Punica granatum* in male rats. J Ethnopharmacol 2012; 140(2): 234-8.
[http://dx.doi.org/10.1016/j.jep.2012.01.003] [PMID: 22285521]

[574] Cekmen M, Otunctemur A, Ozbek E, *et al.* Pomegranate extract attenuates gentamicin-induced nephrotoxicity in rats by reducing oxidative stress. Ren Fail 2013; 35(2): 268-74.
[http://dx.doi.org/10.3109/0886022X.2012.743859] [PMID: 23176634]

[575] Motamedi F, Nematbakhsh M, Monajemi R, *et al.* Effect of pomegranate flower extract on cisplatin-induced nephrotoxicity in rats. J Nephropathol 2014; 3(4): 133-8.
[PMID: 25374882]

[576] Tracy CR, Henning JR, Newton MR, Aviram M, Bridget Zimmerman M. Oxidative stress and nephrolithiasis: a comparative pilot study evaluating the effect of pomegranate extract on stone risk factors and elevated oxidative stress levels of recurrent stone formers and controls. Urolithiasis 2014; 42(5): 401-8.
[http://dx.doi.org/10.1007/s00240-014-0686-8] [PMID: 25085198]

[577] Mestry SN, Gawali NB, Pai SA, *et al.* *Punica granatum* improves renal function in gentamicin-induced nephropathy in rats *via* attenuation of oxidative stress. J Ayurveda Integr Med 2020; 11(1): 16-23.
[http://dx.doi.org/10.1016/j.jaim.2017.09.006] [PMID: 29555255]

[578] Bahuguna YM, Rawat MSM, Juyal V, Gusain K. Evaluation of *Pyracantha crenulata* Roem. for antiurolithogenic activity in albino rats. Afr J Urol 2009; 15(3): 159-66.
[http://dx.doi.org/10.1007/s12301-009-0029-0]

[579] Moriyama MT, Miyazawa K, Noda K, Oka M, Tanaka M, Suzuki K. Reduction in oxalate-induced renal tubular epithelial cell injury by an extract from *Quercus salicina* Blume/*Quercus stenophylla* Makino. Urol Res 2007; 35(6): 295-300.
[http://dx.doi.org/10.1007/s00240-007-0114-4] [PMID: 17882411]

[580] Moriyama MT, Suga K, Miyazawa K, *et al.* Inhibitions of urinary oxidative stress and renal calcium level by an extract of *Quercus salicina* Blume/*Quercus stenophylla* Makino in a rat calcium oxalate urolithiasis model. Int J Urol 2009; 16(4): 397-401.
[http://dx.doi.org/10.1111/j.1442-2042.2009.02268.x] [PMID: 19425219]

[581] Vargas Solis R, Perez Gutierrez RM. Diuretic and urolithiatic activities of the aqueous extract of the fruit of *Randia echinocarpa* on rats. J Ethnopharmacol 2002; 83(1-2): 145-7.
[http://dx.doi.org/10.1016/S0378-8741(02)00091-0] [PMID: 12413721]

[582] Vargas R, Perez RM, Perez S, Zavala MA, Perez C. Antiurolithiatic activity of *Raphanus sativus* aqueous extract on rats. J Ethnopharmacol 1999; 68(1- 3): 335-8.

[583] Ali BH. The effect of treatment with the medicinal plant *Rhazya stricta* decne on gentamicin nephrotoxicity in rats. Phytomedicine 2002; 9(5): 385-9.
[http://dx.doi.org/10.1078/09447110260571607] [PMID: 12222656]

[584] Yokozawa T, Suzuki N, Zheng PD, Oura H, Nishioka I. Effect of orally administered rhubarb extract in rats with chronic renal failure. Chem Pharm Bull (Tokyo) 1984; 32(11): 4506-13.
[http://dx.doi.org/10.1248/cpb.32.4506] [PMID: 6532552]

[585] Alam MM, Javed K, Jafri MA. Effect of *Rheum emodi* (Revand Hindi) on renal functions in rats. J Ethnopharmacol 2005; 96(1-2): 121-5.
[http://dx.doi.org/10.1016/j.jep.2004.08.028] [PMID: 15588659]

[586] Grases F, Masárová L, Costa-Bauzá A, March JG, Prieto R, Tur JA. Effect of "*Rosa Canina*" infusion and magnesium on the urinary risk factors of calcium oxalate urolithiasis. Planta Med 1992; 58(6): 509-12.
[http://dx.doi.org/10.1055/s-2006-961537] [PMID: 1484889]

[587] Tayefi-Nasrabadi H, Sadigh-Eteghad S, Aghdam Z. The effects of the hydroalcohol extract of *Rosa canina* L. fruit on experimentally nephrolithiasic Wistar rats. Phytother Res 2012; 26(1): 78-85.
[http://dx.doi.org/10.1002/ptr.3519] [PMID: 21544885]

[588] Christina AJ, Priya Mole M, Moorthy P. Studies on the antilithic effect of *Rotula aquatica* lour in male Wistar rats. Methods Find Exp Clin Pharmacol 2002; 24(6): 357-9. b
[http://dx.doi.org/10.1358/mf.2002.24.6.693068] [PMID: 12224442]

[589] Chauhan CK, Joshi MJ, Vaidya ADB. Growth inhibition of struvite crystals by the aqueous root extract of *Rotula aquatica.* Indian J Biochem Biophys 2011; 48(3): 202-7.
[PMID: 21793313]

[590] Umesh KG, Christina AJM. Effect of *Rotula aquatica* Lour. on ethylene-glycol induced urolithiasis in rats. Int J Drug Dev & Res 2011; 3(1): 273-80.

[591] Sasikala V, Radha SR, Vijayakumari B. *in vitro* evaluation of *Rotula aquatica* Lour. for antiurolithiatic activity. J Pharma Res 2013; 378-82.
[http://dx.doi.org/10.1016/j.jopr.2013.02.026]

[592] Prashanthi P, Anitha S, Shashidhara S. Effect of *Rotula aquatica* Lour. on experimental kidney stones. Intern J Pharmacogn & Phytochem Res 2015; 7(6): 1142-6.

[593] Vijayakumari B, Sasikala V, Radha SR, Rameshwar HY. *Rotula aquatica* Lour aqueous extract as anti-urolithiatic agent in experimentally induced urolithiatic rat model. Intern J Pharmacogn Phytochem Res 2017; 9(4): 1-6.
[http://dx.doi.org/10.25258/phyto.v9i4.8128]

[594] A V, S A, Kuriakose J, Midhun SJ, Jyothis M, Latha MS. Protective effect of *Rotula aquatica* Lour against gentamicin induced oxidative stress and nephrotoxicity in Wistar rats. Biomed Pharmacother 2018; 106: 1188-94.
[http://dx.doi.org/10.1016/j.biopha.2018.07.066] [PMID: 30119187]

[595] Divakar K, Pawar AT, Chandrasekhar SB, Dighe SB, Divakar G. Protective effect of the hydro-alcoholic extract of *Rubia cordifolia* roots against ethylene glycol induced urolithiasis in rats. Food Chem Toxicol 2010; 48(4): 1013-8.
[http://dx.doi.org/10.1016/j.fct.2010.01.011] [PMID: 20079795]

[596] Joy J, Nair CKK. Amelioration of cisplatin induced nephrotoxicity in Swiss albino mice by *Rubia cordifolia* extract. J Cancer Res Ther 2008; 4(3): 111-5.
[http://dx.doi.org/10.4103/0973-1482.43139] [PMID: 18923202]

[597] Sharma US, Kumar A. Nephroprotective evaluation of *Rubus ellipticus* (Smith) fruits extracts against cisplatin and gentamicin induced renal-toxicity in rats. J Pharm Res 2011; 4(1): 285-7.

[598] Moreira Galdino P, Nunes Alexandre L, Fernanda Pacheco L, *et al.* Nephroprotective effect of *Rudgea*

viburnoides (Cham.) Benth leaves on gentamicin-induced nephrotoxicity in rats. J Ethnopharmacol 2017; 201: 100-7.
[http://dx.doi.org/10.1016/j.jep.2017.02.035] [PMID: 28242383]

[599]   Sathya M, Kokilavani R. Antiurolithiatic activity of ethanolic root extract of *Saccharum spontaneum* on glycolic acid induced urolithiasis in rats. J Drug Deliv Ther 2012; 2(5): 86-9.

[600]   Palani S, Raja S, Kumar SN, Kumar BS. Nephroprotective and antioxidant activities of *Salacia oblonga* on acetaminophen-induced toxicity in rats. Nat Prod Res 2011; 25(19): 1876-80.
[http://dx.doi.org/10.1080/14786419.2010.537269] [PMID: 21848492]

[601]   Jabbar Z, Ali M. An experimental evalution on nephroprotective activity of the flowers of *Salix caprea* (Salicaceae). Intern Res J Pharm 2012; 3(3): 139-42.

[602]   Vargas SR, Perez RMG. Antiurolithiatic activity of *Salix taxifolia* aqueous extract. Pharm Biol 2002; 40(8): 561-3.
[http://dx.doi.org/10.1076/phbi.40.8.561.14655]

[603]   Jeong JC, Hwang WM, Yoon CH, Kim YK. Salviae radix extract prevents cisplatin-induced acute renal failure in rabbits. Nephron J 2001; 88(3): 241-6.
[http://dx.doi.org/10.1159/000045996] [PMID: 11423755]

[604]   Dizaye K. Alleviation of cisplatin-induced nephrotoxicity in albino rats by aqueous extract of *Salvia officinalis*. Iraq J Pharm 12(1): 48-55.

[605]   Patel J, Shanmukha I, Kumar V, Ramachandra Setty S, Rajendra SV. Role of polyphenols in nephroprotective potential of *Samanea saman* (Jacq.) Merr. leaves on experimentally induced renal injury. Indo Am J Pharm Res 2013; 3: 2571-81.

[606]   Gondwe M, Kamadyaapa DR, Tufts M, Chuturgoon AA, Musabayane CT. *Sclerocarya birrea* [(A. Rich.) Hochst.] [Anacardiaceae] stem-bark ethanolic extract (SBE) modulates blood glucose, glomerular filtration rate (GFR) and mean arterial blood pressure (MAP) of STZ-induced diabetic rats. Phytomedicine 2008; 15(9): 699-709.
[http://dx.doi.org/10.1016/j.phymed.2008.02.004] [PMID: 18406590]

[607]   Jose S, Adikay S. Effect of the ethanolic extract of *Scoparia dulcis* in cisplatin induced nephrotoxicity in wistar rats. Indian J Pharm Educ Res 2015; 49(4) (Suppl.): s68-74.
[http://dx.doi.org/10.5530/ijper.49.4s.8]

[608]   Alqasoumi SI. Evaluation of the hepatoprotective and nephroprotective activities of *Scrophularia hypericifolia* growing in Saudi Arabia. Saudi Pharm J 2014; 22(3): 258-63.
[http://dx.doi.org/10.1016/j.jsps.2013.12.001] [PMID: 25061411]

[609]   Mumtaz SMF, Paul S, Bag AK. Effect of *Sechium edule* on chemical induced kidney damage in experimental animals. Bangladesh J Pharmacol 2013; 8: 28-35.

[610]   Bhuvaneswari P, Krishnakumari S. Nephroprotective effects of ethanolic extract of *Sesamum indicum* seeds (Linn.) in streptozotocin induced diabetic male albino rats. Intern J Green Pharm 2012; 6(4): 330-5.
[http://dx.doi.org/10.4103/0973-8258.108249]

[611]   Doddola S, Pasupulati H, Koganti B, Prasad KVSRG. Evaluation of *Sesbania grandiflora* for antiurolithiatic and antioxidant properties. J Nat Med 2008; 62(3): 300-7.
[http://dx.doi.org/10.1007/s11418-008-0235-2] [PMID: 18408896]

[612]   Shah NA, Khan MR, Nigussie D. Phytochemical investigation and nephroprotective potential of *Sida cordata* in rat. BMC Complement Altern Med 2017; 17(1): 388.
[http://dx.doi.org/10.1186/s12906-017-1896-8] [PMID: 28778164]

[613]   Lovkesh B, Vivek B, Manav G. Nephroprotective effect of fresh leaves extracts of *Sida cordifolia* Linn. in gentamicin induced nephrotoxicity in rats. Intern J Res Pharm Sci 2012; 2(2): 151-8.

[614]   Makwana MV, Pandya NM, Darji DN, Desai SA, Bhaskar VH. Assessment of nephroprotective

potential of *Sida cordifolia* in experimental medicine. Scholars Research Library 2012; 4(1): 175-80.

[615] Thounaojam MC, Jadeja RN, Devkar RV, Ramachandran AV. Sida rhomboidea.Roxb leaf extract ameliorates gentamicin induced nephrotoxicity and renal dysfunction in rats. J Ethnopharmacol 2010; 132(1): 365-7.
[http://dx.doi.org/10.1016/j.jep.2010.08.037] [PMID: 20728516]

[616] Yusufoglu HS, Soliman GA, Foudah AI, Abdulkader MS, Ansari MN, Salkini MA. Protective role of aerial parts of *Silene villosa* alcoholic extract against CCl₄-induced cardiac and renal toxicity in rats. Int J Pharmacol 2018; 14(7): 1001-9.
[http://dx.doi.org/10.3923/ijp.2018.1001.1009]

[617] Chen L, Yin H, Lan Z, *et al.* Anti-hyperuricemic and nephroprotective effects of *Smilax china* L. J Ethnopharmacol 2011; 135(2): 399-405.
[http://dx.doi.org/10.1016/j.jep.2011.03.033] [PMID: 21420478]

[618] Prashanth Kumar V, Shashidhara S, Kumar MM, Sridhara BY. Cytoprotective role of *Solanum nigrum* against gentamicin-induced kidney cell (Vero cells) damage *in vitro*. Fitoterapia 2001; 72(5): 481-6.
[http://dx.doi.org/10.1016/S0367-326X(01)00266-0] [PMID: 11429239]

[619] Kushwaha V, Sharma M, Vishwakarma P, Saini M, Bhatt S, Saxena KK. Evaluation of nephroprotective and nephrocurative activity of *Solanum nigrum* on gentamicin induced nephrotoxicity in experimental rats. Int J Basic Clin Pharmacol 2016; 5(1): 74-8.
[http://dx.doi.org/10.18203/2319-2003.ijbcp20160104]

[620] Chinnala HM, Shanigarm S, Elsani MM. Antiurolithiatic activity of the plant extracts of *Solanum virginianum* on ethylene glycol induced urolithiasis in rats. Int J Pharm Biol Sci 2013; 3: 328-34.

[621] Hussain T, Gupta RK, Sweety K, Eswaran B, Vijayakumar M, Rao CV. Nephroprotective activity of *Solanum xanthocarpum* fruit extract against gentamicin-induced nephrotoxicity and renal dysfunction in experimental rodents. Asian Pac J Trop Med 2012; 5(9): 686-91.
[http://dx.doi.org/10.1016/S1995-7645(12)60107-2] [PMID: 22805718]

[622] Patel PK, Patel MA, Vyas BA, Shah DR, Gandhi TR. Antiurolithiatic activity of saponin rich fraction from the fruits of *Solanum xanthocarpum* Schrad. & Wendl. (Solanaceae) against ethylene glycol induced urolithiasis in rats. J Ethnopharmacol 2012; 144(1): 160-70.
[http://dx.doi.org/10.1016/j.jep.2012.08.043] [PMID: 22981722]

[623] Alam Q. Vijayanarayana. Nephroprotective effect of alcoholic extracts of fruits of *Solanum xanthocarpum* against cisplatin-induced nephropathy in rats. Int J Advance Pharm Biol Chem 2013; 2(1): 147-51.

[624] Melzig MF. Goldenrod--a classical exponent in the urological phytotherapy. Wien Med Wochenschr 2004; 154(21-22): 523-7.
[http://dx.doi.org/10.1007/s10354-004-0118-4] [PMID: 15638071]

[625] Khan RA, Khan MR, Sahreen S, Bokhari J. Prevention of CCl₄-induced nephrotoxicity with *Sonchus asper* in rat. Food Chem Toxicol 2010; 48(8-9): 2469-76.
[http://dx.doi.org/10.1016/j.fct.2010.06.016] [PMID: 20550952]

[626] Mathew JE, Joseph A, Srinivasan K, Dinakaran SV, Mantri A, Movaliya V. Effect of ethanol extract of *Sphaeranthus indicus* on cisplatin-induced nephrotoxicity in rats. Nat Prod Res 2012; 26(10): 933-8.
[http://dx.doi.org/10.1080/14786419.2010.534999] [PMID: 21790496]

[627] Varghese R, Moideen MM, Suhail MJM, Dhanapal CK. Nephroprotective effect of ethanolic extract of *Strychnos potatorum* seeds in Rat Models. Res J Pharm Biol Chem Sci 2011; 2(3): 521-9.

[628] Binu TV, Vijayakumari B. *In-vitro* anti urolithiatic activity of *Strychnos potatorum* L.f. South Indian J Biol Sci 2016; 2(1): 174-8.
[http://dx.doi.org/10.22205/sijbs/2016/v2/i1/100388]

[629] Parmar RK, Kachchi NR, Tirgar PR, Desai TR, Bhalodiya PN. Preclinical evalution of anti-urolithiatic

activity of *Swertia chirata* stems. Intern Res J Pharm 2012; 3(8): 198-202.

[630] Sreedevi A, Pavani B, Bharathi K. Protective effect of fruits of *Syzygium cumini* against cisplatin-induced acute renal failure in rats. J Pharm Res 2010; 3(11): 2756-8.

[631] Sanjuna C, Anjali M, Sandhya N, Prasad M, Rohini B, Himabindu J, *et al.* Evaluation of *in vitro* antiurolithiatic activity of *Syzygium cumini* leaves. World J Gastroenterol Hepatol Endosc 2019; 1(1) WJGHE-1-109

[632] Joseph KC, Bharat Parekh B, Joshi MJ. Inhibition of growth of urinary type calcium hydrogen phosphate dihydrate crystals by tartaric acid and tamarind. Curr Sci 2005; 88: 1232-8.

[633] Chaudhary A, Singla SK, Tandon C. Calcium oxalate crystal growth inhibition by aqueous extract of *Tamarindus indica.* Indian J Urol 2008; 24: 105-11.

[634] Ullah N, Azam Khan M, Khan T, Ahmad W. Protective potential of *Tamarindus indica* against gentamicin-induced nephrotoxicity. Pharm Biol 2014; 52(4): 428-34.
[http://dx.doi.org/10.3109/13880209.2013.840318] [PMID: 24417619]

[635] Rathore P, Pendse AK, Handa S, Sharma K, Singh PP. Effectiveness of Tamarind *(Tamarindus indica)* therapy (3 gm and 10 gm) on calcium oxalate and calcium phosphate crystallization using three different methods. Indian J Clin Biochem 1993; 8: 136-43.

[636] Bensatal A, Ouahrani MR. Inhibition of crystallization of calcium oxalate by the extraction of *Tamarix gallica* L. Urol Res 2008; 36(6): 283-7.
[http://dx.doi.org/10.1007/s00240-008-0157-1] [PMID: 19002446]

[637] Sreedevi A, Sravanthi U. Alleviation of cisplatin-induced nephrotoxicity in albino rats by roots of *Catunaregam uliginosa.* Asian J Pharm Clin Res 2016; 9(6): 147-51.
[http://dx.doi.org/10.22159/ajpcr.2016.v9i6.13956]

[638] Venkateswarlu K, Preethi JK, Chandrasekhar KB. Antiurolithiatic activity of ethanolic extract of *Taxillus tomentosus* plant on ethylene glycol and ammonium chloride induced urolithiasis in wistar rats. Indones J Pharm 2016; 27(2): 66-73.
[http://dx.doi.org/10.14499/indonesianjpharm27iss2pp66]

[639] Raju S, Kavimani S, Maheshwara Rao VU, Reddy KS, Kumar GV. Floral extract of *Tecoma stans*: a potent inhibitor of gentamicin-induced nephrotoxicity *in vivo*. Asian Pac J Trop Med 2011; 4(9): 680-5.
[http://dx.doi.org/10.1016/S1995-7645(11)60173-9] [PMID: 21967688]

[640] Kameshwaran S, Thenmozhi S, Vasuki K, Dhanalakshmi M, Dhanapal C. Antiurolithiatic activity of aqueous and methanolic extracts of *Tecoma stans* flower in rats. Int J Pharm Biol Arch 2013; 4(3): 446-50.

[641] Patel BA, Patel PU, Patel RK. *in-vitro* evaluation of anti-lithiatic activity on *Tectona grandis* Linn. seeds. J Pharm Res 2011; 4(6): 1699-700.

[642] Swathi D, Sujatha D, Bharathi K, Prasad KVSRG. Antilithiatic activity of the aqueous extract of the roots of *Tephrosia purpurea* Linn. Pharmacogn Mag 2008; 4(16): S206-11.

[643] Jain A, Nahata A, Singhai AK. Effect of *Tephrosia purpurea* (L.) Pers. leaves on gentamicin-Induced nephrotoxicity in rats. Sci Pharm 2013; 81(4): 1071-87.
[http://dx.doi.org/10.3797/scipharm.1302-09] [PMID: 24482774]

[644] Manna P, Sinha M, Sil PC. . Aqueous extract of *Terminalia arjuna* prevents carbon tetrachloride induced hepatic and renal disorders. Bio Med Central complementary and alternative med 2006; 6(1): 33.

[645] Das K, Pratim Chakraborty P, Ghosh D, Kumar Nandi D. Protective effect of aqueous extract of *Terminalia arjuna* against dehydrating induced oxidative stress and uremia in male rat. Iran J Pharm Res 2010; 9(2): 153-61.
[PMID: 24363722]

[646] Chaudhary A, Singla SK, Tandon C. *in vitro* Evaluation of *Terminalia arjuna* on calcium phosphate and calcium oxalate crystallization. Indian J Pharm Sci 2010; 72(3): 340-5.
[http://dx.doi.org/10.4103/0250-474X.70480] [PMID: 21188043]

[647] Venkateshwarlu E, Sharat Chandra K, Bharat Kumar K, Sharavanabhava BS, Shivakumar R, Venkateswara Rao J. Evaluation of protective effect of different doses of *Terminalia arjuna* bark ethanolic extract on cisplatin induced oxidative nephrotoxicity in rats. Iraqi J Pharm Sci 2014; 23(2): 89-98.

[648] Mittal A, Tandon S, Singla SK, Tandon C. *in vitro* studies reveal antiurolithic effect of *Terminalia arjuna* using quantitative morphological information from computerized microscopy. Int Braz J Urol 2015; 41(5): 935-44.
[http://dx.doi.org/10.1590/S1677-5538.IBJU.2014.0547] [PMID: 26689519]

[649] Mittal A, Tandon S, Singla SK, Tandon C. *in vitro* inhibition of calcium oxalate crystallization and crystal adherence to renal tubular epithelial cells by *Terminalia arjuna*. Urolithiasis 2016; 44(2): 117-25.
[http://dx.doi.org/10.1007/s00240-015-0822-0] [PMID: 26424092]

[650] Mittal A, Tandon S, Singla SK, Tandon C. Cytoprotective and anti-apoptotic role of *Terminalia arjuna* on oxalate injured renal epithelial cells. Cytotechnology 2017; 69(2): 349-58.
[http://dx.doi.org/10.1007/s10616-017-0065-8] [PMID: 28181139]

[651] Mittal A, Tandon S, Singla SK, Tandon C. Modulation of lithiatic injury to renal epithelial cells by aqueous extract of *Terminalia arjuna*. J Herb Med 2018; 63-70.
[http://dx.doi.org/10.1016/j.hermed.2018.01.003]

[652] Upadhyay N, Tiwari SK, Srivastava A, Seth A, Maurya SK. Anti-urolithiatic effect of *Terminalia bellirica* Roxb. fruits on ethylene glycol-induced renal calculi in rats. Indo American J Pharacet Res 2015; 5(5): 2031-40.

[653] Prasad L, Husain Khan T, Jahangir T, Sultana S. Chemomodulatory effects of *Terminalia chebula* against nickel chloride induced oxidative stress and tumor promotion response in male Wistar rats. J Trace Elem Med Biol 2006; 20(4): 233-9.
[http://dx.doi.org/10.1016/j.jtemb.2006.07.003] [PMID: 17098582]

[654] Pawar AT, Gaikwad GD, Metkari KS, Tijore KA, Ghodasara V, Kuchekar BS. Effect of *Terminalia chebula* fruit extract on ethylene glycol induced urolithiasis in rats. Biomed Aging Pathol 2012; 2(3): 99-103.
[http://dx.doi.org/10.1016/j.biomag.2012.07.005]

[655] Tayal S, Duggal S, Bandyopadhyay P, Aggarwal A, Tandon S, Tandon C. Cytoprotective role of the aqueous extract of *Terminalia chebula* on renal epithelial cells. Int Braz J Urol 2012; 38(2): 204-13.
[http://dx.doi.org/10.1590/S1677-55382012000200008] [PMID: 22555028]

[656] Fahmy NM, Al-Sayed E, Abdel-Daim MM, Karonen M, Singab AN. Protective effect of *Terminalia muelleri* against carbon tetrachloride-induced hepato and nephro-toxicity in mice and characterization of its bioactive constituents. Pharm Biol 2016; 54(2): 303-13.
[http://dx.doi.org/10.3109/13880209.2015.1035794] [PMID: 25894213]

[657] Yokozawa T, Chung HY, He LQ, Oura H. Effectiveness of green tea tannin on rats with chronic renal failure. Biosci Biotechnol Biochem 1996; 60(6): 1000-5.
[http://dx.doi.org/10.1271/bbb.60.1000] [PMID: 8695898]

[658] Yokozawa T, Nakagawa T, Kyeoungi M, Eun JC, Shigeya T, Terasawa K. Effect of green tea tannin on cisplatin induced nephropathy in LLC-PK1 cells and rats. J Pharm Pharmacol 1995; 1: 1325-31.

[659] El-Beshbishy HA. Hepatoprotective effect of green tea (*Camellia sinensis*) extract against tamoxifen-induced liver injury in rats. J Biochem Mol Biol 2005; 38(5): 563-70.
[PMID: 16202236]

[660] Leena P, Balaraman R. Effect of green tea extract on cisplatin induced o xidative damage on kidney

and testes of rats. Ars Pharm 2005; 46: 5-18.

[661] Jeong BC, Kim BS, Kim JI, Kim HH. Effects of green tea on urinary stone formation: an *in vivo* and *in vitro* study. J Endourol 2006; 20(5): 356-61.
[http://dx.doi.org/10.1089/end.2006.20.356] [PMID: 16724910]

[662] Khan SA, Priyamvada S, Farooq N, Khan S, Khan MW, Yusufi AN. Protective effect of green tea extract on gentamicin-induced nephrotoxicity and oxidative damage in rat kidney. Pharmacol Res 2009; 59(4): 254-62.
[http://dx.doi.org/10.1016/j.phrs.2008.12.009] [PMID: 19429467]

[663] Khan SA, Priyamvada S, Khan W, Khan S, Farooq N, Yusufi ANK. Studies on the protective effect of green tea against cisplatin induced nephrotoxicity. Pharmacol Res 2009; 60(5): 382-91.
[http://dx.doi.org/10.1016/j.phrs.2009.07.007] [PMID: 19647078]

[664] Abdel-Raheem IT, El-Sherbiny GA, Taye A. Green tea ameliorates renal oxidative damage induced by gentamicin in rats. Pak J Pharm Sci 2010; 23(1): 21-8.
[PMID: 20067862]

[665] Ahn T-G, Kim H-K, Park S-W, Kim S-A, Lee B-R, Han SJ. Protective effects of green tea polyphenol against cisplatin-induced nephrotoxicity in rats. Obstet Gynecol Sci 2014; 57(6): 464-70.
[http://dx.doi.org/10.5468/ogs.2014.57.6.464] [PMID: 25469334]

[666] Mika D, Guruvayoorappan C. The effect of *Thespesia populnea* on cisplatin induced nephrotoxicity. J Cancer Res Ther 2013; 9(1): 50-3.
[http://dx.doi.org/10.4103/0973-1482.110362] [PMID: 23575074]

[667] Khanam S, Mohan NP, Devi K, Sultana R. Protective role of *Tinospora cardifolia* against cisplatin induced nephrotoxicity. J Int Pharm Sci 2011; 3(4): 268-70.

[668] Uppuluri S, Ali SL, Nirmala T, Shanthi M, Sipay B, Uppuluri KB. Nephroprotector activity of hydroalcoholic extract of *Tinospora cordifolia* roots on cisplatin induced nephrotoxicity in rats. Drug Invention Today 2013; 5: 281-7.
[http://dx.doi.org/10.1016/j.dit.2013.09.001]

[669] Sharma M, Pundir J, Vishwakarma P, Goel RK, Saini M, Saxena KL. Evaluation of nephroprotective activity of *Tinospora cordifolia* against gentamicin induced nephrotoxicity in albino rats: an experimental study. Int J Basic Clin Pharmacol 2019; 8(6): 1179-84.
[http://dx.doi.org/10.18203/2319-2003.ijbcp20192181]

[670] Kaur T, Bijarnia RK, Singla SK, Tandon C. *In vivo* efficacy of *Trachyspermum ammi* anticalcifying protein in urolithiatic rat model. J Ethnopharmacol 2009; 126(3): 459-62.
[http://dx.doi.org/10.1016/j.jep.2009.09.015] [PMID: 19781619]

[671] Kaur T, Bijarnia RK, Singla SK, Tandon C. Purification and characterization of an anticalcifying protein from the seeds of *Trachyspermum ammi* (L.). Protein Pept Lett 2009; 16(2): 173-81.
[http://dx.doi.org/10.2174/092986609787316252] [PMID: 19200041]

[672] Palani S, Kumar SN, Gokulan R, Rajalingam D, Senthil Kumar B. Evaluation of nephroprotective and antioxidant potential of *Tragia involucrata*. Drug Discov Today 2009; 1(1): 55-60.

[673] Cyril DG, Landry KS, François KYK, Abou B, Felix YH, Timothée OA. Evaluation of nephroprotective activity of aqueous and hydroethanolic extracts of *Trema guineensis* leaves (Ulmaceae) against gentamicin-induced nephrotoxicity in rats. Int J Biochem Res Rev 2016; 15(2): 1-10.
[http://dx.doi.org/10.9734/IJBCRR/2016/30539]

[674] Balamurugan G, Mohan CJ, Muthusamy P. Protective effect of *Trianthema portulacastrum* Linn leaves on gentamicin induced nephrotoxicity in rats. J Nat Rem 2009; 9: 165-9.

[675] Anand R, Patnaik GK, Srivastava S, Kulshreshtha DK, Dhawan BN. Evaluation of antiurolitiatic activity of *Tribulus terrestris*. Int J Pharmacogn 1992; 32: 217-24.
[http://dx.doi.org/10.3109/13880209409082997]

[676] Anand R, Patnaik GK, Kulshreshtha DK, Dhawan BN. Activity of certain fractions of *Tribulus terrestris* fruits against experimentally induced urolithiasis in rats. Indian J Exp Biol 1994; 32(8): 548-52.
[PMID: 7959935]

[677] Sangeeta D, Sidhu H, Thind SK, Nath R. Effect of *Tribulus terrestris* on oxalate metabolism in rats. J Ethnopharmacol 1994; 44(2): 61-6.
[http://dx.doi.org/10.1016/0378-8741(94)90069-8] [PMID: 7853865]

[678] Nagarkatti DS, Rege N, Mittal BV, Uchil DA, Desai NK, *et al.* Nephroprotection by *Tribulus terrestris*. Update Ayurveda-94. Mumbai, 1994, 41.

[679] Abdel-Kader MS, Al-Qutaym A, Saeedan ASB, Hamad AM, Alkharfy KM. Nephroprotective and hepatoprotective effects of *Tribulus terrestris* L. growing in Saudi Arabia. J Pharm Pharmacogn Res 2016; 4(4): 144-52.

[680] Al-Ali M, Wahbi S, Twaij H, Al-Badr A. *Tribulus terrestris*: preliminary study of its diuretic and contractile effects and comparison with *Zea mays*. J Ethnopharmacol 2003; 85(2-3): 257-60.
[http://dx.doi.org/10.1016/S0378-8741(03)00014-X] [PMID: 12639749]

[681] Joshi VS, Parekh BB, Joshi MJ, Vaidya AD. Inhibition of the growth of urinary calcium hydrogen phosphate dihydrate crystals with aqueous extracts of *Tribulus terrestris* and *Bergenia ligulata*. Urol Res 2005; 33(2): 80-6.
[http://dx.doi.org/10.1007/s00240-004-0450-6] [PMID: 15791467]

[682] Aggarwal A, Tandon S, Singla SK, Tandon C. Diminution of oxalate induced renal tubular epithelial cell injury and inhibition of calcium oxalate crystallization *in vitro* by aqueous extract of *Tribulus terrestris*. Int Braz J Urol 2010; 36(4): 480-8.
[http://dx.doi.org/10.1590/S1677-55382010000400011] [PMID: 20815954]

[683] Arasaratnam V, Sandrasegarampalli B, Senthuran A, Rajendraprasad R. A study of *Tribulus terrestris* extract on risk factors for urinary stone in normal subjects and urolithic patients. J Natl Sci Found Sri Lanka 2010; 38(3): 187-91.
[http://dx.doi.org/10.4038/jnsfsr.v38i3.2308]

[684] Pachana K, Wattanakornsire A, Nanuam J. Application of small caltrops (*Tribulus terrestris*) to inhibit calcium oxalate monohydrate crystallization. Sci Asia 2010; 36: 165-8.
[http://dx.doi.org/10.2306/scienceasia1513-1874.2010.36.165]

[685] Raoofi A, Khazaei M, Ghanbari A. Protective effect of hydroalcoholic extract of *Tribulus terrestris* on Cisplatin induced renal tissue damage in male mice. Int J Prev Med 2015; 6: 11.
[http://dx.doi.org/10.4103/2008-7802.151817] [PMID: 25789143]

[686] Aggarwal A, Singla SK. Priyadarshini, Tandon C. *in vitro* studies on anticalcifying potency of *Tribulus terrestris*. Int J Urol 2010; 17: A211. a

[687] Aggarwal A, Gandhi M, Singh SK, Singla SK, Tandon C. *Tribulus terrestris* extract as curative agent in experimentally induced urolithiasis. 27th. Eur Urol Suppl 2012; 11(1): e861.
[http://dx.doi.org/10.1016/S1569-9056(12)60858-6]

[688] Aggarwal A, Singla SK, Singh SK, Tandon C. Prophylactic effect of *Tribulus terrestris* fruits on experimentally induced urolithiasis in rats. 27th. Eur Urol Suppl 2012; 11(1): e862.
[http://dx.doi.org/10.1016/S1569-9056(12)60859-8]

[689] Kaushik J, Tandon S, Bhardwaj R, Kaur T, Singla SK, Kumar J, *et al.* Delving into the antiurolithiatic potential of *Tribulus terrestris* extract through –*in vivo* efficacy and preclinical safety investigations in Wistar rats. Sci Rep 2019; 9: 1-3.
[http://dx.doi.org/10.1038/s41598-019-52398-w]

[690] Kaushik J, Tandon S, Gupta V, Nayyar J, Singla SK, Tandon C. Response surface methodology based extraction of *Tribulus terrestris* leads to an upsurge of antilithiatic potential by inhibition of calcium oxalate crystallization processes. PLoS One 2017; 12(8): e0183218.

[http://dx.doi.org/10.1371/journal.pone.0183218] [PMID: 28846699]

[691]   Chaudhary SJ, Paranjape AN. Histopathological evaluation of nephroprotective effect of *Trichosanthes dioica* Roxb. on gentamicin induced nephrotoxicity in wistar rats by colorimerty and spectrophotometry. Am J Adv Drug Deliv 2013; 2: 022-38.

[692]   Solomon JA, Ganeshpurkar A, Pandey V, Bansal D, Dubey N. Protective effect of *Trichosanthes dioica* extract against gentamicin induced nephrotoxicity in rats. Pharmacogn Commun 2016; 6(1): 23-7.
[http://dx.doi.org/10.5530/pc.2016.1.4]

[693]   Gupta RK, Swain SR, Murthy PN, Sahoo J, Verma P, Venkateswara Rao C, *et al.* Nephroprotective potential of *Trichosanthes dioica* Roxb. leaves extract against gentamicin-induced nephropathy in albino rats. Asian J Pharmaceut. &. Health Sci 2015; 5(3): 1300-5.

[694]   2019.

[695]   Laroubi A, Touhami M, Farouk L, *et al.* Prophylaxis effect of *Trigonella foenum graecum* L. seeds on renal stone formation in rats. Phytother Res 2007; 21(10): 921-5.
[http://dx.doi.org/10.1002/ptr.2190] [PMID: 17582593]

[696]   Kapase CU, Bodhankar SL, Mohan V, Thakurdesai PA. Therapeutic effects of standardized fenugreek seed extract on experimental urolithiasis in rats. J Appl Pharm Sci 2013; 3(9): 29-35.

[697]   Shekha M, Qadir AB, Ali HH, Selim XE. Effect of fenugreek (*Trigonella foenum-graecum*) on ethylene glycol induced kidney tone in rats. Jordan J Biol Sci 2014; 7(4): 257-60.
[http://dx.doi.org/10.12816/0008248]

[698]   Pradeep SR, Srinivasan K. Alleviation of oxidative stress-mediated nephropathy by dietary fenugreek (*Trigonella foenum-graecum*) seeds and onion (*Allium cepa*) in streptozotocin-induced diabetic rats. Food Funct 2018; 9(1): 134-48.
[http://dx.doi.org/10.1039/C7FO01044C] [PMID: 29068452]

[699]   Khan PJ, Neelam K, Sohel HM. Evaluation of *Coleus barbatus* and *Trigonella foenum-graecum* extracts and their combination on kidney stones in rats. Int J Toxicol Appl Pharmacol 2011; 1(1): 1-5.

[700]   Hilmi SR, Dewan ZF, Kabir AKMN, Islam MM. Comparison of effect of silymarin and ethanol extract of *Trigonella foenum-graecum* on gentamicin induced nephrotoxicity in rats. J Curr Adv Med Res 2019; 6(1): 23-7.
[http://dx.doi.org/10.3329/jcamr.v6i1.40779]

[701]   Hilmi SR, Dewan ZF, Kabir AKMN. Effect of ethanol extract of *Trigonella foenum-graecum* on gentamicin-induced nephrotoxicity in rat. Bangabandhu Sheik Mujib Medical University Journal 2018; 11: 107-11.
[http://dx.doi.org/10.3329/bsmmuj.v11i2.35778]

[702]   Kale RH, Halde UK, Biyani KR. Protective effect of aqueous extract of *Uraria picta* on acetaminophen induced nephrotoxicity in rats. Int J Res Pharm Biomed Sci 2012; 3(1): 110-3.

[703]   Zhang H, Li N, Li K, Li P. Protective effect of *Urtica dioica* methanol extract against experimentally induced urinary calculi in rats. Mol Med Rep 2014; 10(6): 3157-62.
[http://dx.doi.org/10.3892/mmr.2014.2610] [PMID: 25310585]

[704]   McHarg T, Rodgers A, Charlton K. Influence of cranberry juice on the urinary risk factors for calcium oxalate kidney stone formation. BJU Int 2003; 92(7): 765-8.
[http://dx.doi.org/10.1046/j.1464-410X.2003.04472.x] [PMID: 14616463]

[705]   Pandir D, Kara O, Kara M. Cisplatin-induced kidney damage and the protective effect of bilberry (*Vaccinium myrtillus* L.): an experimental study. Turk J Med Sci 2013; 43: 951-6.
[http://dx.doi.org/10.3906/sag-1210-82]

[706]   Ullah N, Khan MA, Rauf A, *et al.* Nephrotoxic effects of *Valeriana wallichii*. Pak J Pharm Sci 2018; 31(1): 37-44.

[PMID: 29348082]

[707] Ntchapda F, Bonabe C, Kemeta Azambou DR, Talla E, Dimo T. Diuretic and antioxidant activities of the aqueous extract of leaves of *Vepris heterophylla* (Engl.) R. Let (Rutaceae) in rats. BMC Complement Altern Med 2016; 16(1): 516.
[http://dx.doi.org/10.1186/s12906-016-1439-8] [PMID: 27964714]

[708] Imafidon CE, Akomolafe RO, Abubakar SA, Ogundipe OJ, Olukiran OS, Ayowole OA. Amelioration of cadmium-induced nephropathy using polyphenol-rich extract of *Vernonia amygdalina* (Del.) leaves in rat model. Open Access Maced J Med Sci 2015; 3(4): 567-77.
[http://dx.doi.org/10.3889/oamjms.2015.120] [PMID: 27275289]

[709] Sreedevi A, Bharathi K, Prasad KVSRG. Effect of *Vernonia cinerea* aerial parts against Cisplatin-induced nephrotoxicity in rats. Pharmacologyonline 2011; 2: 548-55.

[710] Hiremath RD, Jalalpure SS. Effect of hydro-alcoholic extract of *Vernonia cinerea* Less. against ethylene glycol-induced urolithiasis in rats. Indian J Pharmacol 2016; 48(4): 434-40.
[http://dx.doi.org/10.4103/0253-7613.186211] [PMID: 27756957]

[711] Ilhan M, Ergene B, Süntar I, *et al.* Preclinical evaluation of antiurolithiatic activity of *Viburnum opulus* L. on sodium oxalate-induced urolithiasis rat model. Evid Based Complement Alternat Med 2014; 2014: 578103.
[http://dx.doi.org/10.1155/2014/578103] [PMID: 25165481]

[712] Nitin M, Ifthekar S, Mumtaz M. Evaluation of hepatoprotective and nephroprotective activity of aqueous extract of *Vigna mungo* on rifamycin induced toxicity in albino rats. Int J Health Allied Sci 2012; 1(2): 85-91.
[http://dx.doi.org/10.4103/2278-344X.101695]

[713] El-Ashmawy IM, El-Nahas AF, Salama OM. Grape seed extract prevents gentamicin-induced nephrotoxicity and genotoxicity in bone marrow cells of mice. Basic Clin Pharmacol Toxicol 2006; 99(3): 230-6.
[http://dx.doi.org/10.1111/j.1742-7843.2006.pto_497.x] [PMID: 16930296]

[714] Safa J, Argani H, Bastani B, *et al.* Protective effect of grape seed extract on gentamicin-induced acute kidney injury. Iran J Kidney Dis 2010; 4(4): 285-91.
[PMID: 20852368]

[715] Bhargavi K, Ramani ND, Janarthan M, Durraivel S. Evaluation of nephro protective activity of methanolic extract of seeds of *Vitis vinifera* against rifampicin and carbon tetrachloride induced nephrotoxicity in Wistar rats. Indian J Res Pharm Biotech 2013; 1(5): 731-5.

[716] Sharma S, Joshi A, Hemalatha S. Protective effect of *Withania coagulans* fruit extract on cisplatin-induced nephrotoxicity in rats. Pharmacognosy Res 2017; 9(4): 354-61.
[http://dx.doi.org/10.4103/pr.pr_1_17] [PMID: 29263628]

[717] Panda S, Gupta P, Kar A. Protective role of Ashwagandha in cadmium induced hepatotoxicity and nephrotoxicity in male mouse. Curr Sci 1997; 72: 546-7.

[718] Jeyanthi T, Subramanian P. Nephroprotective effect of *Withania somnifera*: a dose-dependent study. Ren Fail 2009; 31(9): 814-21.
[http://dx.doi.org/10.3109/08860220903150320] [PMID: 19925290]

[719] Jeyanthi T, Subramanian P. Protective effect of *Withania somnifera* root powder on lipid peroxidation and antioxidant status in gentamicin-induced nephrotoxic rats. J Basic Clin Physiol Pharmacol 2010; 21(1): 61-78.
[http://dx.doi.org/10.1515/JBCPP.2010.21.1.61] [PMID: 20506689]

[720] Sharma V, Sharma S. Pracheta, Paliwal R, Sharma S. Therapeutic efficacy of *Withania somnifera* root extract in the regulation of lead nitrate induced nephrotoxicity in Swiss albino mice. J Pharm Res 2011; 4(3): 755-8.

[721] Shimmi SC, Jahan N, Baqi N, Rahman Z. Histological evidence of nephroprotective effect of

Ashwagandha (*Withania somnifera*) root extract against gentamicin induced nephrotoxicity in rats. J Enam Med Col 2014; 4(1): 26-30.
[http://dx.doi.org/10.3329/jemc.v4i1.18065]

[722] Kushwaha V, Sharma M, Vishwakarma P, Saini M, Saxena K. Biochemical assessment of nephroprotective and nephrocurative activity of *Withania somnifera* on gentamicin-induced nephrotoxicity in experimental rats. Int J Res Med Sci 2016; 4: 298-302.
[http://dx.doi.org/10.18203/2320-6012.ijrms20160047]

[723] Govindappa PK, Gautam V, Tripathi SM, Sahni YP, Raghavendra HLS. Effect of *Withania somnifera* on gentamicin induced renal lesions in rats. Brazilian J Pharmacog 2019; 29: 234-40.
[http://dx.doi.org/10.1016/j.bjp.2018.12.005]

[724] Grases F, March JG, Ramis M, Costa-Bauz'a A. The influence of *Zea mays* on urinary risk factors for kidney stones in rats. Phytother Res 1993; 7: 146-9.
[http://dx.doi.org/10.1002/ptr.2650070210]

[725] Rathod DV, Fitwe P, Sarnaik D, Kshirsagar SN. *in vitro* anti-lithiatic activity of corn silk of *Zea mays*. Int J Pharm Sci Rev Res 2013; 21(2): 16-9.

[726] Talekar YP, Gund KA, Kale SD, Apte KG, Parab PB. Antiurolithic activity of corn silk extract in rats. Int J Univers Pharm Bio Sci 2013; 2: 65-77.

[727] Sabiu S, O'Neill FH, Ashafa AOT. Membrane stabilization and detoxification of acetaminophen-mediated oxidative onslaughts in the kidneys of Wistar rats by standardized fraction of *Zea mays* L. (Poaceae), *Stigma maydis*. Evid Based Complement Alternat Med 2016; 2016: 2046298.
[http://dx.doi.org/10.1155/2016/2046298] [PMID: 27579048]

[728] Okokon E, Nyong M, Essien G, Nyong E. Nephroprotective activity of husk extract and fractions of *Zea mays* against alloxan-induced oxidative stress in diabetic rats. J Basic Pharmacol Toxicol 2017; 1(3): 1-10.

[729] Okokon JE, Udobang JA, Obot DN, Agu EC. Nephroprotective activity of husk extract of *Zea mays* against gentimicin-induced liver injury in rats. J Med Plant Studies 2019; 7(6): 156-60.

[730] Ajith TA, Nivitha V, Usha S. *Zingiber officinale* Roscoe alone and in combination with α-tocopherol protect the kidney against cisplatin-induced acute renal failure. Food Chem Toxicol 2007; 45(6): 921-7.
[http://dx.doi.org/10.1016/j.fct.2006.11.014] [PMID: 17210214]

[731] Ajith TA, Aswathy MS, Hema U. Protective effect of *Zingiber officinale* roscoe against anticancer drug doxorubicin-induced acute nephrotoxicity. Food Chem Toxicol 2008; 46(9): 3178-81.
[http://dx.doi.org/10.1016/j.fct.2008.07.004] [PMID: 18680783]

[732] Uz E, Karatas OF, Mete E, *et al.* The effect of dietary ginger (*Zingiber officinalis* Rosc) on renal ischemia/reperfusion injury in rat kidneys. Ren Fail 2009; 31(4): 251-60.
[http://dx.doi.org/10.1080/08860220902779921] [PMID: 19462272]

[733] Lakshmi BV, Sudhakar M. Protective effect of *Zingiber officinale* on gentimicin-induced nephrotoxicity in rats. Int J Pharmacol 2010; 6(1): 58-62.
[http://dx.doi.org/10.3923/ijp.2010.58.62]

[734] Shanmugam KR, Ramakrishna CH, Mallikarjuna K, Reddy KS. Protective effect of ginger against alcohol-induced renal damage and antioxidant enzymes in male albino rats. Indian J Exp Biol 2010; 48(2): 143-9.
[PMID: 20455323]

[735] Ramudu SK, Korivi M, Kesireddy N, Chen CY, Kuo CH, Kesireddy SR. Ginger feeding protects against renal oxidative damage caused by alcohol consumption in rats. J Ren Nutr 2011; 21(3): 263-70.
[http://dx.doi.org/10.1053/j.jrn.2010.03.003] [PMID: 20599394]

[736] Ramudu SK, Korivi M, Kesireddy N, *et al.* Nephro-protective effects of a ginger extract on cytosolic

and mitochondrial enzymes against streptozotocin (STZ)-induced diabetic complications in rats. Chin J Physiol 2011; 54(2): 79-86.
[http://dx.doi.org/10.4077/CJP.2011.AMM006] [PMID: 21789888]

[737]   Hamed MA, Ali SA, El-Rigal NS. Therapeutic potential of ginger against renal injury induced by carbon tetrachloride in rats. ScientificWorldJournal 2012; 2012: 840421.
[http://dx.doi.org/10.1100/2012/840421] [PMID: 22566780]

[738]   Nasri H, Nematbakhsh M, Ghobadi S, Ansari R, Shahinfard N, Rafieian-Kopaei M. Preventive and curative effects of ginger extract against histopathologic changes of gentamicin-induced tubular toxicity in rats. Int J Prev Med 2013; 4(3): 316-21.
[PMID: 23626888]

[739]   Al Hroob AM, Abukhalil MH, Alghonmeen RD, Mahmoud AM. Ginger alleviates hyperglycemia-induced oxidative stress, inflammation and apoptosis and protects rats against diabetic nephropathy. Biomed Pharmacother 2018; 106: 381-9.
[http://dx.doi.org/10.1016/j.biopha.2018.06.148] [PMID: 29966984]

[740]   Abdul Hamid Z, Budin SB, Wen Jie N, Hamid A, Husain K, Mohamed J. Nephroprotective effects of *Zingiber zerumbet* Smith ethyl acetate extract against paracetamol-induced nephrotoxicity and oxidative stress in rats. J Zhejiang Univ Sci B 2012; 13(3): 176-85.
[http://dx.doi.org/10.1631/jzus.B1100133] [PMID: 22374609]

CHAPTER 4

Polyherbal Formulations for Nephroprotection, Nephrocuration and Antiurolithiasis

Abstract: In this chapter nephroprotection by polyhedral formulations has been given. These include commercial Cystone of Himalaya Drug Company, Bailva agada, Crashcal, etc. Details of herbal formulations of traditional medicines like Ayurveda, Siddha, Unani, Chinese and Japanese in nephroprotection, nephrocuration and antiurolithiatic activity are also given. These include Triphala Karpa Chooranam and Gokshuradi Polyherbal Ayurvedic Formulation, Amirthathi churnam and Sirupeelai Samoola Kudineer of Sidha medicine, Jawarish zarooni sada of Unani medicine, Takusha and Zhu Ling Tang of Japanese medicine and Wu Ling San of Chinese medicine.

Keywords: Amirthathi Churnam, Bilva agada. Jawarish Zarooni Sada, Crashcal, Cystone, Polyherbal Formulations, Renomet.

INTRODUCTION

As per Ayurveda, having more than two species of medicinal herbs in a formulation is known as polyherbal formulation (PF). Presently a day's PF accomplished its prominence around the world because polyherbal has different benefits that are not accessible in allopathic medications [1].

Tiwari *et al.* [2] explained the impact of PF utilized in experimentally incited urolithiasis. Numerous pharmacological examinations on the medicinal plants utilized in traditional antiurolithic treatment have revealed their remedial potential *in vivo* or *in vitro* models [3]. Generally, every one of the cures is connected and gotten from plants, and their conventional applications are demonstrated to be helpful to mainly diminishing the advancement of urolithiasis without bringing about any side effects. Numerous PF formulations have their mechanism of action for the treatment and management of urolithiasis.

Amirthathi Churna and Nandukkal (Fossil Crab) Churna

Chellakkan *et al.* [4] assessed the action of Amirthathi and Nandukkal churna's of Siddha drugs in the treatment of Nephrolithiasis. Churna is a combination of powdered spices and additionally minerals utilized in Siddha and Ayurvedic medication. The formulation of Amirthathi churna is performed from the 25 homegrown plants and synthetic camphor substances. The roots, leaves, barks, woods, organic products, seeds, blossom, rhizomes, and nutlets of the plants are dried and pummeled to 0.004 mm (powder molecule size) to make Amirthathi churna according to the Pala Thiratha Chuvadi (Tamil medication writing written in palm leaves). Whereas, the Nandukkal churna is prepared from the pooneeru and lime water. After purification, *Aole vera* latex is blended in with the formulation and calcinated according to the methodology of Agasthiar Nandukkal Sootheram. The viability of Amirthathi and Nandukkal churna's has been done by the clinical preliminary for 20 patients between the ages 15 and 75. The urinary tract stones are responsible for renal damage because of the presence of citrate ions in urine which forms a dissolvable complex with Ca^+ and Mg^+. The clinical trial of these formulations against the treatment of nephrolithiasis uncovers the recuperation of ureteric calculus (80%), renal calculus (77%), and vesicle calculus (50%). Subsequently, the utilization of Amirthathi and Nandukkal churna's has shown successful outcomes in the management of urinary tract stones by excretion of citrate ions. The chemical analysis reveals that the components are within the WHO suggested limits. It was seen that these medications would diminish the citrituric impact for a long life expectancy. The role of these churna's utilization as lithotropic specialist has checked in around 20 patients with nephrolithiasis. The clinical evaluation reveals that the symptom of burning micturition, dysuria, haematuria, abdominal pain from loin to groin, back pain, and general symptoms like nausea and vomiting was reduced significantly in all clinical patients. This demonstrated the positive outcomes to eliminate the urinary stones.

Ashmarihara Kashaya and Nagaradi Kashaya

Ashmarihara kashaya is an Ayurvedic preparation. It consists of *Aerva lanata, Carica papaya, Asparagus racemosus* root, *Tribulus terrestris, Crataeva nurvala, Saccharum spontaneum, Oryza sativa, Boerhavia diffusa, Tinospora cordifolia, Achyranthes aspera, Cucumis sativus, Nardostachys jatamansi* and *Hyoscyamus niger*. All the ingredients are mixed with water in 1:16 ratios, boiled and concentrated to quarter, and stored. Nagaradi Kashaya is an Ayurvedic preparation. The ingredients are *Tinospora cordifolia* (6 parts), *Zingiber officinale* (2 parts), *Terminalia chebula* (4 parts). Ashmarihar kashaya and Nagaradi kashaya were studied by Meena *et al.* [5] for its nephroprotective activity in cisplatin and gentamicin initiated nephropathy in Albino rats. Various parameters like serum biochemical parameters, biochemical parameters of kidney homogenate, and histopathological study of the kidney and heart were done to evaluate the action. The outcomes indicated that gentamicin and cisplatin-initiated nephropathy were diminished by using Ashmarihara kashaya in mild to moderate; no activity was observed in Nagaradi kashaya. Interestingly, both Ayurvedic preparations have shown cardioprotective action against cisplatin and gentamicin-initiated cardiotoxicity in rats.

Bilva Agada

Bilvādi agada (BA) [6] is an antivenom formulation indicated in the context of snake venom management. It is also revealed in low potent poisons. It contains *Aegle marmelos* L., *Ocimum sanctum* L., *Pongamia pinnata* L., *Valeriana wallichi* DC., *Cedrus deodara* Roxb.,, *Terminalia chebula* Retz., *Phyllanthus emblica* L., *Terminalia bellirica* (Gaertn.) Roxb., *Piper nigrum* L., *Zinziber officinale* Rosc., *Piper longum* L., *Curcuma longa* L., *Berberis aristata* DC. and goat's urine.

The ingredients of BA possess anti-inflammatory, immunomodulatory, diuretic, anti-toxic properties. Besides, many of them (*A. marmelos, P. pinnata, O. sanctum, P. emblica, T. chebula, T. bellirica, Z.officinale, P. nigrum, C. longa*) have been proven for their nephroprotective activity [7].

Kanna *et al.* [8] assessed the impact of BA in GM-initiated nephrotoxicity in male Wistar rodents. BA treated animals showed a massive change in degrees of urine creatinine, serum creatinine, and potassium levels in urine. There was no much change found in sodium, chloride, serum potassium, phosphorous, calcium and urine sodium, and chloride in every one of the three animal groups. Glomerular blockage, tubular necrosis, interstitial edema interstitial hemorrhage was decreased in bilva treated animal groups. The aftereffects of this investigation demonstrate that BA reduces the GM-initiated nephrotoxicity, and it very well might be because of anti-inflammatory, immunomodulatory, diuretic, and antioxidant properties of medications. Further examinations are important to investigate the specific action of BA in nephroprotection.

Crashcal

A polyherbal formulation Crashcal [9] was checked for its antiurolithiatic action rats by ethylene glycol initiated urolithiasis animal model. All the contents of the formulation have shown excellent antiurolithiatic activity. The formulation had *Dolichos biflorus, Bergenia ligulata, Boerhavia diffusa, Mimosa pudica, Tribulus terrestris, Crataeva nurvala,* Triphala, Asphaltum, Hajrul Yahood Bhasma, *Commiphora mukul* and lupeol as contents of Crashcal. The composition plants have also been reported to demonstrate antioxidant, diuretic, antibacterial and immunomodulation activities.

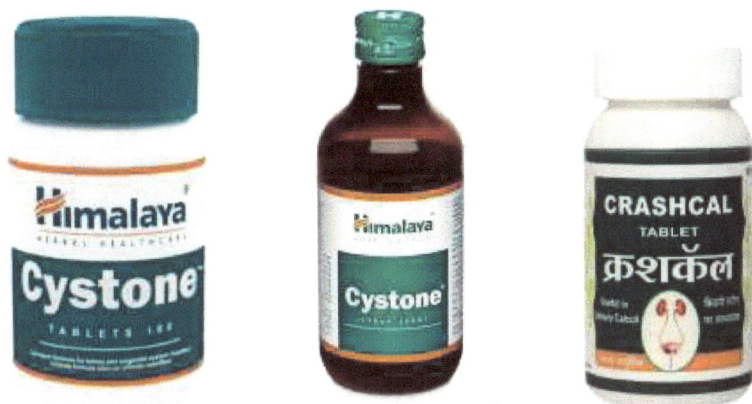

Fig. (1). Some Polyherbal formulations in the market for antiuroliathiasis.

Cystone®

An Ayurvedic polyherbal proprietary medicine Cystone is used in India to treat various urinary disorders, including urolithiasis, and Himalaya Drug Company, India, market it. It is available both in tablet form and syrup form (Fig. **1**).

Each tablet of Cystone contains:

Didymocarpus pedicellata 130 mg, *Saxifraga ligulata* 98 mg, Purple fleabane/ *Veronoia cinerea* 32 mg, *Rubia cordifolia* 32 mg, Lime silicate calx/ Hajrul yahood Bhasma/ Badrashma bhasma 32 mg, *Cyperus scariosus* 32 mg, *Onosma bracteatum* 32 mg, Prickly chaff flower/ *Achyranthes aspera* 32 mg, and Shilajit 26 mg. The tablets were widely prescribed to treat and manage many urinary complications, UTIs, and urolithiasis [10 - 21].

Apart from the antiurolithic effect, cystone also shows various pharmacological actions, including diuretic, antimicrobial, antispasmodic, anti-inflammatory activities. *D. pedicellata* has reported showing diuretic activity. Bergenin and afzelechin are the active principles of *S.lingulata* having astringent actions, making it an effective antimicrobial agent. Bergenin is a diuretic, and it is involved in the control of urolithiasis by glycolic acid induction as well as in the lowering of formation of urinary crystals by crystalloid-colloid balance action. *R. cordifolia* was reported to have diuretic, anti-inflammatory, and antioxidant activity [2].

Cystone has a significant diuretic activity because of its mineral salts in high concentration. It also shows urinary antiseptic and antispasmodic properties. In general, it also causes smooth muscle relaxation. It maintains the cystalloid-colloid imbalance and having an exceptional property of disintegrating the renal stones. In this manner, it relieves the pain and spasm caused by the section of the particles of calculi or the exceptionally acidic urine. Cystone is known to unwind the detrusor muscles and follow up on the mucin in the calculi that predicaments the particles together. It in this manner permits the deteriorating particles to escape with the flow of urine. Drawn out utilization of cystone doesn't adjust the electrolyte balance. It is accordingly valuable in urinary diseases, crystalluria, and other urinary complications [22].

Sengupta [22] tested the protective action of cystone in urinary tract complaints during pregnancy. Cystone demonstrated promising in 100 instances of UTIs seen during 14 weeks to full term of pregnancy. Certain medications are contraindicated in pregnancy. In such cases as opposed to giving antimicrobials or different medications, they suggest utilizing cystone tablets decisively. Cystone is protected, has no poisonous or results, and is very much endured by every patient. As decided from the time taken for the patients to be organism-free and complaint-free, cystone tablets demonstrated accommodating and valuable.

Mitra *et al.* [23] have studied the action of cystone in experimentally actuated urolithiasis in rodents. 3% glycolic acid in the diet is followed for 42 days to initiate oxalate urolithiasis in animals. Glycolic acid treatment brought about the rise in calcium levels, oxalate in the kidney, just as in the total kidney weight. Likewise, the urinary levels of and inorganic phosphorus, oxalate, and calcium were raised. At a dose of 250, 500, and 750 mg/kg b.w. of cystone p.o. for a period of 42 days uncovered a dose-dependent impact in the decrease of lithogenic substances, following glycolic acid prompted urolithiasis. Simultaneous oral treatment with cystone at 500 and 750 mg/kg for 42 days fundamentally switched the glycolic acid prompted urolithiasis, probably by forestalling the urinary supersaturation of lithogenic substances, particularly of oxalate and calcium. The decrease of urinary and kidney oxalate levels by cystone might be because of its inhibitory activity on oxalate blending liver catalyst glycolate oxidase. These perceptions demonstrate that cystone can assume a significant part in avoiding problems related to kidney stone development.

Cystone, significantly active against cisplatin-intiated renal toxicity administered intraperitoneally one hour before cisplatin [24]. At a dose of 500 and 1000 $\mu g/ml$, it also stops lipid peroxidation actuated by cisplatin in renal cortical slices. cystone pre-treated rats with at a dose of 1000 mg/kg i.p. had markedly lower blood urea nitrogen, serum creatinine when compared to cisplatin alone. The animals with cystone lost their body weight when compared to cisplatin alone treated animals on day five. Renal functions like creatinine clearance, urine to serum creatinine ratio showed better improvement when cystone was given one h before cisplatin. However, the decreased WBC count and increased urinary protein excretion caused by cisplatin isn't corrected by the cystone. Rao and Rao [24] suggest that the cystone shows kidney protection from cisplatin-initiated toxicity, and the defense may have resulted through its ability to stop lipid peroxidation.

Kumaran and Patki [25] assessed the safety and efficacy of cystone in patients with urolithiasis by surveying the decrease/removal of renal stones, symptomatic relief, and urinary biochemical parameters. In this investigation, 60 patients with renal calculi sizes between 5 mm and 12 mm were incorporated. Thirty patients got cystone, and the remaining 30 received placebo treatment orally at a dose of two tablets twice day by day for 12 weeks. Patients were assessed at 6 and 12 weeks to alleviate clinical indications just as urine and biochemical parameters. X-ray and an ultrasound assessment were completed on section, a month and a half, and 12 weeks of the investigation. The cystone may expel the stones in eighteen patients. The expected time for removing stone was 12.3 days in patients treated with medicament with a considerable decrease in the calculi size. However, in placebo-treated patients, there was no decline in stone size. There were improvements in clinical indications and haematuria, recurrence of urine, and delicacy in KUB region. Marked lowering in urinary WBC and RBC quantity was seen in patients on cystone alongside the critical reduction in serum uric acid levels.

Bodakhe *et al.* [26] assessed the protective action of cystone in hyperoxaluria-incited CaOx crystal deposition and oxidative stress in urolithiasis. 0.75% ethylene glycol in drinking water for a period of 28 days was given to rodents to prompt urolithiasis with concurrent treatment of cystone at a dose of 500 and 750 mg/kg bw, and different urinary risk components of urolithiasis and antioxidant markers were evaluated. EG treatment leads to raised urine volume and brought down urinary pH, alongside raised urinary discharge of calcium, oxalate, and phosphate in untreated animals. These progressions caused CaOx stone formation, raised lipid peroxidation, and diminished antioxidants in the kidney of untreated rodents. Cystone forestalled these hyperoxaluric appearances and repressed CaOx stone formation in treated rodents at the two doses.

Erickson *et al.* [27] investigated the impact of cystone on kidney stone formation and urinary composition. Investigators recruited ten kidney stone patients for a two-phased study to evaluate the safety and efficacy of cystone for the avoidance of kidney stones. The first phase was designed as a randomized double-blinded cross-over 12-week study for assessing the effect of cystone vs placebo, and the second phase was an open-label one-year study. Results uncovered no marked impact of cystone on the urinary structure. The normal renal stone weight raised as opposed to diminished on Cystone. Like this, this examination doesn't uphold the adequacy of cystone to treat CaOx stone formers

Gokshuradi Kashaya

Siddaram *et al.* [28] evaluated the efficacy of the decoction of *Ricinus cummunis, Zingiber officinale, Tribulus terrestris,* and *Crataeva nurvala* known as Gokshuradi Kashaya with an aim of disintegration, dislodgement, dissolution, and removal of renal stones. A total of thirty patients were randomly selected and were grouped *i.e.* G-I and G-II having 15 patients each. G-I was treated with Gokshuradi decoction at a dose of 45 ml; after food for a period of 45 days, twice daily, G-II was treated with hydrotherapy. After 45 days, Gokshuradi kashaya showed promising relief of pain, dysuria, haematuria, size, and renal calculi.

Gokshuradi Yog Polyherbal Formulation

A polyherbal formulation Gokshuradi Yog is used to manage and treat urolithiasis in the Indian tradition system for centuries. The formulation components with various pharmacological properties include *Tribulus terrestris* shows litholytic, diuretic, antidiabetic, antioxidant, anti-inflammatory, and hepatoprotective activity. *Ricinus communus* was reported for its antioxidant, anti-inflammatory, hepatoprotective and antidiabetic action. *Hygrophila spinosa* was assessed for its anti-inflammatory, diuretic, hepatoprotective, antioxidant, litholytic, antidiabetic and analgesic activities. *Solanum surattense* and *Solanum anguivi* were reported for their litholytic, diuretic, antioxidant, antihyperlipidemic, antioxidative, anti-inflammatory, and hepatoprotective effects [29].

Jawarish Zarooni Sada

Multicomponent formulations were widely used in Unani medicine for the treatment and management of renal diseases. Jawarish Zarooni Sada (JZS) is one such polyherbal formulation having 15 different ingredients prescribed for its nephroprotective and diuretic actions. The diuretic activity of aqueous and ethanolic extracts of JZS at a dose of 300 mg was tested by Afzal *et al.* [30] by calculating the total output of urine, potassium, and sodium levels for six hours. Nephroprotective action of JZS against gentamicin-initiated nephrotoxicity was evaluated by giving JZS with gentamicin at 40 mg/kg, and then the elevation of serum creatinine, serum urea were taken as the parameter nephrotoxicity. JZS showed marked diuretic and nephroprotective effects.

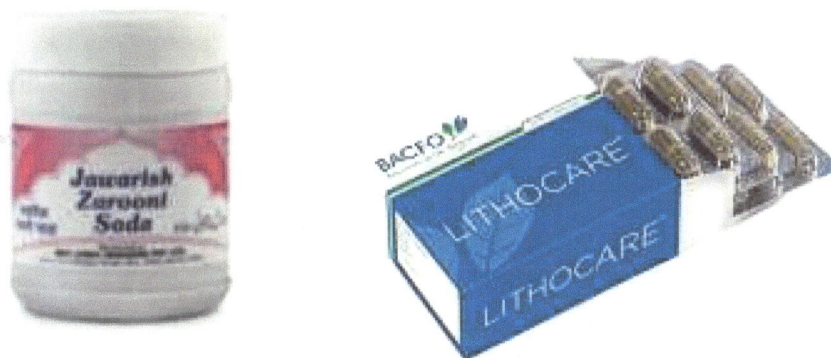

Fig. (2). Some polyherbal formulations in the market for antiurolithiasis.

Lithocare

A polyherbal formulation Lithocare is manufactured by Bacfo Pharmaceuticals India Limited, Noida having different medicinal components including *Boerhaavia diffusa*, *Crataeva nurvala*, and *Asteracantha longifolia* (Fig. **2**). All these plants having scientifically proven therapeutic actions like antioxidant, diuretic, anti-inflammatory, litholytic hepatoprotective, anticancer etc. Lithocare has shown its beneficial actions on ethylene glycol initiated animal models of urolithiasis by eliminating the formation of urinary stones.

Lulat *et al.* [31] explored the defensive impact of Lithocare against ethylene glycol prompted urolithiasis in Wistar rodents. The defensive impact of Lithocarr at a dose of 400 and 800 mg/kg was assessed utilizing ethylene glycol actuated urolithiasis in rodents. Allowing of ethylene glycol in drinking water came about in hypocalcemia, hyperoxaluria, raised renal discharge of phosphate. Supplementation with Lithocare altogether decreased the urinary oxalate, calcium, and phosphate discharge portion conditionally. There was a critical decrease in the levels of oxalate, calcium, CaOx stores in the kidney tissue of rodents given with Lithocare in ethylene glycol treated rodents. There was a marked decrease in urea, creatinine, uric acid, and BUN when Lithocare was given inethylene glycol-treated rodents.

Neeri –KFT

Scientifically proven polyherbal sugar free syrup NEERI KFT is manufactured by AIMIL Pharmaceuticals Ltd., India, and it is used in the treatment and management of different types of urinary disorders like urinary calculi, prostate associated problems, and UTI's. The formulation having different extracts of *Tinospora cordifolia, Boerhavia diffusa,, Nelumbo nucifera, Tribulus terrestris, Butea monosperma, Moringa oleifera, Crataeva nurvala, Vetiveria zizanioides,* and *Amaranthus spinosus..* These extracts are having different phytochemical components like quinolone derivatives, arbutin, bioflavonoids, tannins, glycosides, and several other micronutrients beneficial in the functioning of the uterus, kidneys, prostate gland and urinary bladder. *Boerhaavia diffusa* had shown various actions like diuretic, antioxidant, anticancer, and litholytic, etc [2].

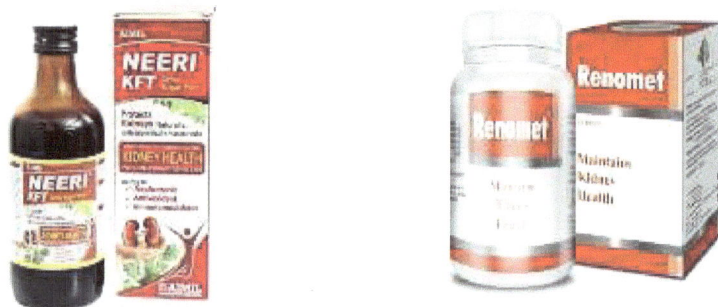

Fig. (3). Some polyherbal formulations in the market for nephroprotection and nephrocuration.

Pashanabhedadi Ghrita

Pashanabhedadi Ghrita (PBG) (Fig. **3**) is an Ayurvedic formulation having different plant extracts including *Bergenia ligulata, Calotropis gigantea, Achyranthes aspera, Oxalis corniculata, Asparagus racemosus, Tribulus terrestris, Solanum indicum, Solanum surattense, Bacopa monnieri, Barleria prionitis, Vetiveria zizanioides, Abrus precatorius, Dendrophthoe falcata, Oroxylum indicum, Crataeva nurvala, Tectona grandis, Hordeum vulgare, Dolichos biflorus, Piper nigrum,* and *Strychnos potatorum.* Gupta *et al.* [32] evaluated the antiurolithiatic activity of PBG against experimentally initiated renal calculi in rats. In this investigation, PBG has been given against ammonium oxalate-rich diet, and gentamicin prompted renal calculi in animals. The test drug was given at a dose of 900 mg/kg for 15 days. Rodents were forfeited on the sixteenth day. Various parameters like serum biochemical, kidney weight, kidney tissue, and histopathology were calculated. Attending treatment of PBG lessens biochemical blood levels, while it altogether constricts lipid peroxidation and raised glutathione peroxidase and glutathione actions. It likewise diminished stone formation uniquely into the renal tubules in number just as size and forestalled harm to the renal tubules. The discoveries showed that PBG is having anti-urolithiatic action against ammonium oxalate-rich diet in addition to gentamicin infusion actuated urolithiasis in rodents.

Renomet

Scientificcaly proven a polyherbal formulation Renomet is having different extracts of *Crataeva nurvala, Tribulus terrestris, Saxifraga ligulata,* and *Dolichos biflorus* used in treatment and management of renal calculi. It significantly reduces the size and formation of renal stones. *Saxifraga ligulata* having properties like antiurolithiatic, diuretic, antioxidant and anti-inflammatory may the presence of phytocompound bergenin. *Tribulus terrestris* showed therapeutic actions like litholytic, diuretic, antioxidant, anti-inflammatory, antidiabetic, hepatoprotective activities due to the presence of specific Saponins, glycosides, flavonoids, alkaloids, etc. *Dolichos biflorus* having scientifically proven antiurolithiatic activity; and the presence of flavonoids and phenolic compounds are responsible for its activity. *Crataeva nurvala* also showed anthelmintic, antioxidant, diuretic, and lithotriptic activity.

Roy *et al*. [33] assessed the safety and efficacy of Renomet, used in the treatment of urolithiasis. Seventy-four patients between 35-60 years old and satisfying inclusion criteria were recruited for the study. Every one of the patients had different stones up to 9 mm in size and had a past history with renal stones carefully eliminated. They were divided into two groups and after taken informed consent, they have given Renomet at the dose of 1 tablet twice day by day for about a month and a half. Patients were approached to report for any results during the treatment time frame. Toward the finish of the trial, patients in the Renomet treated group were discovered to be side effect-free, and about 98% of them had passed the stone.

Rilith

A polyherbal formulation Rilith has different plant extracts, including *Bergenia ligulata, Boerhavia diffusa, Crataeva nurvala, Tribulus terrestris*, and *Withania somnifera*. This formulation was scientifically proven to have antiurolithiatic action on ethylene glycol initiated urolithiasis in rats. *Bergenia ligulata* has diuretic, astringent, antioxidant, and lithotriptic properties, and *Boerhavia diffusa* having diuretic, antioxidant, litholytic, and anticancer properties. *Tribulus terrestirs* has litholytic, diuretic, antioxidant, anti-inflammatory, antidiabetic, hepatoprotective activities while *Withania somnifera* possesses antilithiatic, diuretic properties. *Crataeva nurvala* showed diuretic, antioxidant, anti-inflammatory, anthelmintic, and lithotriptic properties. A mix of an assortment of therapeutic activities makes this polyherbal formulation successful in treating urolithiasis or kidney stone [2].

Joshi *et al* [34] evaluated the antilithiatic effect of Relith on ethylene glycol-initiated lithiasis in male albino rats. The lithiasis was actuated to rodents by oral administration of 0.75v/v ethylene glycolated water for 28 days. Relith at a dose of 500mg/kg was managed orally from first day for preventive regimen and from the fifteenth day for therapeutic regimen. The urinary ionic levels were modified by ethylene glycol, which raised the oxalate, calcium, proteins, and inorganic phosphates in the urine. The Relith fundamentally diminished the raised levels of these particles and protein in the urine. Additionally, the concentrate essentially raised the urinary levels of magnesium. The raised serum creatinine levels of lithiatic rodents were diminished by a prophylactic and therapeutic regimen of concentrate treatment. The histological observations additionally showed improvement after treatment with the concentrate. These perceptions empower to reason that the healing and preventive properties of Relith against ethylene glycol actuated urolithiasis.

Sirupeelai Samoola Kudineer

A polyherbal Siddha system of decoction Sirupeelai Samoola Kudineer (SK), having four medicinal plants used in Southern parts of India for the management and treatment of urolithiasis. Vasanthi *et al.* [35] investigated the action of SK in Sprague-Dawley rats providing ethylene glycol through drinking water and intraperitoneal infusion of sodium oxalate. Renal injury was affirmed by the rise of the formation of thiobarbituric acid reactive substance (TBARS). Co-treatment with SK to urolithiatic rodents for 21 days fundamentally forestalled the rise of renal biomarkers and urinary stone formation in this manner, forestalling renal harm and the development of renal calculi. Allowing Sirupeelai Samoola Kudineer at all doses and cystone re-established the antioxidant (glutathione) levels by forestalling the rise of TBARS in the kidney tissue, which was additionally affirmed by histological changes. SK treatment elevates diuresis, which prompts flushing of the renal stones and keeps up the alkaline environment in the urinary framework which most likely intervenes the antilithiatic action. SK gives primary and practical assurance to the kidneys by upgrading its physiological capacity against stone development and validates its clinical use. SK showed diuretic and antilithiatic potential in ethylene glycol and sodium oxalate incited urolithiasis in rodents. Raised urinary stone markers (uric acid, calcium, oxalate, phosphate and magnesium) in serum and renal tubular enzymes (LDH, ALP, AST, GGT, ALT) in urolithiatic rodents were turned around by SK treatment. SK administration essentially diminished renal stress markers like creatinine, urea, LPO, and raised SOD, GSH, GPx, and levels supporting nephroprotection. SK additionally gives structural and functional protection against ethylene glycol-incited renal stones in rodents, as confirmed by histopathological observations.

Shwadanstradi Ghana Vati

Ashmari or urolithiasis can be treatable and or manageable by using shwadanstradi kashaya was referenced in Chakradatta Ashmari Roga Chikitsa of Ayurveda. The contents of this Ayurvedic medicine are *Tribulus terrestris, Ricinus communis* leaves, *Zingiber officinale* rhizome and *Crataeva nurvala* bark. Nagvenkar *et al.* [36] assessed the role of Shwadanstradi Ghana vati in the treatment of urolithiasis in 30 human patients and shown very significant results in the removal of renal stones in urolithiasis.

Takusha

The traditional Japanese therapeutic medicine, Kampo originated in China and was beneficial in the treatment of a variety of diseases. It is also used for the treatment and management of renal calculi for many years. Yasui *et al.* [37] evaluated the inhibitory impact of the kampo medication takusha on the development of CaOx renal stones instigated by ethylene glycol and vitamin D3 in rats. They additionally explored the impact of Takusha on osteopontin (OPN) articulation, which was recognized as a significant stone matrix protein. The control group rodents were non-treated; the stone group rodents were given ethylene glycol and vitamin D3, and the Takusha group was given Takusha apart from EG and vitamin D3. The rate of renal stone development was lower in the Takusha group than in the stone group; thus, the OPN articulation in the Takusha group was less than in the stone group animals. Takusha was powerful in forestalling oxalate calculi development and OPN articulation in rodents. These discoveries recommend that Takusha forestalls CaOx stone formation.

Takusha and Kagosou

Takusha is a Japanese Kampo medicine containing the rhizome of *Alisma orientale* (Sam.) Juzep, while Kagoso contains herb *Prunella vulgaris* L. Yamaguchi *et al.* [38] analyzed the inhibitory impact of Takusha and Kagosou, a kampo medications on the development of CaOx renal stones actuated by ethylene glycol and one alpha(OH)D3 (1 alpha-D3) in rodents. Wistar strain rats were grouped into four types like G-I is normal control, G-II is stone, G-III is kagosou, and G-IV is takusya. There was no marked difference in urinary oxalate excretion or calcium excretion between the stone and kampo medication received in animal groups. The calcium levels of the kidneys were essentially lower in the takusha than in the other two animal groups of stone and kagosou groups. Takusha was viable in forestalling oxalate stone arrangements in rodents. Kagosou, which had solid inhibitory impact on CaOx stone development and total *in vitro* just as takusha, was not successful against *in vivo* CaOx stone arrangement in rodents. These discoveries propose that takusha forestalls CaOx stone by repressing CaOx stone development and conglomeration.

Triphala Karpa Churna

Triphala Karpa Churna (TKC) is a traditional herbal medicine beneficial in treating renal stones, and churna having different plant extracts including *Phyllanthus emblica, Terminalia chebula, Terminalia bellerica*, Vengai sathu and Karungali sathu. Preclinical testing of TKC shows marked antiurolithiatic activity against CaOx and ethylene glycol initiated urolithiasis animal model. The histopathological study of the kidney and urine analysis shows favorable results comparable to a standard drug of cystone, and there is no renal damage and renal stone formation [39].

Unex

Unex is an herbal diuretic formulation available in capsules manufactured and marketed Unijules Life Sciences, Nagpur, India having different extracts of *Tribulus terrestris* and *Boerhaavia diffusa*. Jarald *et al.* [40] tested the action of unex capsule for its antiurolithiatic action by using ethylene glycol-initiated urolithiasis rat model. Cystone has used a standard drug for effective comparison. Various kidney and urinary parameters like urine pH, urinary volume, and complete urine analysis, serum analysis was performed to evaluate the activity. The results state that giving of unex formulation to rats significantly prevents the formation and growth of renal stones. It also restored all the biochemical parameters to normal.

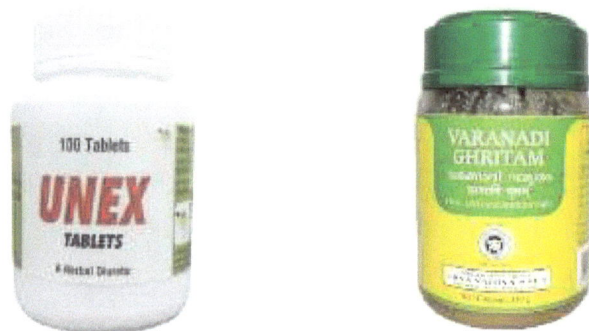

Fig. (4). Some polyherbal formulations in the market for nephroprotection and nephrocuration.

Varunadi Ghrita

The ingredients of Varunadi Ghria (Fig. **4**) are *Crataeva religiosa, Strobilanthus* *ciliatus, Asparagus racemosus, Plumbago zeylanica, Chonemorpha fragrans, Aegle marmelos, Aristolochia braceteolata, Solanum melongena, Aerva lanata, Pongamia pinnata, Holoptelia integrifolia, Premna corymbosa, Terminalia chebula, Moringa oleifera, Desmostachya bipinnata* and *Semecarpus anacardium.* All the ingredients are heated in ghee to prepare the Ghrita. Mandal *et al.* [41] evaluated the nephroprotective effect of Ayurvedic compound formulations 'Varunadi Ghrita' against gentamycin-initiated animal model nephrotoxicity. A total of 36 animals were divided into six groups and weighed. Test drug and vehicles were given to respective groups, after two hours, Gentamicin at a dose of 60 mg./kg. i.p. was given to all groups except the control group for 15 consecutive days. On the 16th day, animals were weighed again and sacrificed by cervical dislocation and severing the jugular veins. Blood samples and kidneys were collected for estimation of serum biochemical parameters and histopathological studies. Accurately weighed kidney tissues were used for the preparation of homogenate for estimation of different biochemical parameters. The result indicated that Varunadi Ghrita having moderate nephroprotective activity.

Varuna Guda

Varuna guda is an Ayurvedic preparation and consists of *Crataeva nurvala* (1 part), *Sacchaarum officinarum* (1 part) and *Bergenia ligulata* (1/100th part). Rani *et al.* [42] assessed the role of Varuna guda in the treatment of urolithiasis by conducting a randomized, single-blind, parallel clinical trial in a total of 36 patients. Based on consideration of various investigational parameters like urine, biochemical examination, USG, and X-ray calculated and taken before and after the treatment with varuna guda. The results clearly stated that the formation of renal calculi, its size, and the number of stones was significantly reduced by using varuna guda and providing symptomatic relief.

Wu Ling San

Wu Ling San (WLS) is a traditional Chinese herbal formula useful in treating and preventing renal stone formation. Tsai *et al.* tested the anthurolithiactic activity [43] in an ethylene glycol-initiated nephrolithiatic rat model. The results cleared that the control group animals were gained the least significant body weight compared to animals of WLS-fed groups. The control group animals had shown decreased calcium levels and then lower serum phosphorus in urine than that WLS-fed rat. The histo pathology examination of kidney sections revealed damage, tubular destruction, and inflammatory reactions in the ethylene glycol-water animal groups. The formation of renal crystals lowered significantly in WLS-fed groups and lowered CaOx crystals in rats.

Zhu Ling Tang

Tsai *et al.* [44] tested a traditional Chinese medicament called Zhu ling tang on experimentally initiated CaOx nephrolithiasis for its antinephrolithiatic activity in ethylene glycol-fed rats. Animals were given 0.75% ethylene glycol for four weeks, resulting in the formation of CaOx crystal in renal tubules and the rate of formation. The size of the stones was compared to the control group animals. Animals received with low-dose of Zhu ling tang have shown decreased serum phosphorus levels compared to the control animal groups. Further, measurement of biochemical parameters exhibited favorable results and confirmed the antinephrolithiatic activity of Zhul ling tang.

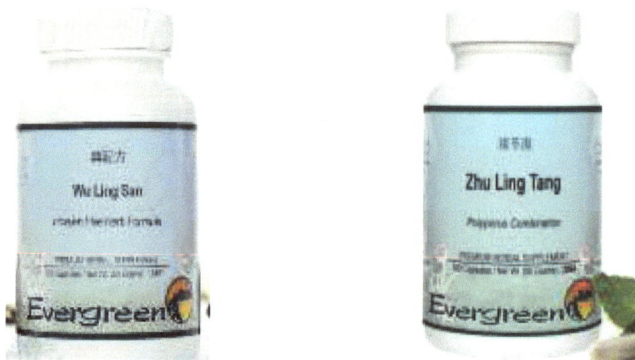

Fig. (5). Some polyherbal formulations in the market for nephroprotection and nephrocuration.

Polyherbal Formulation 1

The PF having aqueous extracts of *Terminalia chebula, Nelumbo nucifera, Zingiber officinale, Hemidesmus indicus, Myristica fragrans, Glycyrrhiza glabra* and *Citrus aurantofolia* was tested by Akila *et al* for its antiurolithiatic activity [45] (Fig. **5**). Albino rats (24 in number) were grouped into four types, and each was having six animals. Group-I is control. Groups-II, III and IV were administered with 0.75% ethylene glycol by gastric lavage and one gram of NH_4Cl in drinking water. Groups-III and IV received PF at a dose of 1 and 2mg/kg bw. In urolithiatic animals, oxalate and calcium, and excretion were significantly increased. Groups III and IV showed increased levels of urinary volume, pH, decreased calcium and oxalate excretion, weight gain, and stone inhibitors. The histoa pathology examination of renal tissues confirmed this result.

Polyherbal Formulation 2

This PF was scientifically proved for its antilithiatic activity against CaOx initiated urolithiasis in animal model. This PF having different extracts of *Plectranthus mollis* Spreng, *Didymocarpus pedicellata*, *Taraxacum officinale*, *Dendrophthoe elastica* Desr, and *Citrus medica*. All these plants were scientifically evaluated for their antiurolitiatic, antioxidant, anticancer, anti-inflammatory, diuretic properties [2].

Polyherbal Formulation 3

This PF prepared aqueous decoction of *Astercantha longifolia, Aerva lanata, Cumimum cyminum, Cucumis sativus, Hemidesmus indicus, Tribulus terrestris,* and *Lagenaria siceraria*. All these extracts were experimentally tested for their antiurolithiatic, antidiabetic, antioxidant, anti-inflammatory, analgesic, diuretic, antimicrobial, and hepatoprotective activities [2].

Polyherbal Formulation 4

This PF was scientifically evaluated for its antiurolithiatic activity on experimentally initiated urolithiasis in animal model. This PF has different plant extracts of *Hemidesmus indicus, Terminalia chebula, Nelumbo nucifera,* and *Zingiber officinale* proven for its different pharmacological actions like antiurolithiatic, hypolipidemic, anti-inflammatory, antioxidant, antidiabetic and hepatoprotective properties [2].

Polyherbal Formulation 5

This PF extracts *Dolichos biflorus, Aerva lanata* and *Musa* tested by Ramachandran *et al.* [46] for its antiurolithiatic activity on 0.75% ethylene glycol initiated urolithiasis animal models for 28 days. Estimation of renal biochemical parameters revealed the significant antiurolithiatic activity.

Polyherbal formulation 6

Baheti and Kadam [47] prepared a polyherbal formulation consisting of extracts of *Didymocarpus pedicellata, Plectranthus mollis, Dendrophthoe elastica, Taraxacum officinale* and *Citrus medica*. This PF was checked for its antiurolithiatic activity on 0.75% ethylene glycol initiated urolithiasis animal models for 28 days at doses of 200, 300, and 400mg/kg, respectively. Estimation of renal biochemical parameters, serum levels, and histopathological studies confirmed the antiurolithiatic activity at a dose of 200 mg/kg bw.

Polyherbal Syrup

This polyherbal syrup has aqueous decoction of *Astercantha longifolia, Aerva lanata, Cucumis sativus, Hemidesmus indicus, Cumimum cyminum, Tribulus terrestris,* and *Lagenaria siceraria*. This syrup was evaluated by Thangarathinam *et al.* [48] for its antiurolithiatic activity against 0.75% ethylene glycol-initiated urolithiasis in rats for 28 days at doses of 100 and 200 mg/kg bw p.o. Estimation of renal biochemical parameters, serum levels, and histopathological studies confirmed the antiurolithiatic activity at a dose of 200 mg/kg bw.

Biherbal Formulation *Bryophyllum pinnatum* (Syn.: *Kalanchoe pinnata*) and *Rotula aquatica*

The biherbal tablets having the extracts of *Bryophyllum pinnatum* and *Rotula aquatica* was scientifically tested by Gilhotra *et al.* [49] for their antiurolithiatic activity by homogenous precipitation *in vitro* method. For this, they were used TRIS buffer at a pH of 7.4 and calcium was estimated by titrimetry and phosphorus by colorimetric analysis methods. In addition, the % inhibition of the test was calculated in comparison with the control.

Purslane, Pumpkin, and Flax Seeds

On hypercholesterolemic rats, Barakat and Mahmoud [50] investigated the renal protective role of seed mixtures obtained from purslane, pumpkin, and flax seeds. This results in increased serum creatinine levels, urea, potassium, and sodium levels, raised serum IgG and IgM levels. Furthermore, the above said poly mixture administration resulted in a marked decrease in lipid parameters and IgM IgG levels and confirmed its renal protective activity.

Biherbal Formulation *Gongronema latifolium* and *Ocimum gratissimum*

Ezeonwu and Dahiru [51] scientifically tested the nephtoprotective role of biherbal formulation having aqueous leaf extracts of *G. latifolium* and *O. gratissimum* on acetaminophen-initiated liver and kidney toxicity in animal models at a doses of 200, 300 and 500 mg/kg bw. Raised levels of ALT, AST, urea, creatinine, triglycerides, and cholesterol were observed. Administration of biherbal formula shown significant results at a dose of 500 mg/kg bw. This study confirmed the use of mixed plant extracts.

Vediuppu Churna and *Aerva lanata*

Selvam *et al.* [52] evaluated the combination of Vediuppu churna and *Aerva lanata* for its antiurolithiatic activity on 0.75% ethylene glycol initiated urolithiasis animal models at doses of 3.5 and 3 mg/kg bw. For 28 days.

Treatment with Vediuppu churna and *Aerva lanata* may decrease urinary excretion levels of oxalate, calcium, uric acid, protein, and phosphorus. Thus, the study confirmed the usage of combination drugs for the treatment of urolithiasis.

CONCLUSION

Polyherbal Formulations is the utilization of more than one species in a herbal preparation. The idea is found in Ayurvedic and other conventional therapeutic frameworks where numerous species in a specific proportion might be utilized to treat sickness. This chapter highlights more than 30 PF's helpful in treating and managing multiple urinary system diseases and disorders. It has always been proved that multiple mixed herbs had synergetic action and a better therapeutic window.

REFERENCES

[1]   Parasuraman S, Thing GS, Dhanaraj SA. Polyherbal formulation: Concept of ayurveda. Pharmacogn Rev 2014; 8(16): 73-80.
[http://dx.doi.org/10.4103/0973-7847.134229] [PMID: 25125878]

[2]   Sharma AK, Tiwari MK, Sharma S, Sharma I, Goyal PK, Barwal A, *et al*. Nephroprotective role of Neeri-kft (a polyherbal formulation) against gentamicin induced nephrotoxicity in experimental rat model: a pre-clinical study. Eur J Pharm Med Res 2016; 3(8): 410-7.

[3]   Aggarwal A, Singla SK, Tandon C. Urolithiasis: phytotherapy as an adjunct therapy. Indian J Exp Biol 2014; 52(2): 103-11.
[PMID: 24597142]

[4]   Chellakkan E, Nainarpandian C, Blessed F, Gnanamanickam VR. Amirthathi churnam and Nandukal chunnam of Siddha formulation and clinical evaluation of nephrolithiasis. J Compl. Med Alternat Med 2018; 6(2): 555688.

[5]   Meena MK, Kushwah HK, Rajagopala M, Ravishankar B. An experimental evaluation on nephroprotective activity of Nagaradi Kashaya AYU 2009; 30(1): 55-61.

[6]   Gupta AV, Upadhyaya Y, Eds. Ashtanga Hridaya. Uttarsthana 36/84, Varanasi: Chaukhambha Sanskrit Sansthan. 2005; 85: p. 585.

[7]   Ramya P, Rajalakshmi I, Indumathy S, Kavimani S. Nephroprotective medicinal plants – A review. Int J Univers Pharm Life Sci 2011; 1: 266-81.

[8]   Kanna S, Hiremath SK, Unger BS. Nephroprotective activity of *Bilvādi agada* in gentamicin induced nephrotoxicity in male Wistar rats. Anc Sci Life 2015; 34(3): 126-9.
[http://dx.doi.org/10.4103/0257-7941.157146] [PMID: 26120225]

[9]   Dixit P, Koti BC, Vishwanathswam AHM. Antiurolithiatic activity of crashcal on ethylene glycol induced urolithiasis in rats. RGUHS J Pharm Sci 2014; 4(1): 30-5.
[http://dx.doi.org/10.5530/rjps.2014.1.6]

[10]   Ghosal KK. Ghose Anima, Sengupta P, Chatterjee S. Cystone in Urinary Tract Infections. Probe (Memphis) 1980; 4: 270.

[11]   Dandia SD, Kalra VB, Pendse AK, Ramdeo IN, Narula I. The preventive action of cystone in oxamide-induced urolithiasis and histochemical changes in the urinary tract–An experimental study in rats. In Pract 1975; 2: 127.

[12]   Garg SK, Singh RC. Role of Cystone in Burning Micturition. Probe (Memphis) 1985; 2: 119.

[13]   Gupta PD, Singh LM. A clinical trial of Cystone tablets in the treatment of various urinary disorders. Probe (Memphis) 1976; 2: 108.

[14]   Pendse AK, Ghosh R, Goyal A, Singh PP. Effect of indigenous drugs on idiopathic hyperoxaluria in stone formers. Asian Med J 1984; 2: 136.

[15]   Prasad RR. The role of cystone in urinary tract infections. In Pract 1980; 12: 685.

[16]   Singh PP, Singh NB, Mand Singh LBK. Effect of cystone treatment on urinary excretion of calcium, oxalic acid and uric acid in stone-formers. Antiseptic 1983; 5: 234. a

[17]   Singh PP, Pendse AK, Goyal A, Ghosh R, Kumawat JL, Srivastava AK. Indian drugs in modern medicine: A study on cystone. ArchMedPrac 1983; 2: 43. b

[18]   Singh PP, Pendse AK, Goyal A. Effectiveness of cystone (a formulation of indigenous products) in urinary calculus disease. Probe (Memphis) 1984; 2: 73.

[19]   Tripathi K, Srivastava PK, Singh RG, Prakash J, Ahmed J. Non-specific urethritis syndrome: A clinical puzzle. Probe 1984; 2: 87-20.

[20]   Trivedi BT, Oza HK, Rajan PS, Pathanwala AD. Cystone in crystalluria and urolithiasis. Probe (Memphis) 1974; 3: 134.

[21]   Saronwalla KC, Rai S, Goyal RS, Gupta ML. Role of cystone tablets in urinary calculi. Antiseptic 1973; 7: 467.

[22]   Sengupta S. Cystone in urinary tract complaints during pregnancy. Med Sr 1987; 27: 8.

[23]   Mitra SK, Gopumadhavan S, Venkataranganna MV, Sundaram R. Effect of cystone, a herbal formulation, on glycolic acid-induced urolithiasis in rats. Phytother Res 1998; 12(5): 372-4. [http://dx.doi.org/10.1002/(SICI)1099-1573(199808)12:5<372::AID-PTR312>3.0.CO;2-X]

[24]   Rao M, Rao MNA. Protective effects of cystone, a polyherbal ayurvedic preparation, on cisplatin-induced renal toxicity in rats. J Ethnopharmacol 1998; 62(1): 1-6. [http://dx.doi.org/10.1016/S0378-8741(98)00003-8] [PMID: 9720605]

[25]   Kumaran MGS, Patki PS. Evaluation of an Ayurvedic formulation (Cystone), in urolithiasis: A double blind, placebo-controlled study. Eur J Integr Med 2011; 3(1): 23-8. [http://dx.doi.org/10.1016/j.eujim.2011.02.003]

[26]   Bodakhe KS, Namdeo KP, Patra KC, Machwal L, Pareta SK. A polyherbal formulation attenuates hyperoxaluria-induced oxidative stress and prevents subsequent deposition of calcium oxalate crystals and renal cell injury in rat kidneys. Chin J Nat Med 2013; 11(5): 466-71. [http://dx.doi.org/10.1016/S1875-5364(13)60085-0] [PMID: 24359768]

[27]   Erickson SB, Vrtiska TJ, Lieske JC. Effect of Cystone® on urinary composition and stone formation over a one year period. Phytomedicine 2011; 18(10): 863-7.

[28]   Siddaram A, Pushkar Y, Seema M. Basalingappa, Verma JP. Clinical study on Gokshuradi kashaya in the management of Urolithiasis (Mutrashmari). Int J Ayurvedic & Herbal Medicine 2012; 2(3): 520-9.

[29]   Shirfule AL, Racharla V, Qadri SSYH, Khandare AL. Exploring antiurolithic effects of gokshuradi polyherbal ayurvedic formulation in ethylene-glycol-induced urolithic rats. Evid Based Complement Alternat Med 2013; 2013: 763720. [http://dx.doi.org/10.1155/2013/763720] [PMID: 23554833]

[30]   Afzal M, Khan NA, Ghufran A, Iqbal A, Inamuddin M. Diuretic and nephroprotective effect of Jawarish Zarooni Sada--a polyherbal unani formulation. J Ethnopharmacol 2004; 91(2-3): 219-23. [http://dx.doi.org/10.1016/j.jep.2003.12.029] [PMID: 15120442]

[31]   Lulat SI, Yadav YC, Balaraman R, Maheshwari R. Antiurolithiatic effect of lithocare against ethylene glycol-induced urolithiasis in Wistar rats. Int J Pharm 2016; 48(1): 78-82.

[PMID: 26997728]

[32] Gupta SK, Baghel MS, Bhuyan C, Ravishankar B, Ashok BK, Patil PD. Evaluation of anti-urolithiatic activity of Pashanabhedadi Ghrita against experimentally induced renal calculi in rats. Ayu 2012; 33(3): 429-34.
[http://dx.doi.org/10.4103/0974-8520.108860] [PMID: 23723654]

[33] Roy A, Adhikari A, Das SK, Banerjee D, De R, Debnath PK. Evaluation of efficacy and safety of renomet, a polyherbal formulation in the treatment of urolithiasis: A double blind randomized study

[34] Joshi N, Joshi M, Shah R, Gajera V. Effect of relith on ethylene glycol induced urolithiasis in rats. Int J Pharma Sci 2012; 3(4): 3018-27.

[35] Vasanthi AHR, Muthulakshmi V, Gayathri V, Manikandan R, Ananthi S, Kuruvilla S. Antiurolithiatic effect of Sirupeelai Samoola Kudineer: A polyherbal Siddha decoction on ethylene glycol-induced renal calculus in experimental rats. Pharmacogn Mag 2017; 13 (Suppl. 2): S273-9.
[http://dx.doi.org/10.4103/pm.pm_454_16] [PMID: 28808392]

[36] Nagvenkar SR, Verlekar MU, Sharma AK. Clinical evaluation of the role of Shwadanstradi ghana vati in the management of Urolithiasis (Mutrashmari). J Ayurveda 2011; 5(2): 5-10.

[37] Yasui T, Fujita K, Sato M, *et al.* The effect of takusha, a kampo medicine, on renal stone formation and osteopontin expression in a rat urolithiasis model. Urol Res 1999; 27(3): 194-9.
[http://dx.doi.org/10.1007/s002400050109] [PMID: 10422821]

[38] Yamaguchi S, Jihong L, Utsunomiya M, *et al.* [The effect of takusha and kagosou on calcium oxalate renal stones in rats]. Hinyokika Kiyo 1995; 41(6): 427-31. [in Japanese].
[PMID: 7645450]

[39] Selvan AT, Jayalaxmi B. Antiurolithiatic activity of Triphala Karpa Chooranam. J Adv Pharm Educ Res 2013; 3(3): 267-72.

[40] Jarald EE, Kushwah P, Edwin S, Asghar S, Patni SA. Effect of Unex on ethylene glycol-induced urolithiasis in rats. Indian J Pharmacol 2011; 43(4): 466-8.
[http://dx.doi.org/10.4103/0253-7613.83124] [PMID: 21845008]

[41] Mandal AK, Dwivedi RR, Manjusha R, Ravishankar B. A comparative study on Vrikka Samrakshanatmaka and Ashmarighna effect of Tiladi kshara and Varunadi ghrita (Nephroprotective and Lithotripsic effect). Ayu 2008; 29(4): 231-4.

[42] Rani M, Agarwal R, Dhiman KS, Sijjoria KK. Role of Varuna guda in the management of Mutrashmari (Urolithiasis) and assessment with imaging techniques. J Ayurveda and Holistic Medicine 2014; 2(2): 27-37.

[43] Tsai CH, Chen YC, Chen LD, *et al.* A traditional Chinese herbal antilithic formula, Wulingsan, effectively prevents the renal deposition of calcium oxalate crystal in ethylene glycol-fed rats. Urol Res 2008; 36(1): 17-24.
[http://dx.doi.org/10.1007/s00240-007-0122-4] [PMID: 18040675]

[44] Tsai CH, Pan T-C, Lai M-T, *et al.* Prophylaxis of experimentally induced calcium oxalate nephrolithiasis in rats by Zhulingtang, a traditional Chinese herbal formula. Urol Int 2009; 82(4): 464-71.
[http://dx.doi.org/10.1159/000218539] [PMID: 19506417]

[45] Akila L, Ashok Kumar P, Nirmala P. Effect of a polyherbal formulation on ethylene glycol induced urolithiasis. Int J Pharma Bio Sci 2011; 2(4): 7-24.

[46] Ramachandran S, Vijayakumar TM, Saisandeep V, Ramsai K, Dhanaraju MD. Antilithiatic activity of poly-herbal extracts on ethylene glycol induced lithiasis in rats. European J Biol Sci 2011; 3(2): 36-9.

[47] Baheti DG, Kadam SS. Antiurolithiatic activity of a polyherbal formulation against calcium oxalate induced urolithiasis in rats. J Adv Pharm Educ Res 2013; 3(1): 31-41.

[48] Thangarathinam N, Jayshree N, Mehta AV, Ramanathan L. Effect of polyherbal formulation on

ethylene glycol induced urolithiasis. Int J Pharm Pharm Sci 2013; 5(3): 116-25.

[49]   Gilhotra UK, Mohan G, Christina AJM. Antilithiatic activity of poly-herbal formulation tablets by in-vitro method. J Appl Pharm Sci 2013; 3(5): 43-8.

[50]   Barakat LA, Mahmoud RH. The antiatherogenic, renal protective and immunomodulatory effects of purslane, pumpkin and flax seeds on hypercholesterolemic rats. N Am J Med Sci 2011; 3(9): 411-7.
[http://dx.doi.org/10.4297/najms.2011.3411] [PMID: 22362450]

[51]   Ezeonwu VU, Dahiru D. Protective effect of bi-herbal formulation of *Ocimum gratissimum* and *Gongronema latifolium* aqueous leaf extracts on acetaminophen-induced hepato-nephrotoxicity in rats. Am J Biochem 2013; 3: 18-23.

[52]   Selvam R, Kalaiselvi P, Govindaraj A, Bala Murugan V, Sathish Kumar AS. Effect of *A. lanata* leaf extract and Vediuppu chunnam on the urinary risk factors of calcium oxalate urolithiasis during experimental hyperoxaluria. Pharmacol Res 2001; 43(1): 89-93.
[http://dx.doi.org/10.1006/phrs.2000.0745] [PMID: 11207071]

CHAPTER 5

Ethnomedicinal Plants for Nephroprotection

Abstract: In recent times usage of traditional medicinal plants has received much-needed attention as sources of bioactive substances and antioxidants, used to treat a wide variety of diseases and disorders of major body organs, including kidney as a nephroprotective. Ethnobotany is how people of particular culture and region make use of the existing traditional knowledge related to plants in their local environments. It is the study of interrelations between humans and herbs/plants; however, the current use of the term implies the study of indigenous or traditional knowledge of plants. The kidney performs crucial functions in the body. It maintains the overall fluid balance in the human body. The kidney regulates and filters the minerals from the blood. It also filters waste materials from food, medications, and toxic substances. Due to the entirety of the indispensable capacities, the kidneys' performance is affected by the poisons they experience. The kidneys are vulnerable to different issues like chronic kidney disease, kidney failure, kidney stones, nephritis, *etc.*, and so on. The present review is an attempt to review the usage of ethnomedicinal plants for nephroprotection by utilizing the different tribal cultures.

This may be useful to researchers who were working in the area nephrology and therapeutics.

Keywords: Ethnobotany, Ethnomedicine, Nephroprotection, Tribal medicine.

INTRODUCTION

The least difficult meaning of ethnobotany is given by the actual word: ethno (individuals) and botany (study of plants). Fundamentally, it is an investigation of how individuals of specific cultures and areas utilize the plants in their nearby surroundings. These utilizations incorporate food, medication, fuel, cover, and in numerous societies, in strict services. In 1895, during a talk in Philadelphia, a botanist named John Harshberger, gave the principal meaning of ethnobotany as the investigation of how local clans utilized plants for food, haven, or dress [1]. One of the best-known modern ethnobotanists– Richard Evans Schultes identified the field of ethnobotany as an interdisciplinary field, combining botany, anthropology, economics, ethics, history, chemistry, and many other areas of study.

Ethnobotanists need to be prepared to ask the following questions:

1. What are the crucial thoughts and originations of individuals living in a specific area about the vegetation encompassing them?

2. What impact does a given climate have on the lives, customs, religion, contemplations, and regular useful issues of individuals considered?

3. In what ways do individuals utilize the nearby plants for food, medication, material culture, and stylized purposes?

4. How much information do individuals have of the parts, capacities, and exercises of plants?

5. How are plant names classified in the language of individuals contemplated, and what can the investigation of these names uncover about the way of life of individuals?

The cutting-edge arrangement of medication actually needs giving reasonable medicament to countless illnesses, despite huge advances made in the revelation of new compounds. A couple of these sicknesses are kidney issues, hepatic issues, viral contaminations, AIDS, rheumatic illnesses [2] and so forth. The accessible, helpful specialists just achieve suggestive alleviation with no impact on the remedial cycle, hence causing the danger of backslide and threat of untoward impacts. An enormous number of populaces experience the ill effects of kidney related issues/infections of obscure starting points. The advancement of nephroprotective medications being a significant pushed territory has attracted the consideration of laborers in the field of normal item research.

ETHNOBOTANY OF NEPHROPROTECTIVE PLANTS

In this chapter, medicinal plants used for curing and prevention of kidney diseases by different ethnic tribes are reviewed. Information is drawn from the published papers in different journals, books and theses. We do not claim to have included all the existing tribal communities of world information about ethnobotanical use of medicinal plants but we rather focused on information easily accessible. A list of plants used by the tribal people prepared which gives the scientific name, part of the plant used, name of the tribal community, local name of the plant, uses and/or mode of use. The precision of botanical identification in this review depends on that from original sources.

Note: Perusers, if it's not too much trouble, note that all material given thus is just data and may not be interpreted as clinical counsel. Perusers ought to counsel fitting wellbeing experts on any matter identifying with their wellbeing and prosperity. The viability of the blossoms and the leaves are at their best, when they are mentioned and culled from the plants after they are completely sprouted on the plant. It is avoided the chance to offer the blossoms culled well ahead of time, in a bud condition to dodge the ill impacts.

Table 1. Ethnobotanical literature review of medicinal plants used for treatment of various liver disease/disorders.

S. No	Plant Name	Part Used	Tribe/Local Community	Local Names (State, Country)	Uses/Mode of Use
1.	*Abelmoschus moschatus* Medik	Seeds	Villagers, elderly persons, traditional healers	Kapukinissa (Srilanka)	Utilized in treatment of kidney sicknesses because of their diuretic impacts. Decoction of beat seeds are professed to be helpful in the management of renal calculi [3]
2.	*Abrus pectorious* L.	Leaves	Local people and herbal practioners	Gurijalu (Warangal, Telangana, India)	Used in the treatment of kidney stones [4]
3.	*Abrus precatorius* L.	Leaves	Local people and traditional healers	Chaning angouba (Manipur, North East India)	Aqueous extract is utilized for treatment of kidney stones [5]
4.	*Abutilon indicum* L.	Root	Villagers, elderly persons, traditional healers	Thuthi (Madurai district, Tamil Nadu, India)	Root powder used as nephroprotective [6]
5.	*Abutilon indicum* L.	Whole plant	Local people and traditional healers	Atibala (Bhopal district, Madhya Pradesh, India)	Used in treatment of kidney stones [7]
6.	*Abutilon indicum* L.	Whole plant	Local people and herbal practioners	Thuthuru benda (Warangal, Telangana, India)	Used in the treatment of kidney stones [4]
7.	*Abutilon indicum* L.	Whole plant	Local people and Traditional healers	Kanghi (Manipur, North East India)	Herb is employed in urinary troubles [5]
8.	*Acacia jacquemontii* Benth.	Whole plant	Local people and Traditional healers	(Pakistan)	Used for the treatment in kidney stone [8]

S. No	Plant Name	Part Used	Tribe/Local Community	Local Names (State, Country)	Uses/Mode of Use
9.	*Acacia nilotica* (L.) Delile	Dry pods, bark	Tribal people, indigenous people and traditional health practitioners	Bana valley, Kotli (Kashmir), Pakistan	The powder of bark and dry pods used for treatment of kidney pains [9]
10.	*Acalypha indica* L.	Leaves	Local people and herbal practioners	Pippanti (Warangal, Telangana, India)	Used in the treatment of kidney stones [4]
11.	*Acalypha indica* L.	Root extract	Villagers, elderly persons, traditional healers	Kuppai meni (Madurai district, Tamil Nadu, India)	Root extract used as kidney protective [6]
12.	*Acer pensylvanicum* L.	Bark	Penobscot, Micmac	Striped maple (New Brunswick, Nova Scotia, Prince Edward Island, Quebec, Ontario, Canada)	Bark used in the form of tea for kidney problems [10]
13.	*Achillea millefolium* L.	Whole plant	Local people and Traditional healers	(Pakistan)	Used for the treatment in kidney stone [8]
14.	*Achillea millefolium* L.	Aerial organs	Local traditional therapists	Boumadaran (Shahrekord, Iran)	Anti-kidney stone effect [11]
15.	*Achyranthes aspera* L.	Leaves, stem	Tribal people, indigenous people and traditional health practitioners	Bana valley, Kotli (Kashmir), Pakistan	Ash of leaves and stem is recommended for treatment of kidney stones [9]

S. No	Plant Name	Part Used	Tribe/Local Community	Local Names (State, Country)	Uses/Mode of Use
16.	*Achyranthes aspera* L.	Leaves, stem, roots	Local people and traditional healers	Apamarg (Bhopal district, Madhya Pradesh, India)	Used in treatment of kidney stones. Root is crushed and taken with water in the morning. Leaves are used in urinary disorders and its whole plant, leaf and seeds are useful in stone disease. The decoction of leaves (25 g) is prepared in 125 ml water and given for 7 days. In case of stone disease, root decoction is given thrice a day for a period of one month [7] [12].
17.	*Achyranthes aspera* L.	Whole plant	Villagers, elderly persons, traditional healers	Nayuruvi (Madurai district, Tamil Nadu, India)	Whole plant extract used for diuretic and didney stones [6]
18.	*Achyranthes aspera* L.	Leaf	Native people, traditional healers, knowledgeable old persons	Uttareni (Anantapur, Andhra Pradesh, India)	Used in the treatment of kidney stones or urolithiasis. 25 ml leaf extract is given twice a day for fifteen days [13]
19.	*Achyranthes aspera* L.	Whole plant	Traditional health practioners, local people	Puthkanda (Hafizabad district, Punjab-Pakistan)	Decoction is used in the treatment of kidney stones [14]
20.	*Achyranthus aspera* L.	Whole plant	Local people and herbal practioners	Utthareni (Warangal, Telangana, India)	Used in the treatment of kidney stones [4]
21.	*Achyranthus aspera* L.	Whol plant	Local people and traditional healers	(Pakistan)	Used for the treatment in kidney stone [8]
22.	*Acorus calamus* L.	Rhizome and root	Villagers, elderly persons, traditional healers	Vasambu (Madurai district, Tamil Nadu, India)	Extract of root and rhizome used for kidney troubles [6]

S. No	Plant Name	Part Used	Tribe/Local Community	Local Names (State, Country)	Uses/Mode of Use
23.	*Actinodaphne angustifolia* (Blume) Nees	Leaves	Local people and traditional healers	Takara (Manipur, North East India)	The decoction of the plant is used in kidney diseases due to stone [5]
24.	*Adiantum capillus-veneris* L.	Flower, Leaf	Local people and traditional healers	Kamar Avizeh (Ilam, Iran)	Used in the treatment of kidney stones [15]
25.	*Adiantum capillus-veneris* L.	Aerial organs	Local traditional therapists	Paresiavashan (Shahrekord, Iran)	Anti-kidney stone effect [11]
26.	*Aegle marmelos* L.	Leaf extract	Villagers, elderly persons, traditional healers	Vilvam (Madurai district, Tamil Nadu, India)	The ground leaves can be used to treat kidney problem [6]
27.	*Aerva javanica* (Burm.f.) Juss. ex Schult.	Whole plant	Native people, traditional healers, knowledgeable old persons	Peddapindiaaku (Anantapur, Andhra Pradesh, India)	Used in the treatment of kidney stones or urolithiasis. 15 g entire plant paste blended in with water and is allowed once every day for 15 days [13].
28.	*Aerva javanica* (Burm. f.) Juss. ex Schult.	Whole plant	Local people and traditional healers	(Pakistan)	Used for the treatment in kidney stone [8]
29.	*Aerva lanata* (L.) Juss.	Leaves	Local people and herbal practioners	Pindi chettu (Warangal, Telangana, India)	Used in the treatment of kidney stones [4]
30.	*Aerva lanata* (L.) Juss.	Roots	Native people, traditional healers, knowledgeable old persons	Kondapindiaaku (Anantapur, Andhra Pradesh, India)	Utilized in the treatment of kidney stones or urolithiasis. Extract of Root decoction or entire plant, allowed twice a day for a month [13]
31.	*Aerva lanata* (L.) Juss.	Whole plant	Traditional healers	Gorakshaganja (India)	Used in management of kidney troubles [16]

(Table 1) cont.....

S. No	Plant Name	Part Used	Tribe/Local Community	Local Names (State, Country)	Uses/Mode of Use
32.	*Aeschynomene indica* L.	Young tender leaves	Local people and traditional healers	Chigonglei (Manipur, North East India)	Taken as salad, cures stone in urinary tract infection. Boiled extract of the leaves with black pepper is prescribed in painful urination [5]
33.	*Ageratum conyzoides* L.	Whole plant	Local people and traditional healers	Mahkua (Bhopal district, Madhya Pradesh, India)	Used in treatment of kidney stones [7]
34.	*Ajuga iva* (L.) Schreb.	Aerial parts	Plant collectors, herbalists, traditional practitioners.	Chendgûra (Izarène, Morocco)	Decoction used in the treatment of urolithiasis [17]
35.	*Alcea flavovirens* (Boiss. & Buhse) Iljin	Leaf	Turkish citizens	Hero (Geçitli Township, Eastern Anatolia Region, Hakkari-Turkey)	Used in treatment of kidney pains [18]
36.	*Alcea hohenackeri* (Boiss. & Huet) Boiss.	Leaf, root	Turkish citizens	Hero (Geçitli Township, Eastern Anatolia Region, Hakkari-Turkey)	Used in treatment of kidney pains [18]
37.	*Alcea hohenackeri* (Boiss. & Huet) Boiss.	Aerial parts, roots, leaf	Native people	Hero (Çatak, Eastern Anatolia Region, Turkey)	One glass of the extract of the plant on an empty stomach in the morning is used in treatment of kidney stones [19]
38.	*Alcea rosea* L. (Syn.: *Althaea rosea* (L.) Cav.)	Leaves, flowers	Local people and traditional healers	Khatmi (Bhopal district, Madhya Pradesh, India)	Used in treatment of kidney stones [7]
39.	*Alhagi maurorum* Medik. (Syn.: *A. camelorum* Fisch.)	Aerial parts	Local people and traditional healers	Kharshotor (Lorestan, Iran)	Used in the treatment of kidney stones [15]
40.	*Alhagi maurorum* Medik. (Syn.: *A. camelorum* Fisch.)	Aerial parts	Traditional healers	Khar Shotor (Urmia, Northwest Iran)	Decoction used in the exertion of kidney stones [20]
41.	*Alhagi maurorum* Medik. (Syn.: *A. camelorum* Fisch.)	Whole plant	Local people and traditional healers	Kharshotor (Kazeroun, Iran)	Used in the treatment of kidney stones [15].

S. No	Plant Name	Part Used	Tribe/Local Community	Local Names (State, Country)	Uses/Mode of Use
42.	*Alhagi maurorum* Medik. (Syn.: *A. camelorum* Fisch.)	Aerial organs	Local traditional therapists	Kharshotor (Shahrekord, Iran)	Anti-kidney stone effect [11]
43.	*Alhagi maurorum* Medik. (Syn.: *A. camelorum* Fisch.)	Roots	Traditional health practioners, local people	Jawansa (Hafizabad district, Punjab-Pakistan)	Decoction is used in the treatment of kidney stones [14]
44.	*Alhagi persarum* Boiss. & Buhse	Aerial parts	Local people and traditional healers	Kharshotor (Persian Gulf, Iran)	Used in the treatment of kidney stones [15]
45.	*Alhagi persarum* Boiss. & Buhse	Flower, pedicel, leaf	Local people and traditional healers	Kharshotor (Kazeroun, Iran)	Used in the treatment of kidney stones [15]
46.	*Alhagi persarum* Boiss. & Buhse.	Pedicel, leaf	Local people and traditional healers	Kharshotor (Ilam, Iran)	Used in the treatment of kidney stones [15]
47.	*Allium akaka* Gmel.	Pedicel	Local people and traditional healers	Loosha (West Azerbaijan, Iran)	Used in the treatment of kidney stones [15]
48.	*Allium akaka* Gmel.	Bulbs, Leaf	Local people and traditional healers	Vallak (Ilam, Iran)	Used in the treatment of kidney stones [15]
49.	*Allium ampeloprasum* L. subsp. *iranicum* Wendelbo	Leaf	Local people and traditional healers	Tare Kouhi (Ilam, Iran)	Used in the treatment of kidney stones [15]
50.	*Allium cepa* L.	Bulbs	Local people and traditional healers	Pyaaz (Bhopaldistrict, Madhya Pradesh, India)	Used in treatment of kidney stones. In case of stone disease, the bulb juice is given 3 times a day for a month [7] [12]
51.	*Allium cepa* L.	Dried bulb	Villagers, elderly persons, traditional healers	Vengayam (Madurai district, Tamil Nadu, India)	Onion juice can reduce the defects of kidney problem [6]
52.	*Allium cepa* L.	Other part	Plant collectors, herbalists, traditional practitioners	Lbesla (Izarène, Morocco)	Raw material used in the treatment of urolithiasis [17]

(Table 1) cont.....

S. No	Plant Name	Part Used	Tribe/Local Community	Local Names (State, Country)	Uses/Mode of Use
53.	*Allium cepa* L.	Bulbs	Local people and traditional healers	Piaz (Khuzestan, Iran)	Used in the treatment of kidney stones [15]
54.	*Allium odorum* L.	Leaves	Muslim Maiba (herbalists)	Yenam nakuppi (Manipur, India)	250 gm of the extract used in treatment of kidney stones. Drink 1 tea glass daily till cure or eat it with salad items as much as possible [21]
55.	*Allium odorum* L.	Leaves	Local people and traditional healers	Yenam nakuppi (Manipur, North East India)	Leaves extract is used in management of painful urination especially urinary tract infections due to stone [5]
56.	*Allium sativum* L.	Other part	Plant collectors, herbalists, traditional practitioners	Toum (Izarène, Morocco)	Raw material used in the treatment of urolithiasis [17]
57.	*Aloe barbadensis* Miller	Leaf, leaf gel	Local people and traditional healers	(Bhopal district, Madhya Pradesh, India)	Used in treatment of kidney stones [7] [12]
58.	*Alpinia officinarum* Han.	Rhizome	Plant collectors, herbalists, traditional practitioners	Khdenjâl (Izarène, Morocco)	Decoction used in the treatment of urolithiasis [17]
59.	*Alternanthera sessilis* (L.) R.Br.ex DC.	Leaves	Villagers, elderly persons, traditional healers	Ponnanganni (Madurai district, Tamil Nadu, India)	Leaf extract used to treat urinary tract infection and kidney troubles [6]
60.	*Alyssum desertorum* Stapf	Seed	Local people and traditional healers	Ghodome (Lorestan, Iran)	Used in the treatment of kidney stones [15]
61.	*Alyssum desertorum* Stapf	Seed	Traditional healers	Ghoddumeh (Urmia, Northwest Iran)	Decoction used in the exertion of kidney stones [20]
62.	*Alyssum pateri* Nyar. subsp. *pateri*	Aerial parts	Turkish citizens	Keselmehmut (Geçitli Township, Eastern Anatolia Region, Hakkari-Turkey)	Decoction is used in the treatment of kidney stones [18]

S. No	Plant Name	Part Used	Tribe/Local Community	Local Names (State, Country)	Uses/Mode of Use
63.	*Amaranthus blitoides* S. Watson	Aerial parts	Local people and traditional healers	Taj khourous (Lorestan, Iran)	Used in the treatment of kidney stones [15]
64.	*Amaranthus blitoides* S.Watson	Aerial parts	Traditional healers	A kind of Taj Khorus (Urmia, Northwest Iran)	Decoction used in the exertion of kidney stones [20]
65.	*Amaranthus caudutus* L.	Leaves	Local people and herbal practioners	Netakoora (Warangal, Telangana, India)	Used in the treatment of kidney stones [4]
66.	*Amaranthus spinosus* L.	Leaves	Local people and herbal practioners	Thotakura (Warangal, Telangana, India)	Used in the treatment of kidney stones [4]
67.	*Amaranthus spinosus* L.	Whole plant	Local people and traditional healers	Kanta chaulai (Bhopal district, Madhya Pradesh, India)	Used in treatment of kidney stones [7]
68.	*Amaranthus spinosus* L.	Leaves	Villagers, elderly persons, traditional healers	Mullukkeerai (Madurai district, Tamil Nadu, India)	Leaf extract used for renal failure [6]
69.	*Amaranthus spinosus* L.	Whole plant	Native people, traditional healers, knowledgeable old persons	Mullathothakoora (Anantapur, Andhra Pradesh, India)	The whole plant ash (3g) mixed with water and is given for one month, twice a day in treatment of kidney stones or urolithiasis [13]
70.	*Amaranthus viridis* L.	Leaves	Local people and herbal practioners	Thotakura (Warangal, Telangana, India)	Used in the treatment of kidney stones [4]
71.	*Amaranthus viridis* L.	Whole plant	Local people and traditional healers	Jangli chaulai (Bhopal district, Madhya Pradesh, India)	Used in treatment of kidney stones. In case of stone disease, fresh leaves curry taken along with food [7] [12].
72.	*Ammi visnaga* (L.) Lam.	Seeds	Plant collectors, herbalists, traditional practitioners	Bachnikha (Izarène, Morocco)	Decoction used in the treatment of urolithiasis [17]
73.	*Amomum subulatum* Roxb.	Seeds	Meitei, Tangkhul, Kabui, Naga, and Mizo	Elaichi (Manipur, North-East India)	Used in treatment of kidney problems [22]

(Table 1) cont.....

S. No	Plant Name	Part Used	Tribe/Local Community	Local Names (State, Country)	Uses/Mode of Use
74.	*Amygdalus arabica* Olivier	Fruit	Local people and traditional healers	Badam Kouhi (Ilam, Iran)	Used in the treatment of kidney stones [15]
75.	*Amygdalus communis* L.	Seed	Local people and traditional healers	Badame Talkh (Khuzestan, Iran)	Used in the treatment of kidney stones [15]
76.	*Anacardium occidentale* L.	Leaves and stem bark	Villagers, elderly persons, traditional healers	Mundiri (Madurai district, Tamil Nadu, India)	Leaf extract lower the risk of kidney stone [6]
77.	*Ananas comosus* L.	Ripe fruit	Local people and traditional healers	Kihom (Manipur, North East India)	In case of bronchitis, asthma and urinary trouble due to stones, ripe fruit extact of the plant is prescribed for management [5].
78.	*Ananas comosus* Merr.	Fruit	Local people and traditional healers	Pineapple (Bhopal district, Madhya Pradesh, India)	Used in treatment of kidney stones [7]
79.	*Anastatica hierochuntica* L.	Aerial parts	Plant collectors, herbalists, traditional practitioners.	Akarbâ (Izarène, Morocco)	Decoction used in the treatment of urolithiasis [17]
80.	*Andrographis paniculata* Nees	Leaves	Local people and traditional healers	Kalmegh (Manipur, North East India)	In case of cold, fever, cough and urinary disorders, boiled leaf extract is preferable for management [5].
81.	*Anethum graveolens* L.	Aerial parts, roots	Turkish citizens	Sıbıt (Geçitli Township, Eastern Anatolia Region, Hakkari-Turkey)	Decoction is used in the treatment of kidney stones [18]
82.	*Anisomeles malabarica* (L.) R.Br. ex Sm.	Whole plant	Villagers, elderly persons, traditional healers	Peyimiratti (Madurai district, Tamil Nadu, India)	Whole plant extract used as nephroprotective [6]
83.	*Anneslea fragrans* Wall.	Dried leaves	Local people and traditional healers	Thingphunchuo (Manipur, North East India)	For management of kidney stones, take boiled leaf extract (10 g in 1 litre) orally three times a day [5].

S. No	Plant Name	Part Used	Tribe/Local Community	Local Names (State, Country)	Uses/Mode of Use
84.	*Anthocephalus cadamba* Miq.	Leaves, flowers	Local people and traditional healers	Kadamba (Bhopal district, Madhya Pradesh, India)	Used in treatment of kidney stones [7]
85.	*Apium graveolens* L.	Whole plant	Caribbean folk medicine practioners, local people	Celery (Trinidad and Tobago, Caribbean)	Kidney tonic [23]
86.	*Apium graveolens* L.	Aerial parts	Plant collectors, herbalists, traditional practitioners.	Krafèss (Izarène, Morocco)	Decoction used in the treatment of urolithiasis [17]
87.	*Apium graveolens* L.	Leaves	Traditional herbalists	Krafess (Rabat-Sal--Kenitra Region, Morocco)	Decoction of the leaves used for treatment of chronic kidney diseases [24]
88.	*Arctium minus* (Hill.) Bernh. subsp. *pubens* (Bab.) Rothm.	Aerial parts, leaf	Native people	Belg gırno, kuncurk,belg misek (Çatak, Eastern Anatolia Region, Turkey)	Aerial parts decoction used in treatment and management of kidney stone by taking one tea glass extract three times a day [19].
89.	*Arctium minus* (Hill.) Bernh.subsp. *pubens* (Bab.) Rothm.	Leaf	Turkish citizens	Nuserk (Geçitli Township, Eastern Anatolia Region, Hakkari-Turkey)	Decoction is used in the treatment of kidney stones [18]
90.	*Arctostaphylos uva-ursi* (L.) Spreng.	Leaf	Algonquin, Blackfoot, Micmac, Salish	Bearberry (All of Canada)	Tea of leaves for kidney problems [10]
91.	*Areca catechu* L.	Nuts	Native people, traditional healers, knowledgeable old persons	Poka (Anantapur, Andhra Pradesh, India)	Nut powder (3g) is used in the treatment of kidney stones or urolithiasis, given twice a day for a week [13].
92.	*Argemone mexicana* L.	Whole plant	Local people and traditional healers	Satyanashi (Bhopal district, Madhya Pradesh, India)	Used in treatment of kidney stones [7]
93.	*Argemone mexicana* L.	Seed	Villagers, elderly persons, traditional healers	Pramma thandu (Madurai district, Tamil Nadu, India)	Seed oil urinary tract infection [6]

(Table 1) cont.....

S. No	Plant Name	Part Used	Tribe/Local Community	Local Names (State, Country)	Uses/Mode of Use
94.	*Argemone mexicana* L.	Roots	Local people and herbal practioners	Rakkisa (Warangal, Telangana, India)	Used in the treatment of kidney stones [4]
95.	*Aristolochia longa* L.	Whole plant	Native people	Bereztem (Rabat, Sale and Temara, Morocco)	The plant dried and crushed to obtain a powder and mixed with the honey is used for treatment of kidney stones [25]
96.	*Artemisia herba-alba* Asso.	Leaves	Plant collectors, herbalists, traditional practitioners.	Chih (Izarène, Morocco)	Decoction used in the treatment of urolithiasis [17]
97.	*Asparagus falcatus* L.	Whole plant	Villagers, elderly persons, traditional healers	Hathavariya (Sri Lanka)	Used in treatment of kidney diseases due to their diuretic effects [3]
98.	*Asparagus racemosus* Willd.	Root	Local people and traditional healers	Nunggarei angouba (Manipur, North East India)	Boiled decoction of the root with sugar is prescribed in urinary troubles due to stone [5]
99.	*Asparagus racemosus* Willd.	Whole plant	Local people and traditional healers	Satawar (Bhopal district, Madhya Pradesh, India)	Used in treatment of kidney stones [7]
100.	*Asphodelus tenuifolius* Cavan	Whole plant	Local people and traditional healers	(Pakistan)	Used for the treatment in kidney stone [8]
101.	*Asteracantha longifolia* Nees	Whole plant	Local people and traditional healers	Talmakhana (Bhopal district, Madhya Pradesh, India)	Used in treatment of kidney stones [7]
102.	*Astragalus hamosus* L.	Fruit	Local people and traditional healers	Nakhonak (Khuzestan, Iran)	Used in the treatment of kidney stones [15]
103.	*Averrhoa carambola* L.	Fruit	Local people and traditional healers	Heinou-Jom (Manipur, North East India)	For treatment of kidney stones, prepare fruit juice by placing 2.8 g silver element into 300 ml fruit juice and drink half tea glass daily for five days [5].

(Table 1) cont.....

S. No	Plant Name	Part Used	Tribe/Local Community	Local Names (State, Country)	Uses/Mode of Use
104.	*Averrhoea carambola* L.	Fruit	Muslim Maiba (herbalists)	Heinoujom (Manipur, India)	300 ml of the extract used in treatment of kidney stones. Drink half tea glass daily for five days [21]
105.	*Azadirachta indica* A. Juss.	Leaves	Villagers, elderly persons, traditional healers	Vembu (Madurai district, Tamil Nadu, India)	Leaves decoction used for renal injury [6]
106.	*Azadirachta indica* A. Juss.	Leaf	Native people, traditional healers, knowledgeable old persons	Vepa (Anantapur, Andhra Pradesh, India)	Leaf ash (2g) with water is given once a day for a month for treatment of kidney stones or urolithiasis [13]
107.	*Azadirachta indica* A.Juss.	All parts	Local people and traditional healers	Neem (Bhopal district, Madhya Pradesh, India)	Used in treatment of kidney stones [7]
108.	*Bacopa monnieri* (L.) Pennell	Leaves	Villagers, elderly persons, traditional healers	Brahmi (Madurai district, Tamil Nadu, India)	Leaf extract used as hepatoprotective and nephroprotective [6]
109.	*Bambusa nutans* Wall.	Shoots	Local people and traditional healers	Ootang (Manipur, North East India)	Drink half tea glass of boiled extract (250 g) daily for seven days, for treatment of kidney stone [5]
110.	*Bambusa nutans* Wall.	Bamboo shoot	Muslim Maiba (herbalists)	Ootang (Manipur, India)	Extract (250 g) is used in treatment of kidney stones by taking daily half tea glass for seven days [21]
111.	*Barleria prionitis* L.	Leaf	Local people and traditional healers	Peeli katsariya (Bhopal district, Madhya Pradesh, India)	Leaf decoction is used to treat stone disease by taking the crushed leaves with curd or buttermilk on an empty stomach early in the morning for 20-21 days [12].

(Table 1) cont.....

S. No	Plant Name	Part Used	Tribe/Local Community	Local Names (State, Country)	Uses/Mode of Use
112.	*Barleria prionitis* L.	Whole plant	Villagers, elderly persons, traditional healers	Katukarandu (Sri Lanka)	Used in treatment of kidney diseases due to their diuretic effects [3]
113.	*Basella alba* L.	Leaf	Native people, traditional healers, knowledgeable old persons	Bacchali (Anantapur, Andhra Pradesh, India)	Leaf extract (25 ml) is given early morning on empty stomach for treatment of kidney stones/urolithiasis [13]
114.	*Bauhinia acuminata* L.	Bark, leaves	Local people and traditional healers	Chingthao (Manipur, North East India)	Bark or leaves decoction is given to cure stones in bladder [5]
115.	*Bauhinia acuminata* L.	Bark, leaves	Local people and herbal practioners	Devachandhanam (Warangal, Telangana, India)	Used in the treatment of kidney stones [4]
116.	*Bauhinia racemosa* Lam.	Leaves, roots, bark	Local people and traditional healers	Kachnar (Bhopal district, Madhya Pradesh, India)	Bark is crushed and given with water for treatment of kidney stones [7] [12]
117.	*Benincasa hispida* (Thunb.) Cogn.	Fruit	Local people and traditional healers	Torobot (Manipur, North East India)	In urinary troubles due to stone and urinary tract infections [5], boiled decoction with sugar is prescribed.
118.	*Benincasa hispida* (Thunb.) Cogn.	Fruit	Local people and herbal practioners	Budidha gummadi (Warangal, Telangana, India)	Used in the treatment of kidney stones [4]
119.	*Benincasa hispida* (Thunb.) Cogn.	Fruit	Native people, traditional healers, knowledgeable old persons	Boodida Gummadi (Anantapur, Andhra Pradesh, India)	Use fruit extract of 50 ml with jaggery, twice a day for a week in treatment of kidney stones or urolithiasis [13].

S. No	Plant Name	Part Used	Tribe/Local Community	Local Names (State, Country)	Uses/Mode of Use
120.	*Berberis aristata* DC.	Rhizome		Daru haldi (Bhopal district, Madhya Pradesh, India)	50 g is boiled in 2 liters of water till reduced to 250 ml. 125 ml is given before a meal and another half after a meal for 15-20 days for treatment if stone disease [12].
121.	*Berberis aristata* DC.	Leaves	Local people and traditional healers	Pambi napu (Manipur, North East India)	Leaves decoction is prescribed for kidney troubles and urinary tract infections [5].
122.	*Berberis integerrima* Bunge	Fruit	Local people and traditional healers	Zereshk (Lorestan, Iran)	Used in the treatment of kidney stones [15]
123.	*Berberis vulgaris* L.	Roots	Mughals, Sheikhs, Mir, Ranas, Pathans, Gujjars, Kiani, Malik and Khawajas.	Kal sunmbal (Bheri, Muzaffarabad, Azad Kashmir, Pakistan)	Root extract is used in treatment of kidney stones [26]
124.	*Bergenia ciliata* (Haw.) Sternb.	Whole plant	Local people and traditional healers	(Pakistan)	Used for the treatment in kidney stone [8]
125.	*Bergenia ligulata* (Haw.) Sternb.	Entire plant, root	Traditional healers	Elephant's Ears (India)	Entire plant juice or powder is prescribed for treatment of urinary problems in Nepal [16] [16]
126.	*Beta vulgaris* L	Roots	Local people and herbal practioners	Beetroot (Warangal, Telangana, India)	Used in the treatment of kidney stones [4]
127.	*Beta vulgaris* L.	Whole plant	Local people and traditional healers	Chukander (Bhopal district, Madhya Pradesh, India)	Used in treatment of kidney stones [7]
128.	*Blumea balsamifera* L.	Leaves	Local people and traditional healers	Nagal Camphor (Manipur, North East India)	Two teaspoons of crushed leaves juice with a glass of water added a bit of local salt "Meitei thum" for the prevention of stone formation [5]

(Table 1) cont.....

S. No	Plant Name	Part Used	Tribe/Local Community	Local Names (State, Country)	Uses/Mode of Use
129.	*Boerhavia diffusa* L.	Whole plant	Local people and traditional healers	Punarnava (Bhopal district, Madhya Pradesh, India)	The whole plant, aerial parts, and roots are used in stone disease. Roots and aerial parts should be collected fresh and crushed to obtain juice and given with honey for the treatment of stone disease. 2 g of whole plant powder is taken with milk or water twice a day for 10-20 days [7] [12].
130.	*Boerhavia diffusa* L.	Roots	Native people, traditional healers, knowledgeable old persons	Atikamamidi (Anantapur, Andhra Pradesh, India)	Roots of *B. diffusa* and *Phyllanthus amarus* (equal portions) pulverized with milk and given once a day for 15 days in the treatment of kidney stones or urolithiasis [13].
131.	*Boerhavia diffusa* L.	Root, leaf	Local people and professional traditional healers	(Palamalai, Eastern Ghats, India)	Used in treatment of kidney stones [27]
132.	*Boerhavia diffusa* L.	Roots	Local people and herbal practioners	Atikamamidi (Warangal, Telangana, India)	Used in the treatment of kidney stones [4]
133.	*Bombax ceiba* L.	Leaves, roots	Local people and traditional healers	Semal (Bhopal district, Madhya Pradesh, India)	Used in treatment of kidney stones [7]
134.	*Bonnaya brachiata* Link & Otto	Whole plant	Local people and traditional healers	Kihommaan (Manipur, North East India)	Urinary stone case [5]
135.	*Bonnaya reptans* (Roxb.) Spreng.	Whole plant	Local people and traditional healers	Lamkihom (Manipur, North East India)	For kidney and urinary complaints because of stone deposition, a boiled decoction of the whole plant is prescribed [5].

S. No	Plant Name	Part Used	Tribe/Local Community	Local Names (State, Country)	Uses/Mode of Use
136.	*Borassus flabellifer* L.	Fruit juice	Local people and herbal practioners	Thati chettu (Warangal, Telangana, India)	Used in the treatment of kidney stones [4]
137.	*Borassus flabellifer* L.	Fruit	Villagers, elderly persons, traditional healers	Panai (Madurai district, Tamil Nadu, India)	Fruit impoves kidney function [6]
138.	*Borassus flabellifer* L.	Fruit	Native people, traditional healers, knowledgeable old persons	Thaati (Anantapur, Andhra Pradesh, India)	Used in the treatment of kidney stones or urolithiasis. Kernel of fruit is given once a day to cure and prevent kidney stones [13]
139.	*Boswellia carterii* Birdw.	Other part	Plant collectors, herbalists, traditional practitioners.	Salabân (Izarène, Morocco)	Decoction used in the treatment of urolithiasis [17]
140.	*Brassica oleracea* L.	Leaves	Plant collectors, herbalists, traditional practitioners.	Krumb (Izarène, Morocco)	Decoction used in the treatment of urolithiasis [17]
141.	*Brassica oleracea* L. var. *capitata* L.	Whole plant	Local people and traditional healers	Patta gobhi (Bhopal district, Madhya Pradesh, India)	Used in treatment of kidney stones [7]
142.	*Brassica rapa* L. subsp. *rapa*	Plant tuber	Local traditional therapists	Shalgham (Shahrekord, Iran)	Anti-kidney stone effect [11]
143.	*Bryophyllum pinnatum* (Lam.) Oken	Leaves	Villagers, elderly persons, traditional healers	Ranakalli (Madurai district, Tamil Nadu, India)	Daily intake of leaf extract and raw leaf for reducing calcium oxalte crystal in kidney [6]
144.	*Bryophyllum pinnatum* (Lam.) Oken	Whole plant	Local people and Traditional healers	(Pakistan)	Used in treatment of kidney stone [8]
145.	*Bryophyllum pinnatum* (Lam.) Oken	Whole plant	Local people and traditional healers	Parnabeej (Bhopal district, Madhya Pradesh, India)	Consumption of leaf decoction twice in a day in case of kidney stone is beneficial [7] [12]

(Table 1) cont.....

S. No	Plant Name	Part Used	Tribe/Local Community	Local Names (State, Country)	Uses/Mode of Use
146.	*Butea monosperma* (Lam.) Taub.	Leaves, flowers	Local people and traditional healers	Palash (Bhopal district, Madhya Pradesh, India)	Used in treatment of kidney stones [7]
147.	*Calendula officinalis* L.	Whole plant	Local people and traditional healers	(Pakistan)	Used in treatment of kidney stone [8]
148.	*Camellia sinensis* (L.) Kuntze	Leaf	Local traditional therapists	Chaye sabz (Shahrekord, Iran)	Anti-kidney stone effect [11]
149.	*Canna indica* L.	Root	Villagers, elderly persons, traditional healers	Kalvaalai (Madurai district, Tamil Nadu, India)	Root extract used as diuretic [6]
150.	*Capparis spinosa* L.	Fruits	Plant collectors, herbalists, traditional practitioners.	Al'Kabbar (Izarène, Morocco)	Decoction used in the treatment of urolithiasis [17]
151.	*Capsella bursa-pastoris* (L.) Medik.	Leaf, fruit	Local people and traditional healers	Hendevane (Lorestan, Iran)	Used in the treatment of kidney stones [15]
152.	*Capsella bursa-pastoris* (L.) Medik.	Whole plant	Local people and traditional healers	Chantruk (Manipur, North East India)	Freshly taken in urinary problems [5]
153.	*Capsella bursa-pastoris* (L.) Medik.	Leaf	Traditional healers	Kiseh Keshish (Urmia, Northwest Iran)	Decoction used in the exertion of kidney stones [20]
154.	*Capsella bursa-pastoris* (L.) Medik.	Aerial parts	Local people and traditional healers	Kise Keshish (Lorestan, Iran)	Used in the treatment of kidney stones [15]
155.	*Capsicum annuum* L.	Fruit	Villagers, elderly persons, traditional healers	Milagai (Madurai district, Tamil Nadu, India)	Raw fruit is used for reducing kidney stone [6]
156.	*Caria papaya* L.	Young fruit	Local people and herbal practioners	Boppayi (Warangal, Telangana, India)	Used in the treatment of kidney stones [4]

S. No	Plant Name	Part Used	Tribe/Local Community	Local Names (State, Country)	Uses/Mode of Use
157.	*Carica papaya* L.	Fruits	Local people and traditional healers	Papita (Bhopal district, Madhya Pradesh, India)	Used in treatment of kidney stones. Its root and fruits are helpful in stone disease. Its recent unripe fruit is cut and unbroken overnight; later it's given to the patient with empty abdomen within the morning for solidifying stones [7] [12]
158.	*Carica papaya* L.	Leaf extract, fruit	Villagers, elderly persons, traditional healers	Pappali (Madurai district, Tamil Nadu, India)	Fruit and leaf extract improves renal function [6]
159.	*Carica papaya* L.	Fruit	Native people, traditional healers, knowledgeable old persons	Parinkaaya (Anantapur, Andhra Pradesh, India)	Used in the treatment of kidney stones. Fruit is eaten to prevent stone formation [13]
160.	*Cassia auriculata* L.	Root	Villagers, elderly persons, traditional healers	Aavaarai (Madurai district, Tamil Nadu, India)	Root extract used as nephroprotective and renal injury [6]
161.	*Cassia fistula* L.	Fruit	Local people and herbal practioners	Rela (Warangal, Telangana, India)	Used in the treatment of kidney stones [4]
162.	*Cedrus deodara* (Roxb. ex D.Don) G.Don	Oil	Kiani, Gujjars, Mir, Mughals, Sheikhs, Ranas, Pathans, Khawajas and Malik	Deodar (Bheri, Muzaffarabad, Kashmir, Pakistan)	Used in management of kidney problems [26]
163.	*Celosia argentea* L.	Whole plant	Local people and traditional healers	Safed murga (Bhopal district, Madhya Pradesh, India)	Used in treatment of kidney stones [7]
164.	*Celosia argentea* L.	Roots	Local people and traditional healers	Haorei-angouba (Manipur, North East India)	Root extract with sugar is preferred in urinary tract and kidney stones [5]

(Table 1) cont.....

S. No	Plant Name	Part Used	Tribe/Local Community	Local Names (State, Country)	Uses/Mode of Use
165.	*Celosia argentea* L.	Seeds, roots	Local people and herbal practioners	Seethajada (Warangal, Telangana, India)	Used in the treatment of kidney stones [4]
166.	*Celtis australis* L.	Leaves	Local people and traditional healers	Heikreng (Manipur, North East India)	Boiled leaf decoction is given in treatment of stone in the urinary tract [5].
167.	*Celtis timorensis* Span.	Aerial parts	Local people and traditional healers	Heikreng (Manipur, North East India)	Drink 1 tea glass of boiled extract twice daily for 10 days for kidney stone [5]
168.	*Celtis timorensis* Span.	Leaves	Muslim Maiba (herbalists)	Heikreng (Manipur, India)	10 gm of the extract used in treatment of kidney stones. Drink 1 tea glass twice daily for 10 days [21].
169.	*Celtis timorensis* Span.	Leaves	Muslim Maiba (herbalists)	Heikreng (Manipur, India)	20 gm of the extract used in treatment of kidney stones. Drink one tea glass daily for seven days [21].
170.	*Centaurea cyanus* L.	Stem, leaf, flower	Local traditional therapists	Gole gandom (Shahrekord, Iran)	Anti-kidney stone effect [11]
171.	*Centella asiatica* (L.) Urban.	Whole plant	Local people and traditional healers	Nungjreng peruk (Manipur, North East India)	Plant juice with sugarcane is given in urinary calculus [5]
172.	*Centella* spp.	Whole plant	Muslim Maiba (herbalists)	Nungjreng peruk (Manipur, India)	20 gm of the extract used in treatment of kidney stones. Drink one tea glass daily for seven days [21]
173.	*Cerasus mahaleb* (L.) Miller	Fruit	Local people and traditional healers	Mahlab (Ilam, Iran)	Used in the treatment of kidney stones [15]
174.	*Cerasus microcarpa* (C.A.Mey.) Boiss.	Fruit	Local people and traditional healers	Albalouye Vahshi (Ilam, Iran)	Used in the treatment of kidney stones [15]
175.	*Cerasus microcarpa* (C.A.Mey.) Boiss.	Fruit	Traditional healers	Albalou (Urmia, Northwest Iran)	Decoction and fresh fruit used in the exertion of kidney stones [20]

(Table 1) cont.....

S. No	Plant Name	Part Used	Tribe/Local Community	Local Names (State, Country)	Uses/Mode of Use
176.	*Cerasus microcarpa* (C.A.Mey.) Boiss.	Fruit	Local people and traditional healers	Albaloo (Lorestan, Iran)	Used in the treatment of kidney stones [15]
177.	*Chenopodium album* L.	Whole plant	Local people and traditional healers	Bethua (Bhopal district, Madhya Pradesh, India)	Used in treatment of kidney stones [7]
178.	*Chenopodium album* L.	Whole plant	Local people and traditional healers	(Pakistan)	Used in the treatment of kidney stone [8]
179.	*Chrysanthemum coronarium* L.	Whole plant	Local people and traditional healers	Guldaudi (Bhopal district, Madhya Pradesh, India)	Used in treatment of kidney stones [7]
180.	*Cichorium intybus* L.	Leaf, pedicel	Local people and traditional healers	Kasni (Persian Gulf, Iran)	Used in the treatment of kidney stones [15]
181.	*Cichorium intybus* L.	Whole plant	Local people and traditional healers	(Pakistan)	Used in treatment of kidney stones [8]
182.	*Cichorium intybus* L.	Aerial parts, leaf	Native people	Kanej (Çatak, Eastern Anatolia Region, Turkey)	Leaf extract is used in treatment of kidney stones. The raw plant is eaten in kidney stones [19]
183.	*Cichorium intybus* L.	Aerial parts	Turkish citizens	Kaniş (Geçitli Township, Eastern Anatolia Region, Hakkari-Turkey)	Decoction is used in the treatment of kidney stones [18]
184.	*Cinnamomum bejolghota* (Buch.-Ham.) Sweet	Bark	Local people and traditional healers	Tezpat (Manipur, North East India)	Bark is useful in the treatment of urinary stone troubles [5]
185.	*Cinnamomum glaucescens* (Nees) Hand-Mazz.	Bark	Local people and traditional healers	Vahmin (Manipur, North East India)	The bark powder is used in management of kidney trouble [5]
186.	*Cinnamomum tamala* L.	Leaves	Local people and traditional healers	Tezpat (Manipur, North East India)	Boiled with *Celtis hamata* Blume and drink in management of kidney stone [5]

S. No	Plant Name	Part Used	Tribe/Local Community	Local Names (State, Country)	Uses/Mode of Use
187.	*Cinnamomum tamala* L.	Leaves	Muslim Maiba (herbalists)	Tezpat (Manipur, India)	5 gm of the extract used in treatment of kidney stones. Take one tea glass twice daily for ten days [21]
188.	*Cinnamomum zeylanicum* Nees	Other part	Plant collectors, herbalists, traditional practitioners.	Qorfa (Izarène, Morocco)	Decoction used in the treatment of Urolithiasis [17]
189.	*Cissus adnata* Roxb.	Leaves	Local people and traditional healers	Kongouyen (Manipur, North East India)	Leaves and root decoction is given in kidney problem due to stone [5]
190.	*Cissus javana* DC.	Leaves	Local people and traditional healers	Kongouyen Laba (Manipur, North East India)	Leaf decoction is given as tonic for treatment of urinary trouble due to stone and to cure the burning sensation during urination [5]
191.	*Cissus quadrangularis* L.	Stem	Villagers, elderly persons, traditional healers	Pirandai (Madurai district, Tamil Nadu, India)	Stem extract used for diabetic kidney disease [6]
192.	*Citrullus colocynthis* (L.) Schrad.	Whole plant	Local people and traditional healers	(Pakistan)	Used in the treatment of kidney stone [8]
193.	*Citrullus colocyunthis* ((L.) Schrad.	Pulp	Villagers, elderly persons, traditional healers	Kumatti (Madurai district, Tamil Nadu, India)	Pulp extract is used for kidney damage [6]
194.	*Citrullus vulgaris* Schrad. ex Eckl. & Zeyh.	Whole plant	Local people and traditional healers	(Pakistan)	Used in the treatment of kidney stone [8]
195.	*Citrus aurantifolia* (Christman) Swingle	Fruits, roots, leaves	Local people and traditional healers	(Pakistan)	Used in the treatment of kidney stone [8]
196.	*Citrus aurantiifolia* (Christm.) Swingle	Fruit	Native people, traditional healers, knowledgeable old persons	Nimma (Anantapur, Andhra Pradesh, India)	Fruit juice with water and honey given daily in the treatment of kidney stones or urolithiasis [13].

S. No	Plant Name	Part Used	Tribe/Local Community	Local Names (State, Country)	Uses/Mode of Use
197.	*Citrus latipes* (Swingle) Tanaka	Fruit	Local people and traditional healers	Heiribob (Manipur, North East India)	The fruit extract with *star fruit,* pinch of salt and honey is prescribed in urinary tract and kidney stone [5]
198.	*Citrus limon* (L.) Brum.f.	Fruits	Plant collectors, herbalists, traditional practitioners.	Lhâmmed (Izarène, Morocco)	Decoction used in the treatment of urolithiasis [17]
199.	*Citrus limon* (L.) Burm.f.	Fruits	Villagers, elderly persons, traditional healers	Elummichai (Madurai district, Tamil Nadu, India)	Lemon juice is used for dehydration and reducing kidney stone [6]
200.	*Citrus sinensis* (L.) Osbeck	Fruits, roots, leaves	Local people and traditional healers	(Pakistan)	Used in the treatment of kidney stone [8]
201.	*Clitoria ternatea* L.	Leaves, flowers	Local people and traditional healers	Aparajita (Bhopal district, Madhya Pradesh, India)	Used in treatment of kidney stones [7]
202.	*Cocos nucifera* L.	Fruits	Villagers, elderly persons, traditional healers	Thennai (Madurai district, Tamil Nadu, India)	Coconut water is used for kidney damage [6]
203.	*Cocos nucifera* L.	Flowers	Native people, traditional healers, knowledgeable old persons	Kobbari (Anantapur, Andhra Pradesh, India)	Flower extract (30 ml) with goat milk and honey (50 ml) is given once a day in the treatment of kidney stones or urolithiasis [13]
204.	*Cocos nucifera* L.	Coconut water	Traditional practitioner's belong to communities of Meitei, Tangkhul, Kabui, Naga, and Mizo	Yubi (Manipur, North-East India)	Used in treatment of kidney problems [22]
205.	*Cocos nucifera* L.	Fruit water	Local people and herbal practioners	Kobbari (Warangal, Telangana, India)	Used in the treatment of kidney stones [4]

S. No	Plant Name	Part Used	Tribe/Local Community	Local Names (State, Country)	Uses/Mode of Use
206.	*Coix lacryma-jobi* L.	Leaves	Local people and Traditional healers	Chang-ning (Manipur, North East India)	Used in management of kidney stones [5]
207.	*Colacasia antiquorum* Schott.	Leaves	Local people and herbal practioners	Chamadumpa (Warangal, Telangana, India)	Used in the treatment of kidney stones [4]
208.	*Coldenia procumbens* L.	Whole plant	Native people, traditional healers, knowledgeable old persons	Hamsapaadi (Anantapur, Andhra Pradesh, India)	Whole plants boiled with *Pedalium microcarpum* Decne in water and decoction is given once a day for 15 days in the treatment of kidney stones or urolithiasis [13].
209.	*Coleus amboinicus* Lour.	Aerial parts, leaf	Traditional healers	Indian mint (India)	Used in management of kidney troubles [16]
210.	*Coleus forskohlii* (Willd.) Briq.	Whole plant	Local people and traditional healers	Patharchur (Bhopal district, Madhya Pradesh, India)	Used in treatment of kidney stones [7]
211.	*Commiphora africana* (A. Rich) Engl.	Other part	Plant collectors, herbalists, traditional practitioners.	Oumm-en-nâs (Izarène, Morocco)	Decoction used in the treatment of urolithiasis [17]
212.	*Cordia grandis* Roxb.	Fruits	Local people and traditional healers	Lamuk (Manipur, North East India)	Fruits are used in the management of urinary trouble due to stone [5]
213.	*Coriandrum sativum* L.	Leaf extract	Villagers, elderly persons, traditional healers	Kothumalli (Madurai district, Tamil Nadu, India)	Leaf juice is used for kidney damage [6]
214.	*Coriandrum sativum* L.	Aerial parts, seeds	Local people and professional traditional healers	(Palamalai, Eastern Ghats, India)	Used in treatment of kidney stones [27]
215.	*Cornus canadensis* L.	Whole plant	Micmac	Bunchberry (All of Canada)	Drinking steeped plant for treatment of kidney problems [10]

S. No	Plant Name	Part Used	Tribe/Local Community	Local Names (State, Country)	Uses/Mode of Use
216.	*Costus speciosus* (Koening) Smith	Roots	Local people and traditional healers	Khongban takhelei (Manipur, North East India)	Root decoction is prescribed in management of urinary and kidney complaints [5]
217.	*Cousinia alexeenkoana* Bornm.	Flower, leaf	Local people and traditional healers	Hezar khar (Lorestan, Iran)	Used in the treatment of kidney stones [15]
218.	*Crataeva religiosa* G. Forst.	Leaves, flowers	Local people and traditional healers	Varun (Bhopal district, Madhya Pradesh, India)	Used in treatment of kidney stones [7]
219.	*Crinum asiaticum* L.	Bulb	Local people and traditional healers	Kanwal (Manipur, North East India)	Prescribed in urinary and kidney complaints [5]
220.	*Crocus sativus* L.	Flowers	Plant collectors, herbalists, traditional practitioners.	Za'âfranelhor (Izarène, Morocco)	Decoction used in the treatment of urolithiasis [17]
221.	*Cucumis melo* L.	Fruits	Local people and traditional healers	Kharbuja (Bhopal district, Madhya Pradesh, India)	Used in treatment of kidney stones [7]
222.	*Cucumis melo* L.	Whole plant	Local people and traditional healers	(Pakistan)	Used in the treatment of kidney stone [8]
223.	*Cucumis melo* L. var. *melo*	Fruit	Native people, traditional healers, knowledgeable old persons	Siddhatum (Anantapur, Andhra Pradesh, India)	Fruit peel paste (5-10 g) is mixed with tender coconut water and given once a day for 15 days for the treatment of kidney stones or urolithiasis [13].
224.	*Cucumis sativus* L.	Whole plant	Local people and traditional healers	(Pakistan)	Used in the treatment of kidney stone [8]
225.	*Cucumis utilissimus* L.	Fruits	Local people and traditional healers	Kakadi (Bhopal district, Madhya Pradesh, India)	Used in treatment of kidney stones [7]
226.	*Cucurbita pepo* L.	Seed	Villagers, elderly persons, traditional healers	Parangi (Madurai district, Tamil Nadu, India)	Seed is used to prevent renal failure [6]

(Table 1) cont.....

S. No	Plant Name	Part Used	Tribe/Local Community	Local Names (State, Country)	Uses/Mode of Use
227.	*Cucurbita* sp.	Seed	Chippewa, Plains Indians	Squash (Quebec, Ontario, Canada)	Seed powder is taken with water for kidney problems [10]
228.	*Cuminum cyminum* L.	Fruits, seeds	Local people and traditional healers	Jeera (Bhopal district, Madhya Pradesh, India)	Used in treatment of kidney stones [7]
229.	*Cuminum cyminum* L.	Fruits	Local people and traditional healers	Jeera (Manipur, North East India)	Boiled decoction is prescribed in urinary and kidney complaints [5]
230.	*Curcuma angustifolia* Roxb.	Whole plant	Local people and traditional healers	Lamthabi (Manipur, North East India)	Used in kidney infection [5]
231.	*Curcuma longa* L.	Rhizomes	Native people, traditional healers, knowledgeable old persons	Pasupu (Anantapur, Andhra Pradesh, India)	Used in the treatment of kidney stones or urolithiasis. Turmeric powder (5g) mixed with jiggery (10g) and given twice a day for one month [13].
232.	*Cydonia oblonga* Mill.	Leaves	Plant collectors, herbalists, traditional practitioners	Ssferjel (Izarène, Morocco)	Decoction used in the treatment of urolithiasis [17]
233.	*Cymbopogon citratus* Stapf	Whole plant	Local people and traditional healers	Hoana (Manipur, North East India)	Whole plant decoction is given orally for stone case [5]
234.	*Cynodon dactylon* (L.) Pers.	Whole plant	Local people and traditional healers	Doob (Bhopal district, Madhya Pradesh, India)	Used in treatment of kidney stones [7]
235.	*Cynodon dactylon* (L.) Pers.	Whole plant	Local people and herbal practioners	Gaddiparaka (Warangal, Telangana, India)	Used in the treatment of kidney stones [4]
236.	*Cynodon dactylon* (L.) Pers.	Roots	Plant collectors, herbalists, traditional practitioners.	Njem (Izarène, Morocco)	Decoction used in the treatment of urolithiasis [17]

S. No	Plant Name	Part Used	Tribe/Local Community	Local Names (State, Country)	Uses/Mode of Use
237.	*Cynodon dactylon* (L.) Pers.	Rhizome	Traditional health practioners, local people	Khanbalgha (Hafizabad district, Punjab-Pakistan)	Decoction is used in the treatment of kidney stones [14].
238.	*Cyperus rotundus* L.	Rhizome	Villagers, elderly persons, traditional healers	Korai (Madurai district, Tamil Nadu, India)	Dried and powdered rhizome is used for removing renal calculi and renal diseses [6]
239.	*Cyperus rotundus* L.	Rhizome, leaf	Local people and professional traditional healers	(Palamalai, Eastern Ghats, India)	Used in treatment of kidney stones [27]
240.	*Cyperus rotundus* L.	Whole plant	Local people and traditional healers	Shembang kaothum (Manipur, North East India)	The decoction of the plant is prescribed in urinary and kidney trouble [5]
241.	*Dactyloctenium aegyptium* P. Beauv.	Whole plant	Traditional health practioners, local people	Madhanagha (Hafizabad district, Punjab-Pakistan)	Paste is used in the treatment of kidney stones [14].
242.	*Datura metel* L.	Fruit	Villagers, elderly persons, traditional healers	Omathai (Madurai district, Tamil Nadu, India)	Fruit is used for kidney damage [6]
243.	*Daucus carota* L.	Whole plant	Local people and traditional healers	Gajar (Bhopal district, Madhya Pradesh, India)	Used in treatment of kidney stones [7]
244.	*Daucus carota* L.	Seeds	Plant collectors, herbalists, traditional practitioners.	Khizzu (Izarène, Morocco)	Decoction used in the treatment of urolithiasis [17]
245.	*Daucus carota* L.	Root, seed	Village peoples of Thoppampatti	Manjal Kilangu (Thoppampatti, Dindigul district, Tamil Nadu, India)	Juice is used in treatment of kidney stones [28]
246.	*Descurainia sophia* (L.) Webb. ex Prantl	Seed	Local people and traditional healers	Khkeshir (Khuzestan, Iran)	Used in the treatment of kidney stones [15]
247.	*Desmodium microphyllum* (Thunb.) DC	Whole plant	Local people and traditional healers	Nuggai Yensil (Manipur, North East India)	The plant decoction is prescribed for urinary complaints due to stone [5]

(Table 1) cont.....

S. No	Plant Name	Part Used	Tribe/Local Community	Local Names (State, Country)	Uses/Mode of Use
248.	*Diospyros peregrina* (Gaertn.) Gurke	Fruits, leaves	Local people and traditional healers	Kala tendu (Bhopal district, Madhya Pradesh, India)	Used in treatment of kidney stones [7]
249.	*Docynia indica* (Colebr.) Decne.	Fruit	Local people and traditional healers	Heitoop (Manipur, North East India)	Sugary infusion kept for two week and given orally for urinary and kidney troubles [5]
250.	*Dolichos biflorus* L.	Whole plant	Local people and traditional healers	Kulthi (Bhopal district, Madhya Pradesh, India)	Used in treatment of kidney stones [7]
251.	*Dolichos biflorus* L.	Whole plant	Local people and traditional healers	(Pakistan)	Used in the treatment of kidney stone [8]
252.	*Dolicos biflorus* L.	Seeds	Local people and herbal practioners	Vulavalu (Warangal, Telangana, India)	Used in the treatment of kidney stones [4]
253.	*Duchesnea indica* (Andr.) Focke	Whole plant	Local people and traditional healers	Heirongkak-laba (Manipur, North East India)	The plant decoction is prescribed for urinary complaints due to stone [5]
254.	*Echinophora platyloba* DC.	Aerial organs	Local traditional therapists	Khosharizeh (Shahrekord, Iran)	Anti-kidney stone effect [11]
255.	*Echinops spinosus* L.	Roots	Plant collectors, herbalists, traditional practitioners.	Tassekra (Izarène, Morocco)	Decoction used in the treatment of urolithiasis [17]
256.	*Eclipta prostrasta* (L.) L.	Aerial parts	Villagers, elderly persons, traditional healers	Karisilankanni (Madurai district, Tamil Nadu, India)	Leaf extract is used in treatment of kidney disorders as nephroprotective [6]
257.	*Enhydra fluctuans* Lour.	Aerial parts	Local people and traditional healers	Komprek-tujombi (Manipur, North East India)	Boiled extract is prescribed in kidney stone [5]
258.	*Enhydra fluctuans* Lour.	Whole plant	Muslim Maiba (herbalists)	Komprektujombi (Manipur, India)	5 gm of the extract used in treatment of kidney stones. Drink 100 ml daily for 7 days [21]

(Table 1) cont.....

S. No	Plant Name	Part Used	Tribe/Local Community	Local Names (State, Country)	Uses/Mode of Use
259.	*Ensete superbum* (Roxb.) Cheesman	Seed	Malamalasar, Kanikars, Malapandaram, Kurichiar, Mulu kuruma, Kurumbar, Kattu naikans, Chola naikans.	Kallu vazha (Parambikulam, Kullathu puzha, Achenkovil, Kerala, India)	Used in treatment of kidney stones [29]
260.	*Epigaea repens* L.	Leaf	Algonquin, Iroquois	Trailing arbutus (Southern Canada)	Infusion of leaves for treatment of kidney stones [10]
261.	*Equisetum arvense* L.	Aerial parts	Turkish citizens	Giyagezık (Geçitli Township, Eastern Anatolia Region, Hakkari-Turkey)	Decoction is used in the treatment of kidney stones [18]
262.	*Equisetum arvense* L.	Aerial parts	Local people and traditional healers	Dome asb (Orumieh, Iran)	Used in the treatment of kidney stones [15]
263.	*Equisetum arvense* L.	Aerial parts	Traditional healers	Dom Asb (Urmia, Northwest Iran)	Decoction used in the exertion of kidney stones [20]
264.	*Equisetum fluviatile* L.	Aerial parts	Turkish citizens	Getgedok (Geçitli Township, Eastern Anatolia Region, Hakkari-Turkey)	Decoction is used in the treatment of kidney stones [18]
265.	*Eucalyptus globulus* Labill.	Leaves	Plant collectors, herbalists, traditional practitioners.	Al' Kalitûs (Izarène, Morocco)	Decoction used in the treatment of urolithiasis [17]
266.	*Eugenia caryophyllata* Thunb.	Flowers	Plant collectors, herbalists, traditional practitioners.	Qronfel (Izarène, Morocco)	Decoction used in the treatment of urolithiasis [17]
267.	*Eupatorium burmanicum* DC.	Leaves	Local people and traditional healers	Langthrei (Manipur, North East India)	Boiled leaves decoction with a pinch of salt may helps in eliminating calculi/stones [5]
268.	*Eupatorium* spp.	Leaves	Muslim Maiba (herbalists)	Kangphal langthrei (Manipur, India)	10 gm of the extract used in treatment of kidney stones. Drink half tea glass twice daily for seven days [21]

(Table 1) cont.....

S. No	Plant Name	Part Used	Tribe/Local Community	Local Names (State, Country)	Uses/Mode of Use
269.	*Euphorbia falcata* L.	Whole plant	Plant collectors, herbalists, traditional practitioners.	Hayyat ennufûs (Izarène, Morocco)	Decoction used in the treatment of urolithiasis [17]
270.	*Euphorbia hirta* L.	Whole plant	Local people and traditional healers	Badi dudhi (Bhopal district, Madhya Pradesh, India)	Used in treatment of kidney stones [7]
271.	*Euphorbia hirta* L.	Whole plant	Native people, traditional healers, knowledgeable old persons	Reddivarinanubalaaku (Anantapur, Andhra Pradesh, India)	Whole plant extract (100 ml) mixed with goat milk (200 ml) given once a day for thirty days in the treatment of kidney stones or urolithiasis [13]
272.	*Euphorbia hirta* L.	Whole plant	Local people and traditional healers	Pakhangleiton (Manipur, North East India)	Boiled with *cumin* seeds in water and is given orally for kidney stone [5]
273.	*Euphorbia hirta* L. [Syn.: *Chamaesyce hirta* (L.) Millsp.]	Whole plant	Caribbean folk medicine practioners, local people	Mal nommée (Trinidad and Tobago, Caribbean)	Used in kidney problems [23]
274.	*Faba vulgaris* Moenchris.	Leaf, seed	Local people and traditional healers	Baghla (Khuzestan, Iran)	Used in the treatment of kidney stones [15]
275.	*Ficus carica* L.	Roots, leaves	Local people and traditional healers	(Pakistan)	Used in the treatment of kidney stone [8]
276.	*Ficus hispida* L. f.	Leaves	Traditional practitioners belong to communities of Meitei, Tangkhul, Kabui, Naga, and Mizo	Ashiheibong/ Perenhei (Manipur,North-East India)	Used in treatment of kidney stones [22]
277.	*Ficus palmata* Forssk.	Fruit, latex	Kiani, Gujjars, Mir, Mughals, Sheikhs, Ranas, Pathans, Khawajas and Malik	Pagwara (Bheri, Muzaffarabad, Azad Kashmir, Pakistan)	Nephroprotective [26]

(Table 1) cont.....

S. No	Plant Name	Part Used	Tribe/Local Community	Local Names (State, Country)	Uses/Mode of Use
278.	*Flemingia strobilifera* (L.) W.T.Aiton	Leaves	Caribbean folk medicine practioners, local people	Kidney bush (Trinidad and Tobago, Caribbean)	Used in kidney problems [23]
279.	*Foeniculum vulgare* Mill.	Seeds	Plant collectors, herbalists, traditional practitioners.	Nafaâ (Izarène, Morocco)	Decoction used in the treatment of urolithiasis [17]
280.	*Foeniculum vulgare* Mill.	Fruits	Traditional practitioner's belong to communities of Meitei, Tangkhul, Kabui, Naga, and Mizo.	Hop (Manipur,North-East India)	Used in treatment of kidney stones [22]
281.	*Foeniculum vulgare* Mill.	Seed	Local traditional therapists	Razianeh (Shahrekord, Iran)	Anti-kidney stone effect [11]
282.	*Fragaria indica* Andrews	Vegetative part	Local people and traditional healers	Heirongkaklaba (Manipur, North East India)	Boiled extract with sugar and is used in treatment of urinary tract and stone case [5]
283.	*Fragaria nilgerrensis* Schltdl. ex J. Gay	Vegetative part	Local people and traditional healers	Samu hongpak laba (Manipur, North East India)	Boiled extract with sugar and is used in treatment of urinary tract and stone case [5]
284.	*Fragaria nilgerrensis* Schltdl. ex J. Gay	Whole plant	Muslim Maiba (herbalists)	Samu khongpak laba (Manipur, India)	5 gm of the extract used in treatment of kidney stones. Drink 100 ml daily till cure [21]
285.	*Fragaria nilgerrensis* Schltdl. ex J. Gay	Whole plant	Muslim Maiba (herbalists)	Samukhongpak laba (Manipur, India)	100 gm of the extract used in treatment of kidney stones. Drink 1 tea glass daily for seven days [21]
286.	*Fraxinus excelsior* L.	Leaf	Local people and traditional healers	Zaban Ghnjeshk (Orumieh, Iran)	Used in the treatment of kidney stones [15].

(Table 1) cont.....

S. No	Plant Name	Part Used	Tribe/Local Community	Local Names (State, Country)	Uses/Mode of Use
287.	*Fraxinus excelsior* L.	Leaf	Traditional healers	Zaban Gonješk (Urmia, Northwest Iran)	Decoction used in the exertion of kidney stones [20]
288.	*Glycyrrhiza glabra* L.	Roots	Plant collectors, herbalists, traditional practitioners.	Arqsûss (Izarène, Morocco)	Decoction used in the treatment of urolithiasis [17]
289.	*Gomphrena celosioides* Mart.	Whole plant	Local people and herbal practioners	Pendlibachali (Warangal, Telangana, India)	Used in the treatment of kidney stones [4]
290.	*Gomphrena celosioides* Mart.	Herb	Tribal communities like Bhilala, Bhil, and Pataya	Chota murga (Jhabua, Madhya Pradesh, India)	Whole plant infusion is given twice a day in kidney disorders [30]
291.	*Gossypium herbaceum* L.	Fruits	Native people, traditional healers, knowledgeable old persons	Patthi (Anantapur, Andhra Pradesh, India)	Raw fruits medium in residual hot coals and pounded with water and given once a day for one week in the treatment of kidney stones or urolithiasis [13].
292.	*Gundelia tourneforti* L.	Pedicel	Local people and traditional healers	Kanghar (Khuzestan, Iran)	Used in the treatment of kidney stones [15]
293.	*Gundelia tournefortii* L.	Leaf, pedicel	Local people and traditional healers	Kanghar (Ilam, Iran)	Used in the treatment of kidney stones [15]
294.	*Gymnema sylvestre* R.Br.	Leaves	Local people and traditional healers	Gudmar (Bhopal district, Madhya Pradesh, India)	Used in treatment of kidney stones [7]
295.	*Haloxylon stocksii* (Boiss.) Benth. & Hook.f.	Whole plant	Local people and traditional healers	(Pakistan)	Used in the treatment of kidney stone [8]
296.	*Haplophyllum buxbaumii* (Poir.) G.Don	Aerial parts	Local people and traditional healers	Sedab (Orumieh, Iran)	Used in the treatment of kidney stones [15]
297.	*Hedychium aurantiacum* Rosc.	Rhizome	Local people and traditional healers	Takhellei angangba (Manipur, North East India)	Boiled rhizome water is given in kidney stone problem [5]

S. No	Plant Name	Part Used	Tribe/Local Community	Local Names (State, Country)	Uses/Mode of Use
298.	*Hedychium aurantiacum* Rosc.	Stem	Muslim Maiba (herbalists)	Takhellei (Manipur, India)	10 gm of the extract used in treatment of kidney stones. Drink 1 tea glass daily for seven days [21]
299.	*Helianthus annuus* L.	Seeds	Local people and traditional healers	Surajmukhi (Bhopal district, Madhya Pradesh, India)	Used in treatment of kidney stones [7]
300.	*Helianthus annuus* L.	Roots	Native people, traditional healers, knowledgeable old persons	Proddutirugudu (Anantapur, Andhra Pradesh, India)	Roots of *H. annus* (20 g) pounded with 100 ml of butter milk and given for 15 days, once a day in the treatment of kidney stones or urolithiasis [13]
301.	*Helianthus annuus* L.	Fresh leaves	Local people and traditional healers	Numitlei (Manipur, North East India)	The juice of the fresh leaves is used in urinary trouble and diseases of kidney [5]
302.	*Helichrysum arenarium* (L.) Moench.	Tubers, aerial parts	Native people	Sevik Altın (Çatak, Eastern Anatolia Region, Turkey)	Prescibed as plant extract (one glass) on an empty stomach early in the morning for treatment of kidney stones [19]
303.	*Helichrysum armenium* DC.	Aerial parts	Native people	Guyazerk (Çatak, Eastern Anatolia Region, Turkey)	Prescibed as plant extract (one glass) on an empty stomach early in the morning for treatment of kidney stones [19]
304.	*Helichrysum pallasii* (Spreng.) Ledeb.	Aerial parts	Native people	Guyazerk (Çatak, Eastern Anatolia Region, Turkey)	Prescibed as plant extract (one glass) on an empty stomach early in the morning for treatment of kidney stones [19]
305.	*Heliotropium strigosum* Willd.	Whole plant	Local people and traditional healers	(Pakistan)	Used in the treatment of kidney stone [8]

(Table 1) cont.....

S. No	Plant Name	Part Used	Tribe/Local Community	Local Names (State, Country)	Uses/Mode of Use
306.	*Hemidesmus indicus* (L.) Schult.	Roots	Local people and traditional healers	Kwa-manbi (Manipur, North East India)	Prescribed in kidney stone [5]
307.	*Herniaria glabra* L.	Whole plant	Traditional herbalists	Harrasslhjar (Rabat-Sale-Kenitra Region, Morocco)	Decoction used for treatment of chronic kidney diseases [24]
308.	*Herniaria hirsuta* L.	Whole plant	Local population of Ain Leuh	Haraste Lahjer (Ain Leuh Region, Middle-Atlas of Morocco)	Used in treatment of kidney stones [31]
309.	*Herniaria hirsuta* L.	Whole plant	Plant collectors, herbalists, traditional practitioners.	Herrastlahjar (Izarène, Morocco)	Decoction used in the treatment of urolithiasis [17]
310.	*Hibiscus sabdariffa* L.	Leaves	Local people and traditional healers	Ambasthika Manipur (Northeastern India)	Decoction is used in treatment of kidney stones [32]
311.	*Hibiscus sabdariffa* L.	Leaves	Local people and traditional healers	Silot sougri (Manipur, North East India)	Decoction is used in treatment of kidney stones [5]
312.	*Homonoia riparia* Lour.	Root	Local people and traditional healers	Tuipui-sulhla (Manipur, North East India)	Root decoction is given in stone in the urinary bladder [5]
313.	*Hordeum vulgare* L.	Seeds	Plant collectors, herbalists, traditional practitioners.	Chaâir (Izarène, Morocco)	Decoction used in the treatment of urolithiasis [17]
314.	*Hyptis suaveolens* (L.) Poit.	Whole plant	Local people and traditional healers	Vilayati tulsi (Bhopal district, Madhya Pradesh, India)	Used in treatment of kidney stones [7]
315.	*Indigofera tinctoria* L.	Roots	Local people and traditional healers	Neem (Manipur, North East India)	Roots are used in urinary and kidney complaints [5]
316.	*Inula viscosa* (L.) Ait.	Leaves	Plant collectors, herbalists, traditional practitioners.	Terrahlâ (Izarène, Morocco)	Decoction used in the treatment of urolithiasis [17]
317.	*Ixora sub-sessilis* Wall. ex G.Don	Fruits, seeds	Local people and traditional healers	Shenglong (Manipur, North East India)	Fruits and seeds are preferred in management of urinary and kidney complaints [5]

S. No	Plant Name	Part Used	Tribe/Local Community	Local Names (State, Country)	Uses/Mode of Use
318.	*Juncus inflexus* L.	Roots	Native people	Pizak (Çatak, Eastern Anatolia Region, Turkey)	Prescibed as plant extract (one glass) on an empty stomach early in the morning for treatment of kidney stones [19]
319.	*Juncus inflexus* L.	Roots	Turkish citizens	Pizak (Geçitli Township, Eastern Anatolia Region, Hakkari-Turkey)	Root decoction is prescribed in the treatment of kidney stones [18]
320.	*Juniperus cummunis* L.	Twig, berry	Gitxsan, Blackfoot, Micmac, Cree	Juniper (All of Canada)	Twig and berry tea for treatment of kidney problems [10]
321.	*Kelussia odoratissima* Mozaff	Stem, leaf	Local traditional therapists	Karafs kouhi (Shahrekord, Iran)	Anti-kidney stone effect [11]
322.	*Knoxia roxburghii* (Spreng) M.A.Rau	Leaves	Local people and traditional healers	Hurim (Manipur, North East India)	Leaf- juice is given for urinary and kidney troubles [5]
323.	*Lamium album* L.	Flower	Local people and traditional healers	Ghazane Sephid (Orumieh, Iran)	Used in the treatment of kidney stones [15]
324.	*Lamium album* L.	Floral branches	Traditional healers	Gazaneh Sefid (Urmia, Northwest Iran)	Decoction used in the exertion of kidney stones [20]
325.	*Larix laricina* (DU Roi) K.Koch	Gum	Cree, Ojibwe, Chippewa	Tamarack (Atlantic Canada)	Chewing of gum for treatment of kidney problems [10]
326.	*Lavandula dentata* L.	Flowers	Plant collectors, herbalists, traditional practitioners.	Lakhzama (Izarène, Morocco)	Decoction used in the treatment of urolithiasis [17]
327.	*Lavandula dentata* L.	Leaves	Traditional herbalists	Khzâma (Rabat-Sal--Kenitra Region, Morocco)	Decoction of the leaves used for treatment of chronic kidney diseases [24]
328.	*Lavandula multifida* L.	Leaves	Plant collectors, herbalists, traditional practitioners.	Kohayla (Izarène, Morocco)	Decoction used in the treatment of urolithiasis [17]

S. No	Plant Name	Part Used	Tribe/Local Community	Local Names (State, Country)	Uses/Mode of Use
329.	*Lawsonia inermis* L.	Leaves	Local people and herbal practioners	Maidhaku (Warangal, Telangana, India)	Used in the treatment of kidney stones [4]
330.	*Lawsonia inermis* L.	Seeds, leaves	Local people and traditional healers	Henna (Bhopal district, Madhya Pradesh, India)	Used in treatment of kidney stones [7]
331.	*Ledum groenlandicum* Oeder	Leaf	Cree, Micmac	Labrador tea (All of Canada)	Leaves infusion for treatment of kidney problems [10]
332.	*Lepidium sativum* L.	Seeds	Plant collectors, herbalists, traditional practitioners.	Habrchad (Izarène, Morocco)	Decoction used in the treatment of urolithiasis [17]
333.	*Lindernia ruellioides* (Colsm) Pennell.	Whole plant	Local people and traditional healers	Kihomman (Manipur, North East India)	The whole plant boiled water with honey or sugar candy given in kidney stone [5]
334.	*Lindernia ruellioides* (Colsm) Pennell	Whole plant	Muslim Maiba (herbalists)	Kihomman (Manipur, India)	5 gm of the extract used in treatment of kidney stones. Drink 100 ml daily till cure [21]
335.	*Lindernia ruellioides* (Colsm) Pennell	Whole plant	Muslim Maiba (herbalists)	Kihomman (Manipur, India)	20 gm of the extract used in treatment of kidney stones. Drink one tea glass daily for seven days [21]
336.	*Linum usitatissimum* L.	Seed	Local people and traditional healers	Katan (Khuzestan, Iran)	Used in the treatment of kidney stones [15]
337.	*Lycopersicum esculentum* Mill.	Flower, leaf, fruit	Local people and traditional healers	Ghoje (Khuzestan, Iran)	Used in the treatment of kidney stones [15]
338.	*Macrotyloma uniflorum* (Lam.) Verdc.	Seeds	Native people, traditional healers, knowledgeable old persons	Ulava (Anantapur, Andhra Pradesh, India)	Seed decoction (100 ml) is given twice a day for one month in the treatment of kidney stones or urolithiasis [13].

S. No	Plant Name	Part Used	Tribe/Local Community	Local Names (State, Country)	Uses/Mode of Use
339.	*Macrotyloma uniflorum* (Lam.) Verdc	Seeds	Local people and professional traditional healers	(Palamalai, Eastern Ghats, India)	Used in treatment of kidney stones [27]
340.	*Magnolia grandifolia* L.	Leaves	Local people and traditional healers	Uthambal (Manipur, North East India)	Stone case [5]
341.	*Mallotus philippensis* (Lan) Muell.-Arg.	Bark	Local people and traditional healers	Ureirom laba (Manipur, North East India)	Boiled decoction is given in urinary tract stone problem [5]
342.	*Mallotus philippinensis* Muell.-Arg.	Leaves	Local people and traditional healers	Kamala (Bhopal district, Madhya Pradesh, India)	Used in treatment of kidney stones [7]
343.	*Mangifera indica* L.	Fruit	Local people and herbal practioners	Mamidi (Warangal, Telangana, India)	Used in the treatment of kidney stones [4]
344.	*Manilkara zapota* (L.) P. Royen	Kernels	Native people, traditional healers, knowledgeable old persons	Sapota (Anantapur, Andhra Pradesh, India)	Kernel paste (3-5 g) mixed with water (50 ml) and given twice a day for one month for the treatment of kidney stones or urolithiasis [13].
345.	*Marrubium vulgare* L.	Leaves	Plant collectors, herbalists, traditional practitioners.	Merriwta (Izarène, Morocco)	Decoction used in the treatment of urolithiasis [17]
346.	*Matricaria chamomilla* L.	Flowers	Plant collectors, herbalists, traditional practitioners.	Mansaniya (Izarène, Morocco)	Decoction used in the treatment of urolithiasis [17]
347.	*Medeola virginiana* L.	Crushed dried berry, leaf, root	Iroquois	Cucumber root (New Brunswick, Nova Scotia, Quebec, Canada)	Chewing raw root for treatment of kidney stones; Berry and leaf infusion also useful for kidney problems [10].
348.	*Medicago sativa* L.	Seeds	Plant collectors, herbalists, traditional practitioners.	Fessa (Izarène, Morocco)	Decoction used in the treatment of urolithiasis [17]

(Table 1) cont.....

S. No	Plant Name	Part Used	Tribe/Local Community	Local Names (State, Country)	Uses/Mode of Use
349.	*Medicago sativa* L. subsp. *sativa*	Whole plant	Turkish citizens	Hespıst (Geçitli Township, Eastern Anatolia Region, Hakkari-Turkey)	Used in treatment of kidney and vesicular swelling, kidney malfunctions [18]
350.	*Melia azedarach* L.	All parts	Local people and traditional healers	Bakain (Bhopal district, Madhya Pradesh, India)	Used in treatment of kidney stones [7]
351.	*Melia azedarach* L.	Leaf	Native people, traditional healers, knowledgeable old persons	Turakavepa (Anantapur, Andhra Pradesh, India)	Fresh leaf extract (50 ml) once a day for 20 days in the treatment of kidney stones or urolithiasis [13]
352.	*Melothria perpusilla* (Blume) Cong.	Whole plant	Local people and traditional healers	Lamthabi (Manipur, North East India)	Decoction of vegetative parts along with honey for kidney infection [5]
353.	*Mentha arvensis* L.	Leaves	Muslim Maiba (herbalists)	Podina/ Nungshi hidak (Manipur, India)	250 gm of the extract used in treatment of kidney stones. Drink half tea glass daily for 3-7 days [21]
354.	*Mentha arvensis* L.	Leaves	Local people and traditional healers	Podina/Nungshi hidak (Manipur, North East India)	Drink half tea glass of fresh infusion of leaves daily for 3-7 days [5]
355.	*Mentha piperita* L.	Whole plant	Local people and herbal practioners	Pudhina (Warangal, Telangana, India)	Used in the treatment of kidney stones [4]
356.	*Mentha rotundifolia* L.	Leaves	Plant collectors, herbalists, traditional practitioners.	Mchichtrô (Izarène, Morocco)	Decoction used in the treatment of urolithiasis [17]
357.	*Meriandra benghalensis* Benth.	Leaves	Local people and traditional healers	Kanghuman (Manipur, North East India)	Used in kidney problems [5]
358.	*Merremia emarginata* (Burm. f.) Hallier f.	Whole plant	Native people, traditional healers, knowledgeable old persons	Yelakachevikoora (Anantapur, Andhra Pradesh, India)	Whole plant extract (50 ml) given twice a day for 15 days in the treatment of kidney stones or urolithiasis [13].

(*Table 1*) *cont.....*

S. No	Plant Name	Part Used	Tribe/Local Community	Local Names (State, Country)	Uses/Mode of Use
359.	*Micromeria biflora* (Buch.-Ham. ex D. Don) Benth.	Whole plant	Local people and traditional healers	(Pakistan)	Used in the treatment of kidney stone [8]
360.	*Mimosa pudica* L.	Whole plant	Caribbean folk medicine practioners, local people	Ti marie, mese marie (Trinidad and Tobago, Caribbean)	Used in Kidney problems [23]
361.	*Mimosa pudica* L.	Whole plant	Local people and traditional healers	Lajwanti (Bhopal district, Madhya Pradesh, India)	Used in treatment of kidney stones [7]
362.	*Mimosa pudica* L.	Roots	Local people and traditional healers	Kangphal- ikaithabi (Manipur, North East India)	Root decoction with the rhizome of nut grass is given to remove kidney stone [5]
363.	*Momordica charantia* L.	Fruit, seeds, leaves	Local people and traditional healers	Karela (Bhopal district, Madhya Pradesh, India)	Used in treatment of kidney stones [7]
364.	*Momordica cochinchinensis* (Lour.) Spreng.	Fruits	Local people and Traditional healers	Karot (Manipur, North East India)	Kidney stone treatment [5]
365.	*Momordica cochinchinensis* (Lour.) Spreng	Seed	Muslim Maiba (herbalists)	Karot (Manipur, India)	1 teaspoonful powder is effective in treatment of kidney stones. Drink (100 ml) a day for 7 days [21]
366.	*Momordica dioica* Roxb.ex Willd.	Fruits	Local people and traditional healers	Kaksa (Manipur, North East India)	Roots are used in urinary complaints [5]
367.	*Moringa oleifera* Lam.	Leaves, fruit pods	Local people and traditional healers	Sahajan (Bhopal district, Madhya Pradesh, India)	Used in treatment of kidney stones [7]
368.	*Moringa oleifera* Lam.	Roots	Native people, traditional healers, knowledgeable old persons	Munaga (Anantapur, Andhra Pradesh, India)	Root bark decoction (30 ml) is given twice a day for 15 days in the treatment of kidney stones or urolithiasis [13].

S. No	Plant Name	Part Used	Tribe/Local Community	Local Names (State, Country)	Uses/Mode of Use
369.	*Morus alba* Roxb.	Leaves, fruit	Indigenous people, tribal people, and traditional health practitioners	Bana Valley, Kotli (Azad Jammu and Kashmir), Pakistan	Nephroprotective [9]
370.	*Musa paradisiaca* L.	Fruits	Local people and traditional healers	Kela (Bhopal district, Madhya Pradesh, India)	Used in treatment of kidney stones [7]
371.	*Musa paradisiaca* L.	Stem	Native people, traditional healers, knowledgeable old persons	Arati (Anantapur, Andhra Pradesh, India)	Pseudo stem extract (50 ml) given once a day for 40 days in the treatment of kidney stones or urolithiasis [13].
372.	*Muscari neglectum* Guss. ex Ten.	Plant bulbs	Local people and traditional healers	Kalaghak (Orumieh, Iran)	Used in the treatment of kidney stones [15]
373.	*Muscari neglectum* Guss. exTen.	Bulb	Traditional healers	Kalaghak (Urmia, Northwest Iran)	Decoction used in the exertion of kidney stones [20]
374.	*Myriogyne minuta* (G.Forst.) Less.	Whole plant	Muslim Maiba (herbalists)	Hakthikhanbi (Manipur, India)	Used in treatment of kidney stones. Drink (100 ml) a day for 7 days [21]
375.	*Myriogyne minuta* Less.	Aerial parts	Local people and traditional healers	Hakthi khanbi (Manipur, North East India)	Whole plant extract with sugar cane juice in equal ratio is useful against stone in the urinary tract [5]
376.	*Nasturtium officinale* (L.) R. Br.	Leaf	Local people and traditional healers	Alafe cheshmeh (Lorestan, Iran)	Used in the treatment of kidney stones [15]
377.	*Nasturtium officinale* (L.) R. Br.	Whole plant	Local people and traditional healers	Allafe Cheshme (Kazeroun, Iran)	Used in the treatment of kidney stones [15]
378.	*Nectaroscordeum tripedale* N. coelzi	Leaf, Plant bulbs	Local people and traditional healers	Piaze Tabestani (Lorestan, Iran)	Used in the treatment of kidney stones [15]
379.	*Nigella sativa* L.	Seeds	Local people and traditional healers	Kalaungi (Bhopaldistrict, Madhya Pradesh, India)	Used in treatment of kidney stones [7]

S. No	Plant Name	Part Used	Tribe/Local Community	Local Names (State, Country)	Uses/Mode of Use
380.	*Nigella sativa* L.	Whole plant	Local people and traditional healers	(Pakistan)	Used in treatment of kidney stones [8]
381.	*Nigella sativa* L.	Seeds	Plant collectors, herbalists, traditional practitioners.	Assânûj (Izarène, Morocco)	Decoction used in the treatment of urolithiasis [17]
382.	*Nigella sativa* L.	Leaf, seed	Local traditional therapists	Siahdaneh (Shahrekord, Iran)	Anti-kidney stone effect [11]
383.	*Noaea mucronata* (Forssk.) Asch & Schweinf.	Flower, leaf	Local people and traditional healers	Nakhone Aroos (Kazeroun, Iran)	Used in the treatment of kidney stones [15]
384.	*Nopalea cochenillifera* (L.) Salm-Dyck.	Flowers	Caribbean folk medicine practioners, local people	Rachette (Trinidad and Tobago, Caribbean)	Used in treatment of kidney stones [23]
385.	*Ocimum basilicum* L.	Leaf, seed	Local people and professional traditional healers	(Palamalai, Eastern Ghats, India)	Used in treatment of kidney stones [27]
386.	*Ocimum gratissimum* L.	Leaves	Local people and traditional healers	Aranya tulsi (Bhopal district, Madhya Pradesh, India)	Used in treatment of kidney stones [7]
387.	*Ocimum tenuiflorum* L. (Syn.: *O. sanctum* L.)	Leaves	Local people and traditional healers	Tulsi (Bhopal district, Madhya Pradesh, India)	Used in treatment of kidney stones [7]
388.	*Olea europaea* L. var. *sativa* (Weston) Lehr.	Leaves	Plant collectors, herbalists, traditional practitioners.	Zitoun, Zabbouj (Izarène, Morocco)	Decoction used in the treatment of urolithiasis [17]
389.	*Ononis spinosa* L.	Petals, roots	Traditional healers	Angosht Arus (Urmia, Northwest Iran)	Decoction used in the exertion of kidney stones [20]
390.	*Ononis spinosa* L.	Plant bulbs, leaf	Local people and traditional healers	Anghoshte Aroos (Orumieh, Iran)	Used in the treatment of kidney stones [15]
391.	*Opuntia ficus-indica* (L.) Mill.	Flowers	Plant collectors, herbalists, traditional practitioners.	Nouwaratlhandiya (Izarène, Morocco)	Decoction used in the treatment of urolithiasis [17]

(Table 1) cont.....

S. No	Plant Name	Part Used	Tribe/Local Community	Local Names (State, Country)	Uses/Mode of Use
392.	*Opuntia ficus-indica* (L.) Mill.	Flowers	Traditional herbalists	Nawarhandia (Rabat-Sale-Kenitra Region, Morocco)	Decoction of the flowers used for treatment of chronic kidney diseases [24]
393.	*Origanum compactum* Benth.	Leaves	Plant collectors, herbalists, traditional practitioners.	Zaâtar (Izarène, Morocco)	Decoction used in the treatment of urolithiasis [17]
394.	*Origanum majorana* L.	Leaves	Plant collectors, herbalists, traditional practitioners.	Merdedouch (Izarène, Morocco)	Decoction used in the treatment of urolithiasis [17]
395.	*Orthosiphon spiralis* (Lour.) Merr.	Leaves	Local people and traditional healers	Warak leikham (Manipur, North East India)	Boiled leaf extract is prescribed in urinary complaints [5]
396.	*Oxalis corniculata* L.	Whole plant	Muslim Maiba (herbalists)	Yensil (Manipur, India)	100 gm of the extract used in treatment of kidney stones. Drink 1 tea glass daily for seven days [21]
397.	*Oxalis corniculata* L.	Leaves, flowers	Traditional practitioner's belong to communities of Meitei, Tangkhul, Kabui, Naga, and Mizo	Yensil (Manipur, North-East India)	Used in treatment of kidney problems [22]
398.	*Oxalis corniculata* L.	Leaves	Local people and traditional healers	Yensil (Manipur, North East India)	Boiled leaf decoction with a pinch of salt may helps in eliminating kidney stones [5]
399.	*Pavetta indica* L.	Roots	Local people and traditional healers	Kukurchura (Manipur, North East India)	Roots are used for urinary and kidney diseases [5]
400.	*Pedalium murex* L.	Leaves and stem	Villagers, elderly persons, traditional healers	Aanai Nerunji (Madurai district, Tamil Nadu, India)	Extract of leaves and stem used to treat kidney stone, kidney damage [6]

S. No	Plant Name	Part Used	Tribe/Local Community	Local Names (State, Country)	Uses/Mode of Use
401.	*Pedalium murex* L.	Fruits	Native people, traditional healers, knowledgeable old persons	Peddapalleru (Anantapur, Andhra Pradesh, India)	Fruit powde (4g) is given with sheep milk once a day for seven days in the treatment of kidney stones or urolithiasis [13].
402.	*Pedalium murex* L.	Whole ripe fruit	Local people and professional traditional healers	(Palamalai, Eastern Ghats, India)	Used in treatment of kidney stones [27]
403.	*Peganum harmala* L.	Flower	Local people and traditional healers	Espand (Persian Gulf, Iran)	Used in the treatment of kidney stones [15]
404.	*Peperomia pellucida* (L.) Kunth	Herb	Tribal communities like Bhilala, Bhil, and Pataya	(Jhabua, Madhya Pradesh, India)	Infusion of the whole plant is given in kidney disorders [30]
405.	*Peperomia rotundifolia* (L.) Kunth	Whole plant	Caribbean folk medicine practioners, local people	Giron fleur, mowon (Trinidad and Tobago, Caribbean)	Used in kidney problems [23]
406.	*Petiveria alliacea* L.	Whole plant	Caribbean folk medicine practioners, local people	Mapourite, kudjuruk (Trinidad and Tobago, Caribbean)	Used in kidney problems [23]
407.	*Petroselinum crispum* (Mill.) Fuss	Leaf, Fruit	Local people and traditional healers	Jaffari (Khuzestan, Iran)	Used in the treatment of kidney stones [15]
408.	*Petroselinum hortense* Hoffm.	Fruit, Leaf	Local people and traditional healers	Jaffari (Kerman, Iran)	Used in the treatment of kidney stones [15]
409.	*Petroselinum sativum* Hoffm.	Aerial parts	Plant collectors, herbalists, traditional practitioners.	Maâdanous (Izarène, Morocco)	Decoction used in the treatment of urolithiasis [17]
410.	*Petroselinum sativum* Hoffm.	Leaves	Traditional herbalists	Màadnous (Rabat-Sal--Kenitra Region, Morocco)	Decoction of the leaves used for treatment of chronic kidney diseases [24]

(Table 1) cont.....

S. No	Plant Name	Part Used	Tribe/Local Community	Local Names (State, Country)	Uses/Mode of Use
411.	*Phyllanthus emblica* L. (Syn.: *Emblica officinalis* Gaertn.)	Fruit	Local people and Traditional healers	Heigru (Manipur, North East India)	Juice extraction is prescribed in kidney stone [5]
412.	*Phyllanthus emblica* L. (Syn.: *Emblica officinalis* Gaertn.)	Fruits	Muslim Maiba (herbalists)	Heigru (Manipur, India)	Used in treatment of kidney stones. Extracted juice is mixed with 250 ml lime water, take 4 spoons orally twice daily for 7 days [21]
413.	*Phyllanthus emblica* L.	Seeds	Local people and herbal practioners	Usiri (Warangal, Telangana, India)	Used in the treatment of kidney stones [4]
414.	*Phyllanthus niruri* L.	Whole plant	Local people and herbal practioners	Nelausiri (Warangal, Telangana, India)	Used in the treatment of kidney stones [4]
415.	*Phyllanthus niruri* L.	Leaves	Villagers, elderly persons, traditional healers	Keela nelli (Madurai district, Tamil Nadu, India)	Leaf extract used as powerful medicine for kidney stone [6]
416.	*Phyllanthus niruri* L.	Fruits, leaves	Local people and traditional healers	Bhui amala (Bhopal district, Madhya Pradesh, India)	Used in treatment of kidney stones [7]
417.	*Phyllanthus urinaria* L.	Whole plant	Local people and traditional healers	Chakpaheikru (Manipur, North East India)	Urinary disorder [5]
418.	*Pimpinella anisum* L.	Seeds	Plant collectors, herbalists, traditional practitioners.	Habbethlawa (Izarène, Morocco)	Decoction used in the treatment of urolithiasis [17]
419.	*Pinus strobus* L.	Bark, needle, twig	Algonquin, Iroquois, Ojibwe, Micmac	White pine (Atlantic Canada)	Tea of plant parts used for kidney and urinary problems [10]
420.	*Piper longum* L.	Leaves	Local people and traditional healers	Taboppi (Manipur, North East India)	Boiled leaf decoction with honey or sugar is given in urinary tract and kidney stone [5]

S. No	Plant Name	Part Used	Tribe/Local Community	Local Names (State, Country)	Uses/Mode of Use
421.	*Piper nigrum* L.	Seed	Muslim Maiba (herbalists)	Gul (Manipur, India)	1 teaspoonful powder is effective in treatment of kidney stones. Drink (100 ml) a day for 7 days [21]
422.	*Piper nigrum* L.	Seeds	Local people and Traditional healers	Gul (Manipur, North East India)	Boiled seed extract is prescribed in kidney stone [5]
423.	*Pityrogramma calomelanos* (L.) Link	Whole plant	Caribbean folk medicine practioners, local people	Fern (Trinidad and Tobago, Caribbean)	Used in Kidney and urinary problems [23]
424.	*Plantago major* L.	Whole plant	Local people and traditional healers	Yempat (Manipur, North East India)	Boiled plants used against urinary and kidney disorder [5]
425.	*Polygonatum multiflorum* Allioni	Root	Local people and traditional healers	Kundalei agouba thondaba (Manipur, North East India)	The root decoction is prescribed in kidney and urinary troubles [5]
426.	*Polygonum aviculare* L.	Aerial parts	Local people and traditional healers	Alaphe Haft Band (Orumieh, Iran)	Used in the treatment of kidney stones [15]
427.	*Polygonum aviculare* L.	Aerial parts	Traditional healers	Alaf Haft Band (Urmia, Northwest Iran)	Decoction used in the exertion of kidney stones [20]
428.	*Pongamia pinnata* (L.) Pierre	Seeds	Native people, traditional healers, knowledgeable old persons	Kaanuga (Anantapur, Andhra Pradesh, India)	Seed powder (25 g) with cow milk (50 ml) and given once a day for 20 days in the treatment of kidney stones or urolithiasis [13]
429.	*Pongamia pinnata* (L.) Pierre	Leaves, roots	Local people and traditional healers	Karanj (Bhopal district, Madhya Pradesh, India)	Used in treatment of kidney stones [7]
430.	*Portulaca oleracea* L.	Whole plant	Local people and traditional healers	Kulfa (Bhopal district, Madhya Pradesh, India)	Used in treatment of kidney stones [7]

(Table 1) cont.....

S. No	Plant Name	Part Used	Tribe/Local Community	Local Names (State, Country)	Uses/Mode of Use
431.	*Potentilla anserina* L.	Whole plant	Local people and traditional healers	Samu khongpak (Manipur, North East India)	Whole plant decoction is prescribed in urinary troubles due to stone [5]
432.	*Pratia nummularia* Kurz.	Whole plant.	Local people and traditional healers	Nungai peruk (Manipur, North East India)	Whole plant decoction is administered in kidney stone [5]
433.	*Prosopis juliflora* Swartz.	Whole plant	Traditional health practioners, local people	Mosquit pod (Hafizabad district, Punjab-Pakistan)	Decoction is used in the treatment of kidney stones [14].
434.	*Prunus domestica* L.	Fruits	Plant collectors, herbalists, traditional practitioners.	Barkuk (Izarène, Morocco)	Decoction used in the treatment of urolithiasis [17]
435.	*Prunus persica* (L.) Batsch.	Fruit	Local people and traditional healers	Heikha (Manipur, North East India)	Two week stored fruit infusion is given orally for urinary troubles [5]
436.	*Punica granatum* L.	All parts, fruits	Local people and traditional healers	Anar (Bhopal district, Madhya Pradesh, India)	Used in treatment of kidney stones [7]
437.	*Pyrus communis* L.	Fruit	Local people and traditional healers	Herme (West Azerbaijan, Iran)	Used in the treatment of kidney stones [15]
438.	*Ranunculus muricatus* L.	Roots	Plant collectors, herbalists, traditional practitioners.	Wdene l'halûf (Izarène, Morocco)	Decoction used in the treatment of urolithiasis [17]
439.	*Ranunculus sceleratus* L.	Whole plant	Local people and traditional healers	Kakyel-khujil (Manipur, North East India)	Urinary disorder [5]
440.	*Raphanus sativus* L.	Rhizome	Local people and herbal practioners	Mullangi (Warangal, Telangana, India)	Used in the treatment of kidney stones [4]
441.	*Raphanus sativus* L.	Roots	Local people and traditional healers	Muli (Bhopal district, Madhya Pradesh, India)	Used in treatment of kidney stones [7]

S. No	Plant Name	Part Used	Tribe/Local Community	Local Names (State, Country)	Uses/Mode of Use
442.	*Raphanus sativus* L.	Tubers	Native people, traditional healers, knowledgeable old persons	Mullangi (Anantapur, Andhra Pradesh, India)	3g of ash from fried tuber pieces with water given once a day in the treatment of kidney stones or urolithiasis [13].
443.	*Raphanus sativus* L.	Roots	Local people and traditional healers	Toroup (Khuzestan, Iran)	Used in the treatment of kidney stones [15]
444.	*Rheum ribes* L.	Aerial parts, roots,	Native people	Revas (Çatak, Eastern Anatolia Region, Turkey)	One glass of the plant extract on an empty stomach early in the morning is used in treatment of kidney stones [19]
445.	*Rhus semialata* Murr.	Shoots, leaves and fruit	Local people and traditional healers	Heimang (Manipur, North East India)	Used in treatment of kidney stones [5]
446.	*Rhus succedana* L.	The powders of the fruits	Local people and traditional healers	Heimang (Manipur, North East India)	Fruits powder with egg are given in kidney problems, urinary complaint due to the stone [5]
447.	*Ricinus communis* L.	Seeds, leaves	Local people and traditional healers	Arandi (Bhopal district, Madhya Pradesh, India)	Used in treatment of kidney stones [7]
448.	*Rosa canina* L.	Fruit	Native people	Şilank (Çatak, Eastern Anatolia Region, Turkey)	Plant extract (one tea glass) is given two times a day for treatment of kidney stones [19]
449.	*Rosa canina* L.	Flower	Local people and traditional healers	Shilan (West Azerbaijan, Iran)	Used in the treatment of kidney stones [15]
450.	*Rosa canina* L.	Fruit	Local people and traditional healers	Nastaran (Orumieh, Iran)	Used in the treatment of kidney stones [15]
451.	*Rosa canina* L.	Fruit	Traditional healers	Nastaran (Urmia, Northwest Iran)	Decoction used in the exertion of kidney stones [20]
452.	*Rosa foetida* Herrm.	Flower, leaf	Local people and traditional healers	Nastaran Zard (Orumieh, Iran)	Used in the treatment of kidney stones [15]

(Table 1) cont.....

S. No	Plant Name	Part Used	Tribe/Local Community	Local Names (State, Country)	Uses/Mode of Use
453.	*Rosa foetida* Herrm.	Petals	Traditional healers	Nastaran Zard (Urmia, Northwest Iran)	Decoction used in the exertion of kidney stones [20]
454.	*Rosa indica* L.	Whole plant	Local people and traditional healers	(Pakistan)	Used in the treatment of kidney stone [8]
455.	*Rosmarinus officinalis* L.	Leaves	Plant collectors, herbalists, traditional practitioners.	Aazir (Izarène, Morocco)	Decoction used in the treatment of urolithiasis [17]
456.	*Rotala baccifera* L.	Whole plant	Local people and traditional healers	Ishingkundo (Manipur, North East India)	The whole plant is prescribed in urinary trouble [5].
457.	*Rotala rotundifolia* (Roxb.) Koehne	Whole plant	Local people and traditional healers	Labook Leiri (Manipur, North East India)	Urinary Troubles [5]
458.	*Rubia tinctorum* L.	Roots	Local people and traditional healers	Ronas (Sistan and Baluchestan, Iran	Used in the treatment of kidney stones [15]
459.	*Rubus ellipticus* Smith	Whole plant	Local people and traditional healers	(Pakistan)	Used in the treatment of kidney stone [8]
460.	*Rubus niveus* Thunb.	Leaves	Local people and traditional healers	Heijampat (Manipur, North East India)	The leaf decoction is useful in urinary problems, for relaxing uterus muscles [5]
461.	*Rumex hastatus* D. Don	Whole plant	Local people and traditional healers	(Pakistan)	Used in the treatment of kidney stone [8]
462.	*Ruta graveolens* L.	Aerial parts	Traditional healers	Sodab (Urmia, Northwest Iran)	Decoction used in the exertion of kidney stones [20]
463.	*Saccharum officinarum* L.	Stem	Local people and traditional healers	Chu (Manipur, North East India)	Used in kidney infections [5]
464.	*Saccharum spontaneum* L.	Roots	Local people and traditional healers	Kans (Bhopal district, Madhya Pradesh, India)	Used in treatment of kidney stones [7]
465.	*Salvia officinalis* L.	Leaves	Plant collectors, herbalists, traditional practitioners.	Assalmiya (Izarène, Morocco)	Decoction used in the treatment of urolithiasis [17]

(Table 1) cont.....

S. No	Plant Name	Part Used	Tribe/Local Community	Local Names (State, Country)	Uses/Mode of Use
466.	*Santalum album* L.	Oil and powder of the wood	Local people and traditional healers	Cha-chandan (Manipur, North East India)	Urinary troubles [5]
467.	*Sarracenia purpurea* L.	Root	Micmac	Purple pitcher plant (Southern Canada)	Drinking steeped root for treatment of kidney problems [10]
468.	*Satureja macrosiphon* Bornm.	Pedicel, leaf	Local people and traditional healers	Marzeh (Lorestan, Iran)	Used in the treatment of kidney stones [15]
469.	*Scyphocephalium ochocoa* Warb.	Bark	Traditional healers	Soghe (Woleu-Ntem province, Gabon)	Local application of bark decoction used in management of kidney cancer [33]
470.	*Senna alexandrina* Mill.	Leaves	Plant collectors, herbalists, traditional practitioners.	Sannâharam (Izarène, Morocco)	Decoction used in the treatment of urolithiasis [17]
471.	*Senna italica* (Syn.*Cassia italica* Mill.)	Whole plant	Local people and traditional healers	(Pakistan)	Used in the treatment of kidney stone [8]
472.	*Sesamum indicum* L.	Seeds	Local people and traditional healers	Thoiding amuba (Manipur, North East India)	Seed oil is given in urinary complaints [5]
473.	*Sesamum orientale* L.	Seeds	Local people and traditional healers	Til (Bhopal district, Madhya Pradesh, India)	Used in treatment of kidney stones [7]
474.	*Sida acuta* Burm.f.	Roots	Local people and traditional healers	Balapatta (North eastern and Southern parts of India)	Used in treatment of kidney stones [32]
475.	*Sida acuta* Burm.f.	Roots	Local people and traditional healers	Uhal (Manipur, North East India)	Roots are used in urinary complaints [5]
476.	*Sida rhombifolia* L.	Whole plant	Local people and traditional healers	Mahabala (India)	Used in treatment of kidney disorders [32]
477.	*Sida rhombifolia* L.	Whole plant	Local people and traditional healers	Uhal (Manipur, North East India)	Used in kidney stones [5]
478.	*Smilax lanceaefolia* Roxb.	Rhizome	Local people and traditional healers	Kukur (Manipur, North East India)	The rhizome is used for curing urinary calculi [5]

(Table 1) cont.....

S. No	Plant Name	Part Used	Tribe/Local Community	Local Names (State, Country)	Uses/Mode of Use
479.	*Smilax ovalifolia* Roxb.	Roots	Local people and traditional healers	Jangli-aushbah (Manipur, North East India)	Roots are used in urinary complaints [5]
480.	*Solanum nigrum* L.	Seeds	Local people and herbal practioners	Buddagasi (Warangal, Telangana, India)	Used in the treatment of kidney stones [4]
481.	*Solanum nigrum* L.	Whole plant	Local people and traditional healers	Makoi (Bhopal district, Madhya Pradesh, India)	Used in treatment of kidney stones [7]
482.	*Solanum nigrum* L.	Fruit, leaf	Kiani, Gujjars, Mir, Mughals, Sheikhs, Ranas, Pathans, Khawajas and Malik	Kach mach (Bheri, Muzaffarabad, Kashmir, Pakistan)	Used in management of kidney problems [26]
483.	*Solanum nigrum* L.	Whole plant	Local people and traditional healers	(Pakistan)	Used in the treatment of kidney stone [8]
484.	*Solanum nigrum* L.	Seeds	Local people and traditional healers	Leipungkhanga (Manipur, North East India)	Seeds are used in the treatment of kidney stone [5]
485.	*Solanum surattense* Burm.f.	Whole plant	Local people and traditional healers	(Pakistan)	Used in the treatment of kidney stone [8]
486.	*Solanum surattense* Burm.f	Whole plant	Local people and traditional healers	Bhatkataiya (Bhopal district, Madhya Pradesh, India)	Used in treatment of kidney stones [7]
487.	*Solanum surattense* Burm.f.	Whole plant	Traditional health practioners, local people	Kundiari (Hafizabad district, Punjab-Pakistan)	Decoction is used in the treatment of kidney stones [14]
488.	*Solanum xanthocarpum* Schrad. & Wendl.	Roots	Local people and herbal practioners	Nelamulakkaya (Warangal, Telangana, India)	Used in the treatment of kidney stones [4]
489.	*Sorghum vulgare* L.	Seeds	Local people and traditional healers	Jwar (Bhopal district, Madhya Pradesh, India)	Used in treatment of kidney stones [7]
490.	*Sphaeranthus indicus* L.	Whole plant	Local people and traditional healers	Gorakhmundi (Bhopal district, Madhya Pradesh, India)	Used in treatment of kidney stones [7]
491.	*Stephania hernandifolia* Walf.	Leaves	Local people and traditional healers	Thangga uriangagangba (Manipur, North East India)	The leaf juice is given in urinary trouble [5]

S. No	Plant Name	Part Used	Tribe/Local Community	Local Names (State, Country)	Uses/Mode of Use
492.	*Suaeda fruticosa* Forssk.	Whole plant	Traditional health practioners, local people	Khaari (Hafizabad district, Punjab-Pakistan)	Whole plant decoction is used in the management of kidney stones [14]
493.	*Syzygium aromaticum* (L.) Merr. & Perry.	Flower bud	Local people and traditional healers	Long (Manipur, North East India)	Boiled extract of flower buds is given in kidney stone [5]
494.	*Syzygium aromaticum* (L.) Merr. & Perry	Inflorescence	Muslim Maiba (herbalists)	Long (Manipur, India)	1 teaspoonful powder is effective in treatment of kidney stones. Drink (100 ml) a day for 7 days [21]
495.	*Syzygium cumini* (L.) Skeels	Fruit pulp	Local people and herbal practioners	Neredu (Warangal, Telangana, India)	Used in the treatment of kidney stones [4]
496.	*Syzygium cuminii* (L.) Skeels	Fruits	Local people and traditional healers	Jamun (Bhopal district, Madhya Pradesh, India)	Used in treatment of kidney stones [7]
497.	*Tagetes erecta* L.	Leaves	Local people and herbal practioners	Banthi (Warangal, Telangana, India)	Used in the treatment of kidney stones [4]
498.	*Tagetes erecta* L.	Leaves, flowers	Local people and traditional healers	Genda (Bhopal district, Madhya Pradesh, India)	Used in treatment of kidney stones [7]
499.	*Tagetes erecta* L.	Leaves	Local people and traditional healers	Sanalei (Manipur, North East India)	The leaf extract is prescribed in kidney troubles [5]
500.	*Tamarindus indica* L.	Leaves	Muslim Maiba (herbalists)	Mange hei (Manipur, India)	20 gm of the extract used in treatment of kidney stones. Drink one tea glass daily for seven days [21]
501.	*Tamarindus indica* L.	Leaves	Local people and traditional healers	Mange hei (Manipur, North East India)	Consumption of boiled leaf decoction helps in eliminating calculi/stones [5]
502.	*Tamarindus indica* L.	Leaves	Local people and herbal practioners	Chintha (Warangal, Telangana, India)	Used in the treatment of kidney stones [4]

(Table 1) cont.....

S. No	Plant Name	Part Used	Tribe/Local Community	Local Names (State, Country)	Uses/Mode of Use
503.	*Tamarix aphylla* (L.) Karst.	Whole plant	Local people and traditional healers	(Pakistan)	Used in the treatment of kidney stone [8]
504.	*Tanacetum polycephalum* (L.) Sch.- Bip.	Aerial organs	Local traditional therapists	Mokhalaseh (Shahrekord, Iran)	Anti-kidney stone effect [11].
505.	*Tanacetum chiliophyllum* (Fisch. & Mey) Sch.- Bip.var. *chiliophyllum*	Aerial parts	Turkish citizens	Bevüjan (Geçitli Township, Eastern Anatolia Region, Hakkari-Turkey)	Decoction of the aerial parts is used in the treatment of kidney stones [18]
506.	*Taraxacum officinale* F.H. Wigg.	Whole plant	Local people and traditional healers	Aranya kasni (Bhopal district, Madhya Pradesh, India)	Used in treatment of kidney stones [7]
507.	*Tephrosia purpurea* (L.) Pers.	Leaves, flowers	Local people and traditional healers	Sarphoka (Bhopal district, Madhya Pradesh, India)	Used in treatment of kidney stones [7]
508.	*Tephrosia purpurea* (L.) Pers.	Whole plant	Malayali tribes of Kolli Hills	Kattu-kolingi (Nammakkal district, Eastern Ghats, Tamilnadu, India)	Used in the treatment of kidney disorders [34]
509.	*Terminalia arjuna* (Roxb.) Wight & Arn.	All parts	Local people and traditional healers	Arjuna (Bhopal district, Madhya Pradesh, India)	Used in treatment of kidney stones [7]
510.	*Terminalia bellerica* (Gaertn.) Roxb.	All parts	Local people and traditional healers	Bahera (Bhopal district, Madhya Pradesh, India)	Used in treatment of kidney stones [7]
511.	*Terminalia chebula* Retz.	Fruits	Plant collectors, herbalists, traditional practitioners.	Hlilije (Izarène, Morocco)	Decoction used in the treatment of urolithiasis [17]
512.	*Teucrium polium* L.	Aerial parts	Turkish citizens	Keselmehmut (Geçitli Township, Eastern Anatolia Region, Hakkari-Turkey)	Used in treatment of kidney pains [18]
513.	*Thunbergia alata* Boj. ex Sims.	Leaves	Local people and traditional healers	Lilha (Manipur, North East India)	Boiled leaf extract is prescribed in urinary tract stones [5]
514.	*Thymelaea lythroides* L.	Leaves	Plant collectors, herbalists, traditional practitioners.	L'metnâne (Izarène, Morocco)	Decoction used in the treatment of urolithiasis [17]

S. No	Plant Name	Part Used	Tribe/Local Community	Local Names (State, Country)	Uses/Mode of Use
515.	*Thymus vulgaris* L.	Aerial parts	Plant collectors, herbalists, traditional practitioners.	Zaîtra (Izarène, Morocco)	Decoction used in the treatment of urolithiasis [17]
516.	*Thymus vulgaris* L.	Leaf, flower	Local traditional therapists	Avishan (Shahrekord, Iran)	Anti-kidney stone effect [11]
517.	*Trachyspermum ammi* (L.) Sprague	Leaf, flower	Local traditional therapists	Zenian (Shahrekord, Iran)	Anti-kidney stone effect [11]
518.	*Tragapogon caricifolius* Boiss.	Whole plant	Local people and traditional healers	Sheng (Lorestan, Iran)	Used in the treatment of kidney stones [15]
519.	*Trianthema portulacastrum* L.	Whole plant	Local people and traditional healers	Safed punarnava (Bhopal district, Madhya Pradesh, India)	Used in treatment of kidney stones [7]
520.	*Trianthema portulacastrum* L.	Whole plant	Local people and traditional healers	(Pakistan)	Used in treatment of kidney stones [8]
521.	*Tribulus terrestris* L.	Whole plant	Local people and traditional healers	(Pakistan)	Used in treatment of kidney stones [8]
522.	*Tribulus terrestris* L.	Leaves	Local people and herbal practioners	Palleru (Warangal, Telangana, India)	Used in the treatment of kidney stones [4]
523.	*Tribulus terrestris* L.	Whole plant	Local people and traditional healers	Gokhru (Bhopal district, Madhya Pradesh, India)	Used in treatment of kidney stones [7]
524.	*Tribulus terrestris* L.	Whole plant extract	Villagers, elderly persons, traditional healers	Nerunjil (Madurai district, Tamil Nadu, India)	Whole plant extract used for kidney stone [6]
525.	*Tribulus terrestris* L.	Herb	Tribal communities like Bhil, Bhilala and Pataya	Bhui Gokhru (Jhabua, Madhya Pradesh, India)	50 ml fresh leaf juice is useful in kidney disorder [30]
526.	*Tribulus terrestris* L.	Roots	Native people, traditional healers, knowledgeable old persons	Palleru (Anantapur, Andhra Pradesh, India)	Used in the treatment of kidney stones or urolithiasis. 50 ml root decoction, given twice a day for 15 days [13]

S. No	Plant Name	Part Used	Tribe/Local Community	Local Names (State, Country)	Uses/Mode of Use
527.	*Tribulus terrestris* L.	Leaves, flowers	Malayali tribes of Kolli Hills	Sirunenunji (Nammakkal district, Eastern Ghats, Tamil Nadu, India)	Used in the treatment of kidney stones [34]
528.	*Tribulus terrestris* L.	Aerial parts	Local people and traditional healers	Kharkhasak (Orumieh, Iran)	Used in the treatment of kidney stones [15]
529.	*Tribulus terrestris* L.	Aerial organs	Local traditional therapists	Kharkhasak (Shahrekord, Iran)	Anti-kidney stone effect [11]
530.	*Tribulus terrestris* L.	Whole ripe fruit	Local people and professional traditional healers	(Palamalai, Eastern Ghats, India)	Used in treatment of kidney stones [27]
531.	*Tribulus terrestris* L.	Aerial parts	Traditional healers	Kharkhasak (Urmia, Northwest Iran)	Decoction used in the exertion of kidney stones [20]
532.	*Tribulus terrestris* L.	Whole plant	Local Healers (Hakims), Farmers	Speena Kunda (Lakki Marwat, Pakistan)	Decoction used in the exertion of kidney stones [35]
533.	*Tribulus terrestris* L.	Whole plant	Local people and traditional healers	Kharkhsak (Kazeroun, Iran)	Used in the treatment of kidney stones [15]
534.	*Trichodesma indicum* (L.) R. Br.	Whole plant	Local people and traditional healers	(Pakistan)	Used for the treatment in kidney stone [8]
535.	*Tridax procumbens* L.	Whole plant	Local people and traditional healers	Ghamra (Bhopal district, Madhya Pradesh, India)	Used in treatment of kidney stones [7]
536.	*Tridax procumbens* L	Leaves	Local people and herbal practioners	Gaddichamanthi (Warangal, Telangana, India)	Used in the treatment of kidney stones [4]
537.	*Trigonella foenum-graecum* L.	Seeds	Local people and traditional healers	Methi (Bhopal district, Madhya Pradesh, India)	Used in treatment of kidney stones [7]
538.	*Tripleurospermum parviflorum* L.	Flower	Local traditional therapists	Babouneh (Shahrekord, Iran)	Anti-kidney stone effect [11]
539.	*Triticum aestivum* L.	Seeds	Local people and traditional healers	Gehu (Bhopal district, Madhya Pradesh, India)	Used in treatment of kidney stones [7]
540.	*Triumfetta rhomboidea* Jacq.	Whole plant	Local people and traditional healers	Chiriyari (Bhopal district, Madhya Pradesh, India)	Used in treatment of kidney stones [7]

S. No	Plant Name	Part Used	Tribe/Local Community	Local Names (State, Country)	Uses/Mode of Use
541.	*Tropaeolum majus* L.	Whole plant	Local people and traditional healers	Nasturtium (Bhopal district, Madhya Pradesh, India)	Used in treatment of kidney stones [7]
542.	*Ulmus minor* Mill.	Roots, leaves	Local people and traditional healers	Vazm (Lorestan, Iran)	Used in the treatment of kidney stones [15]
543.	*Urtica dioica* L.	Leaves	Traditional herbalists	Harriga (Rabat-Sal--Kenitra Region, Morocco)	Decoction of the leaves used for treatment of chronic kidney [24]
544.	*Urtica dioica* L.	Leaf	Local people and traditional healers	Ghazane (West Azerbaijan, Iran)	Used in the treatment of kidney stones [15]
545.	*Utrica dioica* L.	Aerial organs	Local traditional therapists	Gazaneh (Shahrekord, Iran)	Anti-kidney stone effect [11]
546.	*Vernonia cinerea* L.	Whole plant	Local people and traditional healers	Sahadevi (Bhopal district, Madhya Pradesh, India)	Used in treatment of kidney stones [7]
547.	*Vitex agnus-castus* L.	Whole plant	Local people and traditional healers	(Pakistan)	Used in treatment of kidney stones [8]
548.	*Vitis vinifera* L.	Fruits, leaves,	Local people and traditional healers	Angur (Bhopal district, Madhya Pradesh, India)	Used in treatment of kidney stones [7]
549.	*Vitis vinifera* L.	Leaf	Native people, traditional healers, knowledgeable old persons	Draksha (Anantapur, Andhra Pradesh, India)	Lleaf extract (20 ml) is given twice a day for 20 days in the treatment of kidney stones or urolithiasis [13]
550.	*Wedelia chinensis* (Osb.) Merril.	Whole plant	Local people and traditional healers	Chinlengbi (Manipur, North East India)	The whole plant decoction is used for curing urinary trouble due to stone [5]
551.	*Withania somnifera* (L.) Dunal	Fruit	Villagers, elderly persons, traditional healers	Amukkara (Madurai district, Tamil Nadu, India)	Fruit powder is used for kidney stone [6]
552.	*Withania somnifera* (L.) Dunal	Whole plant	Local people and traditional healers	(Pakistan)	Used in the treatment of kidney stone [8]

(Table 1) cont.....

S. No	Plant Name	Part Used	Tribe/Local Community	Local Names (State, Country)	Uses/Mode of Use
553.	*Xanthium strumarium* L.	Roots	Local people and herbal practioners	Chevukaya (Warangal, Telangana, India)	Used in the treatment of kidney stones [4]
554.	*Xanthium strumarium* L.	Whole plant	Local people and traditional healers	Gokhru (Bhopal district, Madhya Pradesh, India)	Used in treatment of kidney stones [7]
555.	*Xanthium strumarium* L.	Roots	Local people and traditional healers	Hameng Sampakpi (Manipur, North East India)	The root decoction in urinary stone [5]
556.	*Xeranthemum longipapposum* Fisch. & C.A.Mey	Aerial parts	Traditional healers	Arus Sahra (Urmia, Northwest Iran)	Decoction used in the exertion of kidney stones [20]
557.	*Xeranthemum longipapposum* Fisch. & C.A.Mey.	Aerial parts	Local people and traditional healers	Aroose sahraei (Orumieh, Iran)	Used in the treatment of kidney stones [15]
558.	*Zea mays* L.	Seeds	Local people and traditional healers	Makai (Bhopal district, Madhya Pradesh, India)	Used in treatment of kidney stones [7]
559.	*Zea mays* L.	Seeds	Local people and traditional healers	(Pakistan)	Used in the treatment of kidney stone [8]
560.	*Zea mays* L.	Silk extract	Native people, traditional healers, knowledgeable old persons	Mokkajonna (Anantapur, Andhra Pradesh, India)	Corn silk (50 ml) extract is given once a day for one month in the treatment of kidney stones or urolithiasis [13].
561.	*Zea mays* L.	Flowers	Plant collectors, herbalists, traditional practitioners.	LahyatAdra (Izarène, Morocco)	Decoction used in the treatment of urolithiasis [17]
562.	*Zea mays* L.	Crested plant	Local people and traditional healers	Zorrat (Lorestan, Iran)	Used in the treatment of kidney stones [15]
563.	*Zea mays* L.	Hebal forelock	Local traditional therapists	Zorat (Shahrekord, Iran)	Anti-kidney stone effect [11]
564.	*Zingiber officinal* Rosc.	Rhizome	Plant collectors, herbalists, traditional practitioners.	Sekinjbîr (Izarène, Morocco)	Decoction used in the treatment of urolithiasis [17]

S. No	Plant Name	Part Used	Tribe/Local Community	Local Names (State, Country)	Uses/Mode of Use
565.	*Zingiber officinale* Rosc.	Tuber	Villagers, elderly persons, traditional healers	Zingiber (Madurai district, Tamil Nadu, India)	Extract of Rhizome is used for renal failure [6]
566.	*Zingiber officinale* Rosc.	Rhizome	Traditional practitioner's belonging to communities of Meitei, Tangkhul, Kabui, Naga, and Mizo	Sing (Manipur, North-East India)	Used in treatment of kidney problems [22]
567.	*Ziziphus lotus* (L.) Lam.	Fruits	Plant collectors, herbalists, traditional practitioners.	Nbeg (Izarène, Morocco)	Decoction used in the treatment of urolithiasis [17]
568.	*Ziziphus lotus* (L.) Lam.	Fruits, leaves	Traditional herbalists	Nbeg (Rabat-Sal--Kenitra Region, Morocco)	Decoction used for treatment of chronic kidney diseases [24]
569.	*Zizyphus lotus* (L.) Lam.	Fruit	Local population of Ain Leuh	Nbeg, Cedra (Ain Leuh Region, Middle-Atlas of Morocco)	Used in treatment of kidney stones [31]
570.	*Zygophyllum gaetulum* Emb. & Maire	Aerial parts	Plant collectors, herbalists, traditional practitioners.	Al'âggaya (Izarène, Morocco)	Decoction used in the treatment of urolithiasis [17]

CONCLUSION

Numerous therapeutic plants depicted above have been generally utilized exclusively or in mix for the treatment of assortment of kidney diseases and disorders. This review hopefully will help to find out the effective and safe plant for the treatment of kidney disorders. However, the active ingredients in the herbal formulations are not well defined. It is therefore important to know the active component and their molecular interactions, which will help to analyse the therapeutic efficacy of the product so that it can be standardized and commercialized by pharma companies. Pre-clinical and clinical investigation of traditional medicinal plants for hepatoprotective activity may provide valuable leads for the development of safe and effective drugs.

REFERENCES

[1]   Harshberger J. The purpose of Ethnobotany. Bot Gaz 1896; 21: 146-54.

[http://dx.doi.org/10.1086/327316]

[2]   Mohammad A. Text book of Pharmacognosy. New Delhi: SBS publishers 1994; pp. 8-14.

[3]   Amarasiri SS, Attanayake AP, Arawwawala LDAM, Jayatilaka KAPW, Mudduwa LKB. Protective effects of three selected standardized medicinal plant extracts used in Sri Lankan traditional medicine in adriamycin induced nephrotoxic Wistar rats. J Ethnopharmacol 2020; 259112933
[http://dx.doi.org/10.1016/j.jep.2020.112933] [PMID: 32428654]

[4]   Mahender T, Sai Sreeja A, Anvesh M, Ramakrishna D, Meghana M. Ethnobotanical survey of medicinal plants used in the treatment of urolithiasis in Warangal rural, Telangana, India. World J Pharm Res 2020; 9(4): 427-37.

[5]   Mikawlrawng K, Kumar S, Vandana R. Current scenario of urolithiasis and the use of medicinal plants as antiurolithiatic agents in Manipur (North East India): a review. Int J Herb Med 2014; 2(1): 1-2.

[6]   Sundaram SS, Suresh K, Sundaram SP. Traditional knowledge of medicinal plants used to treat kidney related diseases in selected areas of Madurai district, Tamil Nadu, India. Faslnamah-i Giyahan-i Daruyi 2019; 7(4): 250-3.

[7]   Agarwal K, Varma R. Some ethnomedicinal plants of Bhopal district used for treating stone diseases. Intern J Pharmacy and Life 2012; 3(1)

[8]   Nasim MJ, Bin Asad MH, Durr-e-Sabih , *et al.* Gist of medicinal plants of Pakistan having ethnobotanical evidences to crush renal calculi (kidney stones). Acta Pol Pharm 2014; 71(1): 3-10.
[PMID: 24779189]

[9]   Amjad MS. Ethnobotanical profiling and floristic diversity of Bana Valley, Kotli (Azad Jammu and Kashmir), Pakistan. Asian Pac J Trop Biomed 2015; 5(4): 292-9.
[http://dx.doi.org/10.1016/S2221-1691(15)30348-8]

[10]   Ghayur MN, Janssen LJ. Nephroprotective drugs from traditionally used Aboriginal medicinal plants. Kidney Int 2010; 77(5): 471-2.
[http://dx.doi.org/10.1038/ki.2009.507] [PMID: 20150946]

[11]   Abbasi N, Rafieian-Kopaei M, Karami N, Abbaszadeh S, Bahmani M. Medicinal plants for treatment kidney stones, An ethnobotany study in Shahrekord. Egypt J Vet Sci 2019; 50(2): 145-9.
[http://dx.doi.org/10.21608/ejvs.2019.14057.1090]

[12]   Agarwal K, Varma R. Ethnobotanical study of antilithic plants of Bhopal district. J Ethnopharmacol 2015; 174: 17-24.
[http://dx.doi.org/10.1016/j.jep.2015.08.003] [PMID: 26253579]

[13]   Lakshmi NV. Antilithiatic ethnomedicinal plants used by the native people of Anantapur district, AP. Intern J Res Applied. Natural and Social Sci 2014; 2(7): 61-6.

[14]   Umair M, Altaf M, Abbasi AM. An ethnobotanical survey of indigenous medicinal plants in Hafizabad district, Punjab-Pakistan. PLoS One 2017; 12(6)e0177912
[http://dx.doi.org/10.1371/journal.pone.0177912] [PMID: 28574986]

[15]   Mohsenzadeh A, Ahmadipour S, Eftekhari Z. A review of medicinal herbs affects the kidney and bladder stones of children and adults in traditional medicine and ethno-botany of Iran. Pharm Lett 2015; 7(12): 279-84.

[16]   Srivastava AK, Kaushik D, Shrivastava AK, Lal VK. Nephroprotective ethno-medicinal action of selected Indian medicinal plants. Int J Pharm Sci Drug Res 2017; 9(2): 44-54.

[17]   Benkhnigue O, Zidane L, Douira A. Treatment of urinary treatment of urolithiasis: Ethnobotanical study of plants used by the population bordering the forest of Izarène. Ethnobot Res Appl 2020; 19: 1-5.

[18]   Kaval I, Behçet L, Cakilcioglu U. Ethnobotanical study on medicinal plants in Geçitli and its surrounding (Hakkari-Turkey). J Ethnopharmacol 2014; 155(1): 171-84.
[http://dx.doi.org/10.1016/j.jep.2014.05.014] [PMID: 24911339]

[19] Mükemre M, Behçet L, Çakılcıoğlu U. Ethnobotanical study on medicinal plants in villages of Çatak (Van-Turkey). J Ethnopharmacol 2015; 166: 361-74.
[http://dx.doi.org/10.1016/j.jep.2015.03.040] [PMID: 25819616]

[20] Bahmani M, Zargaran A. Ethno-botanical medicines used for urinary stones in the Urmia, Northwest Iran. Eur J Integr Med 2015; 7(6): 657-62.
[http://dx.doi.org/10.1016/j.eujim.2015.09.006]

[21] Ahmed MM, Singh KP. Traditional knowledge of kidney stones treatment by Muslim Maiba (herbalists) of Manipur, India. Not Sci Biol 2011; 3(2): 12-5.
[http://dx.doi.org/10.15835/nsb325735]

[22] Deb L, Laishram S, Khumukcham N, *et al.* Past, present and perspectives of Manipur traditional medicine: A major health care system available for rural population in the North-East India. J Ethnopharmacol 2015; 169: 387-400.
[http://dx.doi.org/10.1016/j.jep.2014.12.074] [PMID: 25895884]

[23] Lans CA. Ethnomedicines used in Trinidad and Tobago for urinary problems and diabetes mellitus. J Ethnobiol Ethnomed 2006; 2(1): 45.
[http://dx.doi.org/10.1186/1746-4269-2-45] [PMID: 17040567]

[24] El Hachlafi N, Chebat A, Bencheikh RS, Fikri-Benbrahim K. Ethnopharmacological study of medicinal plants used for chronic diseases treatment in Rabat-Sale-Kenitra region (Morocco). Ethnobot Res Appl 2020; 20: 1-23.
[http://dx.doi.org/10.32859/era.20.2.1-23]

[25] Khouchlaa A, Bakri Y, Tijane M. Ethnobotanical study on the Bereztem Plant (*Aristolochia longa*) used in the treatment of some diseases in the cities of Rabat, Sale and Temara (Morocco). J Materials and Environmental Sci 2018; 9(6): 1914-21.

[26] Ahmed MJ, Akhtar T. Indigenous knowledge of the use of medicinal plants in Bheri, Muzaffarabad, Azad Kashmir, Pakistan. Eur J Integr Med 2016; 8(4): 560-9.
[http://dx.doi.org/10.1016/j.eujim.2016.01.006]

[27] Silambarasan R, Ayyanar M. An ethnobotanical study of medicinal plants in Palamalai region of Eastern Ghats, India. J Ethnopharmacol 2015; 172: 162-78.
[http://dx.doi.org/10.1016/j.jep.2015.05.046] [PMID: 26068426]

[28] Sivasankari B, Anandharaj M, Gunasekaran P. An ethnobotanical study of indigenous knowledge on medicinal plants used by the village peoples of Thoppampatti, Dindigul district, Tamilnadu, India. J Ethnopharmacol 2014; 153(2): 408-23.
[http://dx.doi.org/10.1016/j.jep.2014.02.040] [PMID: 24583241]

[29] Vasundharan SK, Jaishanker RN, Annamalai A, Sooraj NP. Ethnobotany and distribution status of *Ensete superbum* (Roxb.) Cheesman in India: A geo-spatial review. J Ayurvedic and Herbal Med 2015; 1(2): 54-8.

[30] Wagh VV, Jain AK. Status of ethnobotanical invasive plants in western Madhya Pradesh, India. S Afr J Bot 2018; 114: 171-80.
[http://dx.doi.org/10.1016/j.sajb.2017.11.008]

[31] Akdime H, Boukhira S. EL Mansouri LEL, Youbi Amal HEL, Bousta D. Ethnobotanical study and traditional knowledge of medicinal plants in Ain Leuh Region (Middle-Atlas of Morocco). Am J Adv Drug Deliv 2015; 3: 248-63.

[32] Abat JK, Kumar S, Mohanty A. Ethnomedicinal, phytochemical and ethnopharmacological aspects of four medicinal plants of Malvaceae used in Indian traditional medicines: A review. Medicines (Basel) 2017; 4(4): 75.
[http://dx.doi.org/10.3390/medicines4040075] [PMID: 29057840]

[33] Ngoua-Meye-Misso RL, Sima-Obiang C, Ndong JD, *et al.* Medicinal plants used in management of cancer and other related diseases in Woleu-Ntem province, Gabon. Eur J Integr Med 2019; 29100924

[http://dx.doi.org/10.1016/j.eujim.2019.05.010]

[34]   Muthuraja R, Nandagopalan V, Thomas B, Marimuthu C. An ethno-botanical survey of medicinal plants used by Kolli Malayalis of Nammakkal district, Eastern Ghats, Tamil Nadu, India. European J Environ Ecol 2014; 1(1): 33-43.

[35]   Ullah S, Rashid Khan M, Ali Shah N, Afzal Shah S, Majid M, Asad Farooq M. Ethnomedicinal plant use value in the Lakki Marwat District of Pakistan. J Ethnopharmacol 2014; 158(Pt A): 412-22. [http://dx.doi.org/10.1016/j.jep.2014.09.048] [PMID: 25448507]

CHAPTER 6

Nephroprotective, Nephrocurative and Antiurolithiatic Phytochemicals

Abstract: Several phytoconstituents are useful in nephroprotection, nephrocuration, and antiurolithiasis. In this chapter, the details of phytoconstituents that have nephroprotective, nephrocurative, and antiurolithaitic properties are given. These include allicin, andrographolide, berberine, betulin, capsaicin, carnosine, carvacrol, catechin, celastrol, cerpegin, chlorogenic acid, chrysin, crocin, curcumin, diosmin, edarabone, ellagic acid, epicatechin, esculentoside A, ferulic acid, flavoxicid, ginsenosides, glycyrrhizin, glycyrrhizic acid, hypericin, kaempferol, kolaviron, lacidipine, licochalcone A, lipoic acid, lupeol, luteolin, lycopene, made cassoside, naringin, naringenin, paeonal, picroliv, proteins, quercetin, resveratrol, rutin, safranol, saponins, silibinin, taraxasterol, thymol, thymoquinone, xanthorrhizol and zingerone.

Keywords: Antiurolithiasis, Nephroprotection, Nephrocurative, Phytochemicals.

INTRODUCTION

Several phytoconstituents are useful in nephroprotection, nephrocuration, and antiurolithiasis. The antiurolithiatic phytocompounds include flavonoids like kaempferol, quercetin, saponins like solasodine, alkaloids like berberine, crocin, khellin, tannins, phenolic compounds, other organic, inorganic compounds and plant proteins like glycosaminoglycans, etc. Triterpenes help in the dissolution of oxalate crystals and demonstrate the antioxidant effect. Citrate and magnesium have a complex structure with calcium and critical supersaturation; magnesium destabilizes CaOx stone grip renal epithelial cells by pre-covering the stones. Flavonoids fundamentally forestall crystallization by the cancer prevention agent, mitigating and antimicrobial properties [1].

Pentacyclic triterpenes can successfully treat CaOx urolithiasis through different actions like cell reinforcement, calming, diuretic, and ACE inhibition. A portion of the pentacyclic triterpenes that show promising exercises incorporate lupeol, oleanolic corrosive, betulin, and taraxasterol. Lobine *et al.* [2] explained the role of pentacyclic triterpenes in the treatment of hypercalciuria. In the following pages, phytoconstituents that have nephroprotective, nephrocurative, and antiurolithaitic properties are given. Agents ameliorating or augmenting gentamicin nephrotoxicity were reviewed by Ali [3]. Ridzuan *et al.* [4] surveyed the defensive job of plant-based compounds in cisplatin-actuated nephrotoxicity. Finally, Zeng *et al.* [5] investigated the defensive assignments of flavonoids, and flavonoid-rich plant removes against urolithiasis.

PHYTOCHEMICALS WITH NEPHROPROTECTIVE, NEPHROCURATIVE AND ANTIUROLITHIATIC PROPERTIES

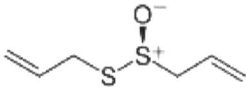

Allicin

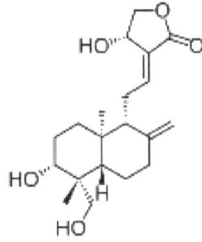

Andrographolide

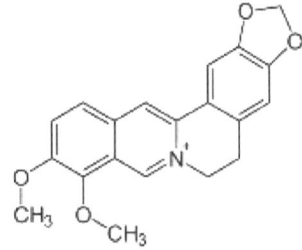

Berberine

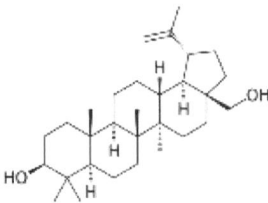

Betulin

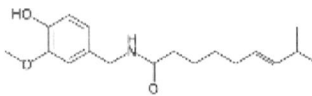

Capsaicin

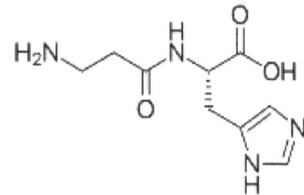

Carnosine

Cont.....

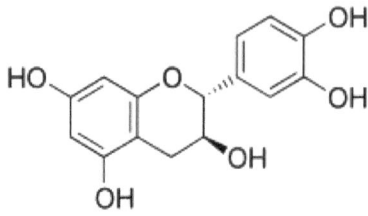

Catechin

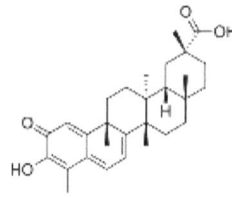

Celastrol

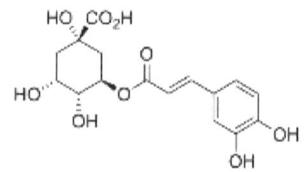

Chlorogenic acid

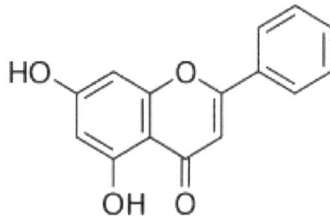

Chrysin

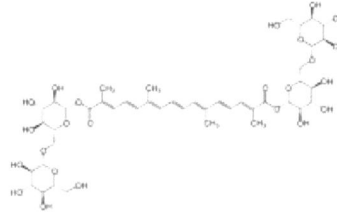

Crocin

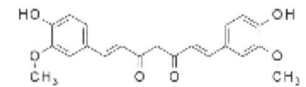

Curcumin

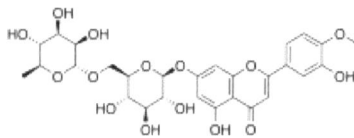

Diosmin

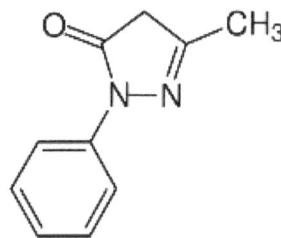

Edarabone

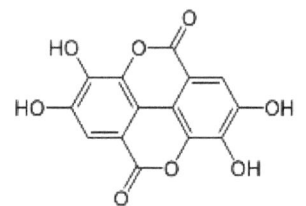

Ellagic acid

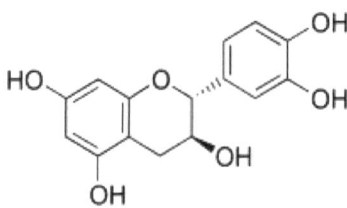

Epicatechin

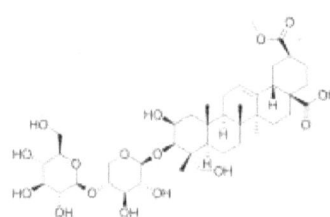

Esculentoside A

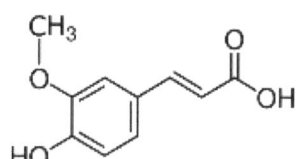

Ferulic acid

Cont.....

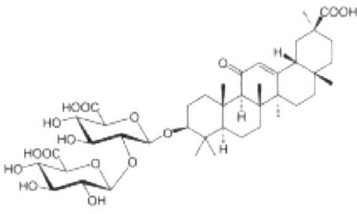

Glycyrrhizin

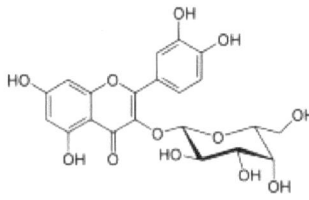

Hyperin

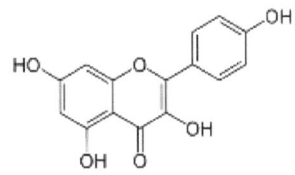

Kaempferol

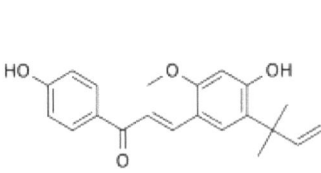

Licochalcone A

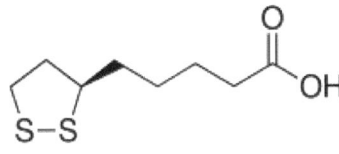

Lipoic acid

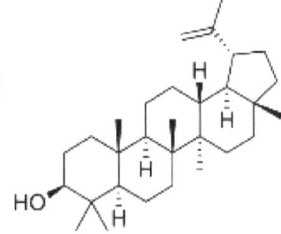

Lupeol

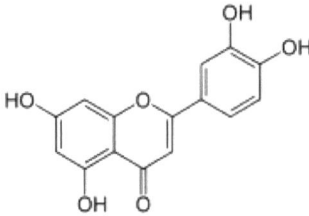

Luteolin

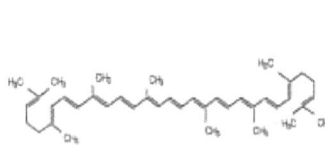

Lycopene

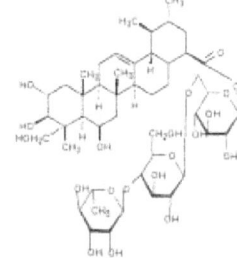

Madecassoside

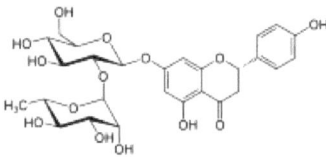

Naringin

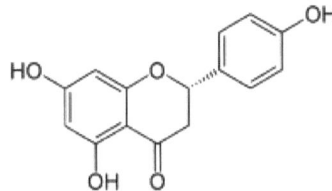

Naringenin

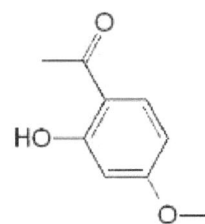

Paeonol

Cont.....

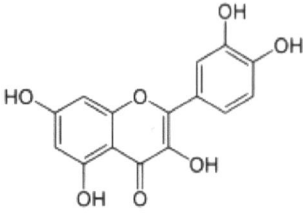

Quercetin

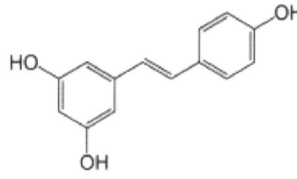

Resveratrol

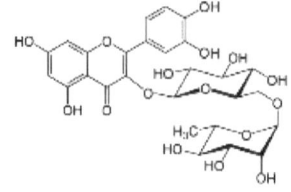

Rutin

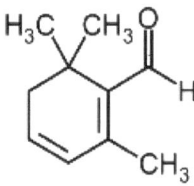

Safranal

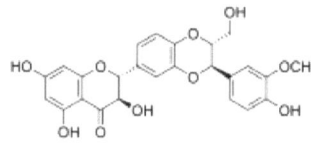

Silibinin

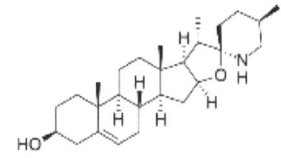

Solasodine

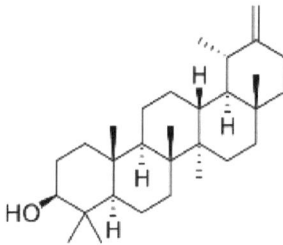

Taraxasterol

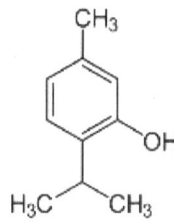

Thymol

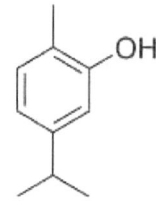

Carvacrol

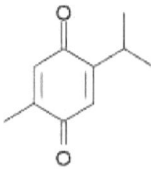

Thymoquinone

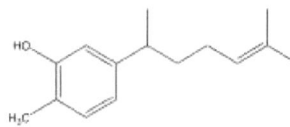

Xanthorrhizol

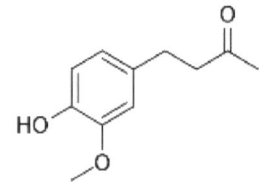

Zingerone

Allicin and Ascorbic Acid

Abdel-Daim *et al.* [6] assessed the cancer prevention and mitigating impacts of allicin and ascorbic acid (AA) and examined the nephroprotective adequacy of their mix against cisplatin (CDDP)- prompted inebriation. Rodents were partitioned into seven groups: control, allicin at a dose of 10 mg/kg for a period of 14 days, AA at a dose of 20 mg/kg for a period of 14 days, CDDP at 7 mg/kg as a solitary portion on the seventh trial day), CDDP-allicin, CDDP-AA, and CDDP-allicin-AA (at the previously mentioned dosages). The injection of CDDP prompted stamped bodyweight reduction and renal harm, shown by a massive rise in serum urea, creatinine, and uric acid levels and critical decreases in serum Na, Ca, and phosphorus fixations, notwithstanding extreme modifications in serum and renal tissue levels of tumor putrefaction factor-α in correlation with control rodents. Besides, CDDP-inebriated rodents displayed fundamentally higher lipid peroxidation, just as lower levels of decreased glutathione and exercises of glutathione peroxidase, SOD, and catalase proteins in the renal tissue, contrasted and controlled rodents. The intake of allicin or AA altogether decreased the CDDP-prompted changes in all the previously mentioned boundaries. Curiously, allicin accomplished equivalent nephroprotection to AA in most evaluated limits; notwithstanding, the reclamation of ordinary serum and renal tissue convergences of these boundaries were more continuous in the CDDP-AA bunch. Both allicin and AA showed critical nephroprotective impacts against CDDP inebriation, and their mix displayed preferred insurance over either specialist alone. Their cell reinforcement and mitigating exercises presumably intervene in these outcomes.

Andrographolide

Andrographolide is a natural bicyclic diterpenoid from *Andrographis paniculata*, a principal constituent in many Ayurvedic medications helpful in treating and managing liver problems. Supekar and Pagar [7] evaluated the nephroprotective activity of Andrographolide. Different doses like 100, 200, and 400 mg/kg doses were used to study nephroprotective action from the results of toxicity studies. The gentamicin incited strategy is utilized for the appraisal of the nephroprotective action and to check the nephrotoxicity. Na^+, K^+, and Cl^- particle focus in urine were dictated by utilizing the autoanalyzer. The treatment of gentamicin and andrographolide at 400 mg/kg has expanded the urine output fundamentally; urinary centralization of Na^+, K^+, and Cl^- particles were the boundaries of the investigation. The gentamicin and andrographolide at 400mg/kg b.w. have shown great nephroprotective, whereas100 and 200 mg/kg portion has shown moderate nephroprotective action.

Berberine

An isoquinoline alkaloid berberine, found in nature as the principal constituent of a few plants with restorative use in kidney stone illness. Bashir and Gilani [8] assessed its antiurolithic activity and investigated the potential basic mechanism(s). Berberine was tried *in vitro* for the cancer prevention agent impact and *in vivo* for its antiurolithiatic and diuretic consequences for a rodent model of CaOx urolithiasis. Berberine displayed fixation subordinate (50-150μg/ml) cell reinforcement impact against ferrous-ascorbate actuated lipid peroxidation in rodent kidney homogenate with intensity marginally higher than the reference cancer prevention agent, butylated hydroxytoluene. In rodents, berberine (5-20 mg/kg) expanded urine yield joined by expanded pH and Na(+) and K(+) discharge and diminished Ca^{2+} discharge, like hydrochlorothiazide. CaOx initiated urolithiasis was prompted in male rodents by adding 0.75% ethylene glycol in drinking water, berberine at a dose of 10mg/kg forestalled just as wiped out CaOx stones in renal tubules and secured against pernicious impacts of lithogenic treatment including weight reduction, debilitated renal capacity, and oxidative pressure, showed as expanded MDA, and protein carbonyl substance drained GSH and diminished cancer prevention agent catalyst exercises of the kidneys. In rodents, berberine at 10mg/kg diminished Ca^{2+} discharge and expanded urine volume and pH. Aftereffects of this investigation propose the presence of antiurolithic impacts in berberine against CaOx stones intervened through a mix of diuretic, urinary alkalinizing, antioxidant, and hypocalciuric results.

Domitrović *et al.* [9] explored the helpful action of berberine against cisplatin (CP)-initiated nephrotoxicity in mice. Berberine was controlled at everyday dosages of 1, 2, and 3 mg/kg by gavage for two progressive days, 48 h after CP infusion, i.p. at a dose of 13 mg/kg. Mice were forfeited 24 h after the last portion of berberine. Histopathological changes and the increment in serum creatinine and BUN instigated by cisplatin were fundamentally improved by berberine in a portion subordinate way. Moreover, oxidative/nitrosative pressure, proven by the expansion in renal 4-HNE, 3-NT, CYP2E1, and heme oxygenase articulation, was altogether diminished. Furthermore, the expression of NF-κB, TNF-α, COX-2, and inducible iNOS was extraordinarily stifled by berberine, showing the restraint of incendiary reaction. Treatment of CP-inebriated creatures with berberine likewise fundamentally diminished the outflow of p53, active caspase-3 just as autophagy marker LC3B in the kidneys.

Betulin

Dinnimath *et al.* [10] assessed the beneficial effect of betulin obtained from *Aerva lanata* on nephrolithiasis. Urolithiasis initiated by 0.75% v/v ethylene glycol model was used to study the antiurolithiatic activity using male Wistar albino rats. Animals were grouped and divided into five and each having six. An identical portion was determined from their yield in light of the LD50 of the plant extricate at a dose of 2 g/kg b.w. Betulin was used at a quantity of 2 mg/kg b.w/day orally as a test dose for 28 days. The urine volume was discovered to be fundamentally raised in rodents treated by betulin. Urine microscopy uncovered a critical decrease in calculi size and fundamentally improved discharge of phosphate, oxalate, and calcium through the raised levels of magnesium. Scanning electron microscopy of kidney areas has uncovered a decrease in the calculi in treated creatures. Serum examination has encountered a critical decline in the amounts of BUN and creatinine in treated rodents.

Capsaicin

Shimeda *et al.* [11] revealed the action of dietary antioxidants and capsaicin against cisplatin-initiated nephrotoxicity and lipid peroxidation and in rats. Allowing cisplatin resulted in a rise in kidney weight as a percentage of the total body weight, urine output, serum creatinine, and BUN compared to the control rats. It also showed notable decreases in the kidney GSH content, SOD activity, and increased MDA production by comparing the values at 0 h. After seven days of capsaicin and cisplatin treatments, the renal damage recovered to significant normal levels. In addition, capsaicin diminished the SOD activities and the rise of MDA content.

Carnosine

Soliman ·*et al.* [12] explored the antioxidant role of carnosine, a dipeptide molecule made up of the amino acids beta-alanine and histidine, in protecting the kidney in a test model. Gentamicin-inebriated rodents showed early kidney work disappointment as blood creatinine and blood urea were fundamentally expanded following one and fourteen days. Experimental evidence proposed a part of receptive oxygen species in gentamicin-prompted nephrotoxicity. The histopathological assessment uncovered degenerative changes in glomeruli and tubules. An ultrastructural study showed glomerular changes, some degeneration of both distal and gathering tubules. The proximal tubules showed stamped levels of changes and rot. Enzymatic histochemical investigations of gentamicin allowed rodents to uncover stamped rise of LDH and hindrance of SDH, ALP, ACP, and ATPase. Blood creatinine and urea were standardized in the carnosine-gentamicin bunch following one and fourteen days. Primary and enzymatic histochemical pictures were extraordinarily enhanced. The instrument by which carnosine protectively affects GM-instigated nephrotoxicity was credited to its numerous activities: twofold antioxidant, protein atom assurance, evacuation of hurtfully changed ones, and actuation insusceptible framework safeguarding of film smoothness, and cytosolic buffering. Carnosine, in this way, offers a guarantee of enhancing gentamicin nephrotoxicity.

Catechin

Green tea is generally burned-through in China, Japan, Morocco, and Korea. Because of the rich antioxidants like flavonoids, tannins, and phenolic acids, green tea applies different impacts on wellbeing, like anticancer, antiatherosclerotic impact, etc [5]. It was well to help that the antiurolithiasis action to remember green tea on the urinary stone was likewise shown in a past examination [13]. In the analysis, green tea treatment astoundingly diminished CaOx stone development, osteopontin (OPN, a significant solvent protein part of CaOx stone) articulation, and renal cylindrical cell apoptosis, while expanded SOD movement in rodent kidney tissues contrasted and a stone gathering [14]. The group probably set forward that the bar of NF-κB initiation (a supportive of incendiary cytokine which could deal with the outflow of other provocative cytokines just as actuate human aortic endothelial cell demise and apoptosis) by cancer prevention agents in green tea may represent its enemy of apoptotic movement in a urolithiasis rodent model [15, 16].

Intraperitoneal ferric nitrilotriacetate to rodents and mice brings about iron-initiated free extreme injury and malignancy in kidneys. Chopra *et al.* [17] examined the impact of catechin, a bioflavonoid with cancer prevention agent potential, on Fe-NTA-prompted nephrotoxicity in rodents. One hour after an i.p. infusion of Fe-NTA at a dose of 8 mg iron/kg, a checked decay of renal engineering, renal capacity, and extreme oxidative pressure was noticed. Pretreatment of animals with catechin particularly constricted renal brokenness, decreased raised thiobarbituric acid reacting substances (TBARS), reestablished the exhausted renal cell reinforcement catalysts, and standardized the renal morphological modifications.

Z Zhai *et al.* [18] analyzed *in vitro* and *in vivo* antiurolithiatic activity of catechin. *in vitro* explore, allowing catechin at a dose of 0.4 μL/mL in NRK-52 cells presented to CaOx monohydrate stones at 80 μg/cm^2 forestalled the progressions in mitochondrial layer potential and articulation of SOD, 4-HNE, lipid peroxidation items, cytochrome c and cut caspase 3. Furthermore, in *in vivo* study, the mitochondrial breakdown and increment of OPN, MDA, and 8-hydroxy-2'-deoxyguanosine (8-OHdG, the overall marker for observing DNA harm) articulation initiated by EG in kidneys of rodents were decreased by low-portion at a dose of 2.5 mg/kg bw each day for 14 days and high-portion dose at 10 mg/kg bw for 14 days of catechin [19]. Consequently, the exploration information suggested that renal calcium crystallization in NRK-52 cells and rodents could be forestalled by catechin by diminishing the level of COM-prompted mitochondrial injury [20].

Nephrotoxicity is perceived as a genuine issue influenced by ongoing cadmium openness. The unevenness between revolutionary age and end is an essential factor in the commencement and movement of renal injury brought about by this heavy metal. Wongmekiat *et al.* [21] researched the reasonable assurance by catechin, characteristic phenolic cell reinforcement, against cadmium nephrotoxicity and explained its likely component in male Wistar rodents. Following a month of treatment, rodents presented to cadmium showed a stamped ascend in blood urea nitrogen and creatinine, a fall in creatinine freedom, and renal pathologies like serious rounded harm, apoptosis, and unusual mitochondrial structure. Massive expansions in MDA, nitric oxide, and tumor rot factor-alpha, while decreases in cell reinforcement thiols, SOD, and catalase, were likewise recognized in the kidney tissues of cadmium-inebriated rodents. These adjustments were related to mitochondrial brokenness as upheld by an expansion in mitochondrial responsive oxygen species creation and decreased mitochondrial film potential. Treatment with catechin altogether constricted every one of the progressions brought about by cadmium. These discoveries recommend that catechin successfully secures the kidney against the harmful impact of cadmium, probably through its cell reinforcement, hostile to aggravation, and mitochondrial insurance.

Celastrol

Celastrol is a characteristic bioactive compound extricated from the roots of *Tripterygium wilfordii* Hook. f. It shows immunosuppressive, calming, and cancer prevention agent exercises. Boran *et al.* [22] assessed the remedial capability of celastrol in cisplatin-actuated nephrotoxicity. A rodent kidney epithelial cell line NRK-52E was pretreated with the ideal groupings of celastrol (50 nm, 100 nm, 200 nm, and) for 24 h. Then, the cells were treated with 50 µM cisplatin for a further 24 h to see whether cisplatin caused something similar or less poisonous than the vehicle control animal groups. Oxidative pressure boundaries were assessed by estimating the glutathione (GSH) and protein carbonyl (PC) levels and by evaluating the chemical exercises of glutathione peroxidase (GPx), glutathione reductase (GR), catalase (CAT), and SOD compounds. Improved the level of protein carbonylation and raised GSH substance of the cells were observed in Celastrol pretreatment. Moreover, celastrol pretreatment improved the GR and CAT exercises. Be that as it may, no critical contrast was seen in GPx and SOD exercises.

Cerpegin

It is a bioactive pyridinone alkaloid from the tuberous roots of *Ceropegia bulbosa* var. *lushii* used to manage kidney stones. The tuberous root also contains polyphenols, steroids, albuminoids, fats, potassium, and sugars. Monika *et al.* [23] described the cerpegin. The antiurolithiatic activity of cerpegin was assessed by using a modified *in vitro* model. The separated compound cerpegin showed the most remarkable disintegration of the two kinds of stones (CaOx and calcium phosphate) in contrast with all the concentrates tried. Cystone was discovered to be more compelling.

Chlorogenic Acid

Chlorogenic acid (CGA), a polyphenolic compound, is the ester of caffeic acid, and quinic acid shows excellent antioxidant and anti-inflammatory properties. Ye *et al.* [24] examined the defensive impacts and action of CGA on lipopolysaccharide (LPS)- instigated intense kidney injury (AKI). Treatment of CGA effectively improved LPS-actuated renal capacity and obsessive harm. Besides, CGA portion conditionally smothered LPS-incited blood urea nitrogen (BUN), creatinine levels, and inflammatory cytokines TNF-α, IL-6, and IL-1β in serum and tissue. The overall proteins' appearance of the TLR4/NF-κB signal pathway was surveyed by western blot technique. CGA portion conditionally constricted LPS-instigated kidney histopathologic changes, serum BUN, and creatinine levels. CGA likewise smothered LPS-incited TNF-α, IL-6, and IL-1β creation both in serum and kidney tissues. Moreover, CGA essentially repressed the LPS-actuated articulation of phosphorylated NF-κB p65 and IκB, just as the statement of TLR4 signal.

Chrysin

Chrysin is also known as 5,7-dihydroxyflavone, found in many plants, having multiple biological activities, such as anti-inflammatory and antioxidant properties. Sultana *et al.* [25] examined the defensive adequacy of chrysin against cisplatin-incited nephrotoxicity. Pretreatment with chrysin fundamentally lessened cisplatin-initiated renal oxidative harm by decreasing the DNA harm and harmfulness markers, for example, BUN, lipid peroxidation, creatinine, and xanthine oxidase movement, joined by an increment in enzymatic (glutathione peroxidase, catalase, glutathione reductase, and glutathione-S-transferase) and non-enzymatic (diminished glutathione) cell reinforcement status. Histological discoveries further validated the defensive viability of chrysin, which decreased cisplatin-prompted renal harm.

Crocin

Yarijani *et al.* [26] assessed the defensive impact of crocin against gentamicin-incited nephrotoxicity in male Wistar rodents. Allowing gentamicin brought about massive expansions in plasma creatinine and urea-nitrogen focuses and renal

330 An Introduction to Nephroprotective Plants

tissue MDA level and reduced renal tissue ferric lessening/cancer prevention agent power (FRAP) level. Crocin diminished plasma creatinine, urea-nitrogen fixations, and tissue MDA level. However, it expanded the degree of tissue FRAP. Likewise, gentamicin prompted cell harm, including glomerular decay, cell desquamation, cylindrical putrefaction and fibrosis, epithelial edema of proximal tubules, vascular clog, and perivascular edema, which were all mostly recuperated by crocin.

Curcumin

Curcumin is a significant yellow pigment from the rhizomes of *Curcuma longa* L., broadly utilized as a flavor and shading specialist in a few food varieties, just as beautifying agents and medications. Venkatesan *et al.* [27] researched the impact of curcumin on Adriamycin (ADR) nephrosis in rodents. The outcomes show that ADR-prompted kidney injury was surprisingly forestalled by treatment with curcumin. Treatment with curcumin extraordinarily ensured against ADR-actuated proteinuria, albuminuria, hypoalbuminemia, and hyperlipidemia. Likewise, curcumin repressed ADR-actuated expansion in the urinary discharge of N-acetyl-beta-D-glucosaminidase (a marker of renal cylindrical injury), fibronectin, and glycosaminoglycan, and plasma cholesterol. Curcumin reestablished renal capacity in ADR rodents, as decided by the increment in GFR. Likewise, the information exhibited curcumin secured against ADR-instigated renal injury by smothering oxidative pressure and expanding kidney glutathione content and glutathione peroxidase movement. In like way, curcumin annulled ADR-invigorated kidney microsomal and mitochondrial lipid peroxidation.

Antunes *et al.* [28] reported the impacts of pre-treatment with two dietary cancer prevention agents, curcumin at a dose of 8 mg kg-1 bw or selenium at an amount of 1 mg kg-1 bw cisplatin-instigated lipid peroxidation and nephrotoxicity in Wistar rodents. Cisplatin supplying brought about a critical decrease in body weight, and higher urinary volumes were seen in all gatherings treated with this antitumor medication. The rodents treated with cisplatin showed consumption of renal glutathione, expanded lipid peroxidation, and an increment in serum creatinine levels. The allowing of curcumin or selenium alone did not expand lipid peroxidation contrasted with the benchmark group. Three days after curcumin or selenium in addition to cisplatin medicines, the renal harm initiated by cisplatin didn't recuperate at a critical measurable level. This examination recommends that the regular cancer prevention agent's curcumin or selenium did not offer security against cisplatin-actuated nephrotoxicity and lipid peroxidation in grown-up Wistar rodents.

The formation of free radicals in the kidney cortex assumes a significant part in the pathogenesis of gentamicin (GM) nephrotoxicity, and curcumin has been affirmed to have a solid cancer prevention agent activity. Along these lines, Ali *et al*. [29] pointed toward testing the conceivable defensive or palliative impact of curcumin on GM nephrotoxicity. Curcumin was given to rodents at an oral portion of 200 mg/kg/day for ten days. GM was additionally infused intramuscularly at a dose of 80 mg/kg/day during the most recent six days of the treatment is a part of these rodents. Nephrotoxicity was assessed histopathologically by light microscopy and biochemically by estimating the centralizations of creatinine and urea in serum, and diminished glutathione (GSH) fixation and SOD movement in the renal cortex. The grouping of GM in the renal cortex was estimated microbiologically. GM fundamentally expanded the convergences of urea and creatinine by around 111 and 97%, individually. GM treatment decreased cortical GSH focus by about 31% and the movement of SOD by about 27%. Curcumin essentially moderated these impacts. Segments from saline and curcumin-treated rodents showed typical proximal tubules.

Notwithstanding, the kidneys of GM-treated rodents had a moderate level of rot. The level of putrefaction seemed reduced when GM was given all the while with curcumin. The grouping of gentamicin in the renal cortex of the rodents given gentamicin along with curcumin was lower than that gentamicin alone. The outcomes recommended that curcumin had enhanced the histopathological and biochemical records of nephrotoxicity in rodents.

Constant hyperglycemia in diabetes prompts the overproduction of free radicals, and the proof is expanding that these add to the improvement of diabetic nephropathy. Sharma *et al*. [30] inspected the impact of curcumin on renal capacity and oxidative stress in streptozotocin (STZ)- prompted diabetic rodents. Streptozotocin-infused rodents showed critical expansions in blood glucose, polyuria, and abatement in body weight contrasted and age-coordinated with control rodents. Following a month and a half, diabetic rodents likewise showed renal brokenness, as confirmed by diminished creatinine and urea freedom and proteinuria, alongside a stamped expansion in oxidative pressure, as dictated by lipid peroxidation and exercises of antioxidant enzymes. Ongoing treatment with curcumin fundamentally lessened both renal brokenness and oxidative stress in diabetic rodents.

He *et al*. [31] assessed the renoprotective impacts of curcumin treatment in gentamicin-prompted AKI. The rodents treated with gentamicin showed stamped weakening of renal capacity, along with more significant levels of neutrophil gelatinase-related lipocalin (NGAL) and kidney injury molecule 1 (KIM-1) in the plasma as contrasted and the controls. Animals that went through irregular treatment with curcumin showed critical upgrades in practical renal boundaries. Treatment with curcumin altogether lessened renal rounded harm, apoptosis, and oxidative stress. Curcumin treatment applied anti-apoptosis and against oxidative impacts by up-directing Nrf2/HO-1 and Sirt1 articulation. Their information exhibits that curcumin shields the kidney from gentamicin-actuated AKI by enhancing oxidative pressure and apoptosis of renal cylindrical cells, hence giving a desire to improve gentamicin-prompted nephrotoxicity.

Hashish and Elgaml [32] assessed the hepatoprotective and nephroprotective action of curcumin against copper harmfulness in rodents. Changes were seen in hepatic marker chemicals like AST, ALT, ALP, and GGT, other than the complete serum protein, urea, and creatinine. The centralization of liver and kidney cell reinforcements like CAT, SOD, diminished GS), and MDA was estimated. An expansion in liver marker proteins, urea, creatinine, and the MDA substance was identified after openness to $CuSO_4$. Then, the exercises of serum all-out protein, hepatic and renal cell reinforcements were diminished. The post-treatment and co-treatment of curcumin lightened changes in all biochemical boundaries.

Ismail *et al.* [33] researched the nephroprotective impact of curcumin against acetaminophen (APAP)- actuated nephrotoxicity in rodents. APAP-prompted nephrotoxicity was evident by a huge increment of lipid peroxidation as MDA, NO, PC substance, and IL-1β. In addition, TNFα, joined by a considerable decline in SOD, CAT, GPx exercises, and GSH content, were seen in the kidney tissues. Furthermore, the cytochrome P2E1 (CYP2E1) and inducible nitric oxide synthase (iNOS) quality articulation proportions showed a critical rise in the kidney tissues. Oral allow of curcumin (100 mg/kg,b.wt.) improved these unfriendly impacts and showed nephroprotective action against APAP harmfulness. The nephroprotective movement of curcumin could be ascribed to the renal cancer prevention agent balance guideline, the down-guideline of CYP2E1 and iNOS gene articulations, and the improvement of IL-1β and TNF-α level.

Alkuraishy *et al.* [34] assessed the nephroprotective impact of curcumin in gentamicin-initiated nephrotoxicity. Rodents treated with gentamicin showed nephrotoxicity confirmed by a critical height in serum creatinine, blood urea, KIM-1, MDA, cystatin-C sera levels. Curcumin treatment prompts a considerable decrease of blood urea, serum creatinine contrasted, and the gentamicin bunch. Curcumin likewise decreased MDA, KIM-1, and cystatin-C sera levels altogether contrasted with and gentamicin group.

Curcumin and α-Tocopherol

Palipoch *et al.* [35] researched the conceivable defensive role of curcumin and α-tocopherol against cisplatin-actuated nephrotoxicity in rodents. Pre-treatment with joined curcumin and α-tocopherol displayed altogether decreased MDA levels and upgraded exercises of SOD and catalase contrasted and the cisplatin-treated gathering. It improved BUN just as creatinine levels and kidney histopathology. In addition, quality articulations of NADPH oxidase were diminished, though p38-MAPK quality articulations were not huge contrasted and the cisplatin-treated gathering. Consolidated curcumin and α-tocopherol can decrease cisplatin-instigated nephrotoxicity through the conceivable restraint of NADPH oxidase, bringing about kidney capacity and histology progress.

Diosmin

Diosmin is chemically diosmetin 7-O-rutinoside, a flavone glycoside found in *Teucrium gnaphalodes* L'Her. (Lamiaceae), and also isolated from citrus peels [36]. In neuronal cells, mitigating and against apoptotic exercises of diosmin have been as of now announced. In a recent animal study, kidney weight, urinary pH, all-out urinary protein, urinary calcium, phosphorus, serum potassium, sodium, magnesium, creatinine, uric acid, and blood urea nitrogen levels (hazard variables of stone arrangement) altogether diminished. In contrast, urinary volume, urinary magnesium, potassium, sodium, creatinine, uric acid, and serum calcium levels (inhibitors of stone development) surprisingly expanded in two diosmin gatherings at 0.75% v/v EG + 2% w/v NH_4Cl^+ diosmin 10 or 20 mg/kg bw for 15 days when contrasted with the gathering just treated with EG and NH_4Cl [37]. It appeared to be that the counter urolithiatic action of diosmin was like the standard medication cystone, and the group deciphered this to its cell reinforcement, mitigating impacts just as defensive consequences of microcirculation

Edarabone

Satoh *et al.* [38] explored the impacts of a novel free radical scavenger, 3-methy--1-phenyl-pyrazolin-5-one called edarabone, on murine proximal rounded cell (PTC) harm incited by openness to cisplatin *in vitro* and on renal capacity in an *in vivo* model of cisplatin-instigated intense renal disappointment. Edarabone restrained cisplatin-prompted (40 μM, 24 h) cytotoxicity in a concentration-dependent way (10^{-5} to 10^{-3} M). Edarabone additionally constricted cisplatin-actuated mitochondrial transmembrane likely misfortune and ROS creation of PTCs. In the *in vivo* study, male Wistar rodents were cotreated with cisplatin at 5 mg/kg, i.p. and edarabone at 1 or 5 mg/kg, i.v. Impacts of edarabone on the kidney were analyzed five days after treatment. Cisplatin brought about renal brokenness, renal rounded harm, mitochondrial harm, renal protein oxidation, and cylindrical apoptosis. The above changes were constricted by edarabone treatment. Along these lines, edarabone displayed cytoprotective impacts in PTCs and renoprotective impacts against cisplatin.

Ellagic Acid

Atessahin *et al.* [39] researched the conceivable defensive part of antioxidant therapy with ellagic acid on cisplatin-incited nephrotoxicity utilizing biochemical and histopathological approaches. Grown-up male Sprague-Dawley rodents were being used for the investigation. Allowing cisplatin to rodents instigated a checked renal disappointment, described by huge expansions in plasma creatinine, urea, and calcium focuses. Cisplatin likewise initiated oxidative pressure, as shown by expanded kidney tissue groupings of MDA and lowered GSH peroxidase and catalase exercises. Besides, treatment with cisplatin caused checked rounded rot, degeneration and desquamation, luminal cast development, karyomegaly, cylindrical dilatation, interstitial mononuclear cell penetration, and between rounded haemorrhagia. Ellagic acid uniquely decreased raised levels of urea, calcium, and creatinine and balanced the detrimental impacts of cisplatin on oxidative pressure markers. Similarly, ellagic acid improved cisplatin-prompted obsessive changes, including cylindrical corruption, degeneration, karyomegaly, rounded dilatation when contrasted with the cisplatin alone group.

Epicatechin

By the similar structural activities, epicatechin can repress renal calculi like catechin too. Unequivocally, Grases *et al.* [40] analyzed that treatment with epicatechin at a dose of 100 mg/L in drinking water for a period of 24 days adequately forestalled the formation of intratubular calcification in the kidneys of rodents enhanced with 0.8% v/v EG in addition to 1% w/v NH_4Cl over the most recent eight days. The outcomes may be ascribed with the impacts of epicatechin on keeping away from hyperoxaluria-prompted peroxidative harm to kidney tissues and the papillary tip epithelium, additionally smother the development of kidney stones [41].

Esculentoside A

Esculentoside A (EsA) extracted from the Indian pokeweed balances the invulnerable reaction, cell multiplication, and apoptosis just as calming impacts. Acute kidney injury (AKI) is a significant clinical issue related to high bleakness and mortality. Chen *et al.* [42] examined the defensive impacts of EsA on LPS-prompted AKI in mice. The defensive impacts of EsA were assessed by recognizing kidney histological change, creatinine and BUN levels, and incendiary cytokine creation. The outcomes showed that EsA altogether weakened LPS-instigated kidney histological change, just as BUN and creatinine levels. EsA additionally hindered LPS-incited TNF-α, IL-1β, and IL-6 creation.

The treatment of EsA essentially stifled LPS-prompted NF-κB enactment. Likewise, EsA up-managed the declaration of PPAR-γ in a dose-dependent way. EsA shielded mice adequately from LPS-actuated AKI by PPAR-γ, which therefore hindered LPS-initiated incendiary reaction.

Ferulic Acid

Ferulic acid, chemically (2E)-3-(4-hydroxy-3-methoxyphenyl)prop-2-enoic acid found in plant cell walls and phenolic. Zhao *et al.* [43] assessed the counter urolithiatic impact of ferulate on ethylene glycol-actuated kidney stones in a rodent model. Five groups of grown-up male Sprague-Dawley rodents (6 rodents in each group) were utilized in this examination. G-I rodents filled in as expected control. Renal analytics was instigated through ethylene glycol at 0.75% v/v in drinking water to all rodents for 28 days aside from those in G-I. Before ethylene glycol treatment, ferulate was given orally to rodents in G-III and IV at portions of 40 and 80 mg/kg, separately. Rodents in G-V (positive control) were treated with standard medication, cystone at a part of 750 mg/kg before ethylene glycol administration, while G-II rodents got no treatment. Kidney tissue and blood serum were tested following 28 days and utilized for biochemical and histopathological investigations. Rodents in G-II showed critical expansions in oxidative pressure design, as seen in huge decreases in GSH, SOD, GPx, and CAT levels, and a considerable rise in lipid peroxidation (LPO), compared with the ordinary benchmark group.

Notwithstanding, renal analytics arrangement and oxidative pressure were fundamentally restrained by ferulate treatment in G-III and IV. Histopathological discoveries upheld these outcomes. Ferulate applies anti-urolithiatic impact through restraint of oxidative stress.

Sepsis-incited intense kidney injury is liable for 70-80% mortality in escalated care patients because of raised degrees of endotoxin, Lipopolysaccharide (LPS) brought about by gram-negative contaminations. Mir *et al.* [44] examined the impact of ferulate on LPS-prompted acute kidney injury in mice models and comprehend the defensive action required to give proof to ferulate in the treatment of kidney injury. BALB/c mice were treated with ferulate at 50 mg/kg and 100 mg/kg doses after LPS incitement (10 mg/kg). Toward the finish of the mediation, the creators decided the convergences of serum creatinine and blood urea nitrogen, provocative cytokines, and histopathological changes in creatures. Additionally, the overall protein articulation level of the TLR4 interceded NF-κB flagging pathway was concentrated in kidney tissues. Ferulate-treated mice showed upregulation of antioxidant defenses and concealment of fiery occasions by repressing TLR-4 interceded NFκB actuation. Be that as it may, LPS alone managed bunch, brought about immediate renal harm with expanded degrees of blood urea nitrogen, a humble expansion in creatinine, diminished cell reinforcement protections, and the arrival of incendiary cytokines. The histopathological examination likewise uncovered the defensive activity of the ferulate against sepsis-initiated fibrosis and renal harm.

Flavocoxid

Flavocoxid, a medicated mixture having flavonoids like baicalin, extricated from *Scutellaria baicalensis*, and catechin from *Acacia catechu*, showed a solid and intense cell reinforcement action. The action of flavocoxid on the morphological and biochemical changes instigated *in vivo* by Cd in mice kidney was assessed by Micali *et al.* [45]. Cd treatment alone essentially expanded urea nitrogen and creatinine, iNOS, MMP-9, and pERK 1/2 articulation and protein carbonyl; decreased GSH, GR, and GPx; and initiated primary and ultrastructural changes in the glomeruli and the cylindrical epithelium. Following 14 days of treatment, flavocoxid supply decreased urea nitrogen and creatinine, iNOS, MMP-9, and pERK 1/2 articulation and protein carbonyl; expanded GSH, GR, and GPx; and showed clear safeguarding of the glomerular and rounded construction and ultrastructure.

Ginsenosides from *Panax Ginseng*

Panax ginseng is extraordinary; its constituents upgrade renal capacity. Identification of its viability and components of activity against drug-incited nephrotoxicity, just as the particular constituents intervening this impact, have as of late arose as a fascinating exploration region zeroing in on the kidney defensive adequacy of *P. ginseng*.

Ginsenosides, the remarkable constituents and auxiliary metabolites of the *Panax* species, have been known to be the pharmacologically dynamic elements of ginseng. Baek *et al.* [46] have fostered another prepared ginseng, called Sun ginseng (SG), which has an expanded measure of the red ginseng special ginsenosides (RGUG). This newly prepared ginseng diminished cisplatin-actuated nephrotoxicity more than white ginseng in both *in vitro* and *in vivo* frameworks in their past examinations. Baek *et al.* [47] confined and described dynamic standards through action-guided fractionation. Ginsenosides Rh4 and Rk3 altogether diminished the cisplatin-prompted nephrotoxicity in LLC-PK1 cells in a portion subordinate way [46].

Park *et al.* [48] explored the impact of microwave-helped preparing on the defensive impact of ginseng and recognize ginsenosides that are dynamic against cisplatin-actuated kidney harm to assess the capability of utilizing ginseng in the administration of nephrotoxicity. The LLC-PK1 cell harm by cisplatin was essentially diminished by treatment with microwave-handled ginseng (MG) and ginsenosides Rg3, Rg5, and Rk1. Diminished articulation of p53 and c-Jun N-terminal kinase proteins by cisplatin in LLC-PK1 cells was uniquely improved after Rg3 and Rg5/Rk1 treatment. Furthermore, raised articulation of divided caspase-3 was essentially decreased by ginsenosides Rg5, Rk1, and significantly more noteworthy power, Rg3. Besides, MG and its division containing dynamic ginsenosides showed defensive impacts against cisplatin-prompted nephropathy in mice. Creators found ginsenosides Rg3, Rg5, and Rk1 produced during the warmth treatment of ginseng improve renal harm by managing aggravation and apoptosis.

Han *et al.* [49] examined the kidney defensive impact of fermented black ginseng (FBG) and its active part ginsenoside 20(S)- Rg3 against cisplatin-prompted harm in pig kidney (LLC-PK1) cells. It zeroed in on surveying the role of mitogen-actuated protein kinases as significant components in kidney security. The decreased cell suitability initiated by cisplatin was fundamentally recuperated with FBG removal and ginsenoside 20(S)- Rg3 portion conditionally. The cisplatin-prompted raised protein levels of phosphorylated c-Jun N-terminal kinase (JNK), p53, and separated caspase-3 were diminished after cotreatment with FBG extricates or ginsenoside 20(S)- Rg3. The raised level of apoptotic LLC-PK1 cells incited by cisplatin treatment was essentially revoked by cotreatment with FBG and the ginsenoside 20(S)- Rg3. FBG and its major ginsenoside 20(S)- Rg3 improved cisplatin-incited nephrotoxicity in LLC-PK1 cells by impeding the JNK-p53-caspase-3 flagging cascade.

Li *et al.* [50] investigated the likely defensive impact of ginsenoside Rg5, an uncommon ginsenoside produced during steaming ginseng, on cisplatin-initiated nephrotoxicity in a mouse test model. The potential systems fundamental this nephroprotective impact were additionally researched. Rg5 was given at portions of 10 and 20 mg/kg for 10 successive days. On Day 7, a solitary nephrotoxic portion of cisplatin (25 mg/kg) was infused to mice. Cisplatin administration brought about renal brokenness as proven by expansion in serum creatinine and blood urea nitrogen (BUN) levels. What's more, cisplatin expanded the degree of MDA and 4-hydroxynonenal (4-HNE), the creators of lipid peroxidation, and drained glutathione (GSH) substance and SOD movement in renal tissues. These impacts were related to the fundamentally expanded degrees of cytochrome P450 E1 (CYP2E1), 4-hydroxynonenal (4-HNE), tumor rot factor (TNF)- α, interleukin (IL)- 1β, atomic factor-kappa B (NF-κB) p65, and cyclooxygenase-2 (COX-2) in renal tissues. Be that as it may, pretreatment with ginsenoside Rg5 essentially lessened the renal brokenness, oxidative stress, and aggravation reaction incited by cisplatin. Moreover, ginsenoside Rg5 supplementation repressed apoptotic pathways by expanding Bcl-2 and diminishing Bax articulation levels. The histopathological assessment further affirmed the nephroprotective impact of Rg5. On the whole, these outcomes propose that Rg5-intervened easing of cisplatin-prompted nephrotoxicity might be identified with its antioxidant, hostile to apoptotic and mitigating effects.

Baek *et al.* [46] assessed the defensive impact of ginsenosides Rk3 and Rh4 on kidney works and explain their cancer prevention impact utilizing *in vitro* and *in vivo* models of cisplatin-incited intense renal disappointment. The *in vitro* test showed that KG-KH (50 µg/mL) essentially expanded cell reasonability (4.6-crease), SOD action (2.8-overlap), and glutathione reductase action (1.5-overlay); however, diminished responsive oxygen species age (56%) contrasted with cisplatin control cells. KG-KH (6 mg/kg, per os) likewise essentially restrained renal edema (87% kidney file) and brokenness (71.4% blood urea nitrogen, 67.4% creatinine) contrasted with cisplatin control rodents. Of note, KG-KH fundamentally recuperated the kidney levels of catalase (1.2-crease) and SOD (1.5-overlay).

Ginsenosides from *Panax vietnamensis*

Vu-Huynh *et al.* [51] tracked down that steamed Vietnamese ginseng (*Panax vietnamensis*) could fundamentally diminish the kidney harm of cisplatin in an *in vitro* model utilizing porcine proximal rounded LLC-PK1 kidney cells. From handled ginseng under advanced conditions (120 °C, 12 h), creators disconnected seven mixtures (20(R,S)- ginsenoside Rh2, 20(R,S)- ginsenoside Rg3, ginsenoside Rk1, ginsenoside-Rg5, and ocotillol genin) that showed kidney-defensive potential against cisplatin harmfulness. By contrasting the half recuperation focus (RC50), the R type of ginsenoside, Rh2, and Rg3, had RC50 upsides of 6.67 ± 0.42 µM Vu-Huynh *et al.* [51] tracked down that steamed Vietnamese ginseng (Panax vietnamensis) could altogether lessen the kidney harm of cisplatin in an *in vitro* model utilizing porcine proximal cylindrical LLC-PK1 kidney cells. From handled ginseng under enhanced conditions (120 °C, 12 h), creators disconnected seven mixtures (20(R,S)- ginsenoside Rh2, 20(R,S)-ginsenoside Rg3, ginsenoside Rk1, ginsenoside-Rg5, and ocotillol genin) that showed kidney-defensive potential against cisplatin harmfulness. By looking at the half recuperation focus (RC50), the R type of ginsenoside, Rh2 and Rg3, had RC50 upsides of 6.67 ± 0.42 µM and 8.39 ± 0.3 µM, individually, while the S types of ginsenoside, Rh2 and Rg3, and Rk1, had more fragile defensive impacts, with RC50 going from 46.15 to 88.4 µM. G-Rg5 and ocotillol, the normal saponin of Vietnamese ginseng, had the most noteworthy RC50 (180.83 ± 33.27; 226.19 ± 66.16, individually). Prepared Vietnamese gingseng (PVG), just as those mixtures, can improve kidney harm due to cisplatin toxicity. And 8.39 ± 0.3 µM, individually, while the S types of ginsenoside, Rh2 and Rg3, and Rk1, had more fragile defensive impacts, with RC50 going from 46.15 to 88.4 µM. G-Rg5 and ocotillol, the commonplace saponin of Vietnamese ginseng, had the most noteworthy RC50 (180.83 ± 33.27; 226.19 ± 66.16, individually). Prepared Vietnamese gingseng (PVG), just as those mixtures, can improve kidney harm due to cisplatin's harmfulness.

Glycyrrhizin (or Glycyrrhizic Acid or Glycyrrhizinic Acid)

Polyuria in rodents with gentamicin-initiated intense renal disappointment was related to the down-guideline of renal aquaporin 2 in the internal and external renal medulla, and cortex. Glycyrrhizin at 200 mg/kg/day permitted reestablished the statement of aquaporin 2 with resembled changes in urine yield. The progressions in renal utilitarian boundaries (creatinine leeway, urinary osmolality, and sans solute reabsorption), going with intense renal disappointment, were mostly reestablished after glycyrrhizin organization. Histological changes in rodents with gentamicin-actuated extreme renal disappointment were likewise repealed by glycyrrhizin therapy [52].

Glycyrrhizic acid (GA) additionally reduced sepsis-incited intense kidney injury by improving the neurotic changes, diminishing the degrees of blood urea nitrogen, creatinine, and expanding the endurance pace of rodents with AKI altogether. The creation of incendiary cytokines, like TNF-α, IL-1β, and IL-6, was especially repressed by GA. Besides, GA repressed the result of nitric oxide and prostaglandin E2 and articulation levels of instigated nitric oxide synthase and cyclooxygenase-2 in kidney tissues. GA likewise stifled the apoptosis in kidney tissue prompted by AKI and hindered the initiation of the NF-κB flagging pathway [53].

7-Hydroxy-4'-Methoxyisoflavone and 7-Hydroxy-2',4', 5'-Trimethoxyiso flavone and From Kidneywood Tree *Eysenhardtia Polystachya*

The diuretic and antilithiatic action of 7-hydroxy-4'-methoxyisoflavone and 7-hydroxy-2',4',5'-trimethoxyisoflavone was investigated by Perez *et al.* [54] in rodents by noticing stone development (tentatively initiated by implantation of a zinc plate in the urinary bladder) and urine production. A critical lessening in urinary stone size was seen in rodents treated with the mixtures as contrasted and animals in the control group. The mixtures additionally raised 24 h urine volume in rodents as contrasted with the control creatures not getting the test compounds.

Hyperin

Hyperin (quercetin-3-glucoside) is chemically 2-(3,4-Dihydroxyphenyl)--,7-dihydroxy-4-oxo-4H-chromen-3-yl D-glucopyranoside, a flavonoid from families of Guttiferae, Ericaceae, and Celastraceae that has been appeared to have different natural impacts, for example, anticancer, antioxidant and anti-inflammatory etc. Gong *et al.* [55] examined the defensive impacts and effect of hyperin on LPS-incited AKI in mice. ELISA technique is used for the measurement of TNF-α, IL-6, and IL-1β levels. The impacts of hyperin on blood urea nitrogen (BUN) and serum creatinine were likewise distinguished. Moreover, the declaration of TLR4, NF-κB, and NLRP3 was recognized by western blot technique. The outcomes showed that hyperin altogether restrained LPS-incited TNF-α, IL-6, and IL-1β creation. The degrees of BUN and creatinine were additionally stifled by hyperin. Moreover, LPS-initiated TLR4 articulation and NF-κB actuation were likewise repressed by hyperin. Also, treatment of hyperin portion conditionally restrained LPS-actuated NLRP3 flagging pathway

Kaempferol

It is a natural flavonoid. Langeswaran *et al.* [56] assessed the restorative ramifications of kaempferol on histopathological and ultrastructural changes against mercuric chloride (HgCl$_2$)- instigated nephrotoxicity in a rodent model. Kaempferol at a dose of 100 mg/kg b.w orally was allowed once every day until the finish of the examination (45 days post-acceptance of nephrotoxicity) to HgCl$_2$-actuated nephrotoxicity in rodents. Toward the finish of the exploratory period, urinary marker chemicals, lipid profile, histopathological, and electron microscopical examinations were evaluated in control and experimental animals. HgCl$_2$ - inebriation showed modified degrees of lipid profiles, a critical decrease in urinary marker catalysts in renal cells, and harm in renal tissues, which sign the HgCl$_2$-incited nephrotoxicity. The treatment with kaempferol standardized the modified degrees of urinary marker compounds, lipid boundaries, histopathology, as wells as electron microscopical changes brought about by HgCl$_2$.

RhoA/Rho-related snaked loop framing protein serine/threonine kinase (ROCK) has shown up as a possible remedial objective in various infections due to its forestalling activity on different chemicals giving cell reinforcement and cytoprotective activity. Movement and pathophysiology of diabetic nephropathy have additionally shown likely inclusion of oxidative stress and inflammatory pathways. Sharma *et al.* [57] researched the impact of kaempferol on hyperglycemia-prompted enactment of RhoA kinase and related provocative flagging course. The creators zeroed in on examining sub-atomic systems for kaempferol through *in vitro* testing, utilizing rodents (NRK-52E) and human renal rounded epithelial cells (RPTEC). Kaempferol repressed hyperglycemia-actuated initiation of RhoA and diminished oxidative stress, favorable to inflammatory cytokines (TNF-α and IL-1β) and fibrosis (TGF-β1 articulation, extracellular grid protein articulation) NRK-52E and RPTEC cells.

Kolaviron

Kolaviron is a biflavonoid from seeds of Bitter kola (*Garcinia kola*). Ayepola *et al.* [58] assessed the renal defensive impact kolaviron (KV), a seed extract having a combination of five flavonoids, in diabetes-incited nephrotoxic rodents. In the diabetic rodents, adjustments in cell reinforcement guards like an increment in lipid peroxidation, glutathione peroxidase (GPX) movement, and a decline in catalase (CAT) action, glutathione (GSH) levels and oxygen extremist absorbance limit (ORAC) were noticed. There was no distinction in the SOD movement. Diabetes enlistment expanded apoptotic cell demise and the degrees of interleukin (IL)- 1β and tumor corruption factor (TNF)- α with no impact on IL-10. KV treatment of diabetic rodents reestablished the exercises of cell reinforcement catalysts, diminished lipid peroxidation, and expanded ORAC and GSH focus in renal tissues. KV treatment of diabetic rodents likewise smothered renal IL-1β. The advantageous impacts of kolaviron on diabetes-incited kidney injury might be its inhibitory activity on oxidative pressure, IL-1β creation, and apoptosis.

Alabi *et al.* [59] and Alabi and Akomolafe [60] researched the defensive role of KV against Diclofenac (DF)- actuated hepatic and renal harmfulness in rodents. Diclofenac caused massive expansion in the plasma levels of creatinine and urea and exercises of liver proteins, including bilirubin level, favorable to provocative markers, and plasma prostaglandin E2 (PGE2). It likewise caused a considerable modification in renal and hepatic PGE2, lipid peroxidation, cell reinforcements, and hematological lists. These poisonous impacts were affirmed by histological examinations and levels of provocative penetration (myeloperoxidase). In any case, KV essentially forestalled or diminished the unfavorable impacts of DF in the plasma, liver, and kidney of the rodents pretreated with KV before DF administration.

Licochalcone A

Licochalcone A, a natural phenol isolated from the roots of licorice (*Glycyrrhiza glabra*), has been accounted for its anti-cancer, anti-inflammatory, and antimalarial actions. Utilizing a mouse model of LPS-initiated AKI, Hu and Liu [61] examined the defensive impacts and activity of Licochalcone A on LPS-instigated AKI in mice. LPS-incited kidney injury was surveyed by identifying kidney histological investigation, blood urea nitrogen (BUN), and creatinine levels. ELISA identified the creation of inflammatory cytokines TNF-α, IL-6, and

IL-1β in serum and kidney tissues. The western blot technique estimated the initiation of NF-κB. Licochalcone A conditionally lessened LPS-prompted kidney histopathologic changes, serum BUN, and creatinine levels. Licochalcone A likewise stifled LPS-incited TNF-α, IL-6, and IL-1β creation both in serum and kidney tissues. Moreover, Licochalcone A essentially repressed LPS-initiated NF-κB enactment.

Lipoic Acid

Lipoic acid is an organosulfur constituent from octanoic acid used in the treatment of diabetic neuropathy. Adriamycin, which is generally utilized in the treatment of different neoplastic conditions, applies harmful consequences for a few organs. Adriamycin nephrotoxicity has been as of late recorded in an assortment of animal models. Malarlodi *et al.* [62] examined the impact of lipoic acid on the nephrotoxic capability of Adriamycin. The examination was completed for albino rats. Intravenous infusions of Adriamycin brought about diminished exercises of the glycolytic catalysts; hexokinase, phosphoglucoisomerase, aldolase and lactate dehydrogenase in the rodent renal tissue. The gluconeogenic catalysts, glucose-6-phosphatase and fructose-1,6-diphosphatase, showed a decrease in their exercises on adriamycin administration. The transmembrane catalysts, specifically the Na^+, K^+-ATPase, Ca^{2+}-ATPase, Mg^{2+}-ATPase, and the brush-line compound ALP, showed lessening in their practices. This decline in the exercises of ATPases and ALP recommends basolateral and brush-line layer harm. Diminished activities of the TCA cycle catalysts isocitrate dehydrogenase, succinate dehydrogenase, and malate dehydrogenase propose a misfortune in mitochondrial capacity and trustworthiness. Nephrotoxicity was apparent from the expanded discharges of N-acetyl-beta-D-glucosaminidase and gamma-glutamyl transferase in the pee of Adriamycin-managed rodents. These unsettling biochemical influences were adequately neutralized on pre-treatment with lipoic acid, which achieved an increment in the exercises of glycolytic chemicals, ATPases, and the TCA cycle proteins. Then again, the gluconeogenic chemicals showed a further diminishing in their exercises on lipoic acid pretreatment. LA pretreatment likewise reestablished the conditioning of the urinary compounds to typical.

Lupeol

It is also known as Fagarasterol, a pentacyclic triterpenoid from many plants like *Mangifera indica, Parasenegalia visco, Camellia japonica,* etc., having a variety of pharmacological actions, including anti-urolithiasis. Anand *et al.* [63] isolated lupeol from *C. nurvala*. Antiurolithiatic action of lupeol was evaluated in rodents by noticing the weight of the stone, biochemical examination of serum and urine, and histopathology of bladder and kidney. Lupeol forestalled the development of vesical calculi as well as decreased the size of the preformed stones.

Examinations were attempted by Malini *et al.* [64] to contemplate the role of lupeol in CaOx experimental rodent urolithiasis. A 2% ammonium oxalate solution was managed by gastric intubation for prompting hyperoxaluric conditions in grown-up male rodents of Wistar strain. The span of treatment was for 15 days. This brought about expanded urinary discharge of oxalate related to a decrease in citrate and glycosaminoglycans. The urinary marker chemicals which show renal tissue harm, specifically - lactate dehydrogenase, inorganic pyrophosphatase, ALP, gamma-glutamyl transferase, beta-glucuronidase, and N-acetyl beta-D glucosaminidase, were discovered to be raised. Administration of Lupeol at 25 mg/kg body weight/day diminished the renal discharge of oxalate. It additionally declined the degree of renal cylindrical harm as proven by the diminished levels of the above-said enzymes in urine. Such a decrease will probably be gainful in limiting the affidavit of stone-shaping constituents in the kidney, which gives the antilithiatic impact.

The cytoprotective activity of lupeol obtained from the stem bark of *C. nurvala* against free toxic radicals has been researched by Baskar *et al.* [65]. Glycolate, an inducer of stone deposition, fundamentally raised the renal tissue levels of calcium, oxalate, phosphorus, and magnesium in calculogenic rodents and achieved an astounding lessening in kidney oxalate level. The increment in lipid peroxidation and SOD activity, related to diminished catalase action and glutathione (GSH) level, is the remarkable highlights seen in tissues of stone framing rodents. Thus, lupeol administration instigated a great diminishing in kidney oxalate level. Furthermore, it was compelling in balancing the free extreme harmfulness by achieving a critical lessening in peroxidative levels and an expansion in cancer prevention agent status.

Sudhakar *et al.* [66] investigated the efficacy of lupeol and its ester lupeol linoleate in trial hyperoxaluria. Hyperoxaluria was incited in male Wistar rodents with 0.75% ethylene glycol in drinking water for 28 days. An increment in an oxidative milieu in hyperoxaluria was apparent by expanded lipid peroxidation (LPO) and diminished enzymic and non-enzymic cell reinforcements. The lessening in the exercises of renal catalysts exemplified the harm initiated by oxalate, which is associated emphatically with expanded LPO and expanded oxalate amalgamation. The microscopic renal examination further stressed the oxalate-prompted harm. These biochemical and histological abnormalities were constricted with test compound treatment.

Administration of lupeol, betulin to hyperoxaluric rodents limited the tubular damage and decreased the markers of stone formation in the kidneys. In this association, lupeol was discovered to be more viable than betulin [67].

Vidya *et al*. [68] assessed the viability of lupeol and its ester, lupeol linoleate, against CaOx urolithiasis in rodents. Allowing pyridoxine lacking diet regimen having 3% glycolate for 21 days prompted expanded discharge of stone shaping constituents like calcium, uric acid, and oxalate. Stone formation and ensuing renal tubular harm brought about expanded discharge of ALP, gamma-glutamyl transferase, lactate dehydrogenase, beta-glucuronidase, and N-acetyl glucosaminidase alongside decreased fibrinolytic proteins. A decrease in the urinary inhibitory variables magnesium and glycosaminoglycans was likewise noticed. Treatment with lupeol and lupeol linoleate reduced the degree of tubular harm as confirmed from diminished enzymuria and limited the discharge of stone shaping constituents.

Luteolin

Luteolin is a 3',4',5,7-Tetrahydroxyflavone extracted from *Reseda luteola* L, having a reported antioxidant activity. Domitrović *et al*. [69] explored the impacts of luteolin against cisplatin (CP)-incited kidney injury in mice. Luteolin at dosages of 10mg/kg was managed intraperitoneally when day by day for three days following a single i.p. infusion of CP at 10 or 20 mg/kg. Mice were forfeited 24h after the last portion of luteolin. The CP treatment essentially expanded serum creatinine and blood urea nitrogen and instigated pathohistological changes in the kidneys. Renal oxidative/nitrosative stress was confirmed by diminished glutathione levels and grew 4-hydroxynonenal and 3-nitrotyrosine arrangement just as CYP2E1 articulation. The CP organization set off an incendiary reaction in mice kidneys through the initiation of atomic factor-NF-κB and overexpression of tumor rot factor-alpha (TNF-α) and cyclooxygenase-2 (COX-2). At the same time, the expansion in renal p53 and caspase-3 articulation showed apoptosis of cylindrical cells. The administration of luteolin fundamentally diminished histological and biochemical changes prompted by CP, diminished platinum levels, and smothered oxidative/nitrosative pressure, irritation, and apoptosis in the kidneys. These outcomes propose that luteolin is a viable nephroprotective specialist, potentially decreasing Pt aggregation in the kidneys and enhancing CP-prompted nephrotoxicity.

Lycopene

Lycopene is a carotenoid hydrocarbon generally extracted from tomatoes, carrots, papaya, etc. Atessahin *et al*. [70] examined the impacts of lycopene on cisplatin-prompted nephrotoxicity and oxidative stress in Sprague-Dawley rodents.

Permitted intake of cisplatin to rodents incited a significant renal disappointment, described by a critical expansion in plasma creatinine and urea focuses. Na^+ and K^+ levels of rodents who got cisplatin alone were not altogether unique contrasted with the benchmark group; however, they had higher kidney MDA, and lower decrease glutathione focuses glutathione peroxidase and catalase exercises. Lycopene administration created enhancement in biochemical files of nephrotoxicity in both plasma and kidney tissues when contrasted with bunch 2; pre-treatment with lycopene being more assertive.

Karahan *et al*. [71] researched the conceivable defensive impacts of lycopene against gentamicin-instigated renal harm in male Sprague-Dawley rodents. Permitted intake of gentamicin to rodents actuated a checked renal disappointment, described by a critical expansion in plasma creatinine and urea fixations. The animals treated with gentamicin alone showed a fundamentally higher kidney MDA and lower GSH-Px an.d CAT exercises yet unaffected GSH focuses when contrasted and the benchmark group. Pre-treatment with lycopene created an improvement in biochemical lists of nephrotoxicity in plasma. In any case, little changes were seen in the kidney MDA and GSH levels and GSH-Px and CAT exercises when contrasted and the gentamicin treated gathering. The histological designs of the proximal renal tubules showed comparative examples. Then again, administration of synchronous lycopene to rodents delivered enhancement in MDA and GSH levels and GSH-Px and CAT exercises when contrasted and gentamicin bunch. Furthermore, synchronous lycopene was found to lessen the level of kidney tissue harm in histopathological discoveries. These outcomes show that particularly synchronous lycopene treatment may have enhanced biochemical files and oxidative pressure boundaries against gentamicin-initiated nephrotoxicity; however, pre-medicines with lycopene had no gainful consequences for these boundaries.

Yilmaz *et al*. [72] examined the conceivable defensive role of lycopene on Adriamycin (ADR)-actuated heart and kidney harmfulness utilizing biochemical and histopathological approaches. The degrees of MDA and decreased glutathione in both the heart and kidneys were higher in the animals treated with ADR alone than in the control group and were lower in the gatherings directed with lycopene than in the ADR alone gathering. Albeit catalase (CAT) action in the heart was higher in the ADR alone group than in the control group, it was lower in the kidneys. Specifically, treatment with lycopene post-infusion standardized both cardiovascular and kidney CAT exercises. In heart and kidney tissues, glutathione peroxidase (GSH-Px) exercises were not essentially extraordinary between all animal groups. Massive expansions in the degrees of plasma creatinine and urea were seen in the ADR bunch when contrasted with the control group, and these increments were standardized by lycopene treatment. Heart and renal histopathological changes were seen in the ADR group when contrasted with the normal group. Conversely, these histopathological changes showed up almost typical in the animals treated with lycopene pre-and post-infusion.

Madecassoside

Madecassoside is a pentacyclic triterpene obtained from *Hydrocotyle asiatica* L./*Centella asiatica*, shows various properties like antiinflammatory and antioxidative actions. Doxorubicin (DOX), a typical chemotherapeutic medication, has been accounted for to prompt mixed poisonous results, including renal harmfulness. Su *et al*. [73] explored this speculation by bringing Madecassoside and DOX into the culture of the Human Proximal Tubule Cells HK-2 and mice model. *in vivo* study exhibited that Madecassoside at 12mg/kg treatment for about fourteen days constricted DOX-prompted renal injury through securing renal capacity, recuperating antioxidant action, hindering Bax, p-ERK1/2, NF-κB p65, iNOS articulation, and expanding Bcl-2 articulation. Comparative discoveries were gotten *in vitro* concentrates with the treatment of DOX as well as Madecassoside. Further investigations with the use of iNOS inhibitor and ERK1/2 kinase inhibitor demonstrated that the inhibitory impacts of MA on DOX-actuated apoptosis and aggravation might be interceded by the concealment of the initiation of separated caspase-3, ERK1/2 pathways, NF-κB p65, and NO creation.

Naringin

Naringin is a 4',5,7-Trihydroxyflavanone-7-rhamnoglucoside found in citrus fruits. Fe-NTA, an iron chelate incites intense proximal tubular putrefaction as an outcome of lipid peroxidation and oxidative tissue harm that in the end prompts a high frequency of renal adenocarcinomas in rodents. Singh *et al*. [74] researched the impact of Naringin, with cancer prevention agent potential, on Fe-NT--instigated nephrotoxicity in rodents. One hour after a solitary intraperitoneal (i.p.) infusion of Fe-NTA at 8 mg iron/kg bw, a stamped weakening of renal design and renal capacity was noticed. Fe-NTA instigated a critical renal oxidative pressure, exhibited by raised thiobarbituric acid responding substances and decrease in exercises of renal catalase, SOD, and glutathione reductase. Pre-treatment of animals with Naringin, 60 min before Fe-NTA intake particularly lessened renal brokenness; morphological modifications diminished raised thiobarbituric acid reacting substances and reestablished the exhausted renal cell reinforcement proteins.

Rhabdomyolysis-initiated myoglobinuric intense renal disappointment represents around 10-40% of all instances of extreme renal disappointment. Responsive oxygen intermediates have been shown to assume an etiological part in myoglobinuric renal disappointment. Singh *et al*. [75] researched the impact of naringin with antioxidant potential in glycerol-incited ARF in rodents. Glycerol treatment brought about a significant renal oxidative stress and fundamentally unhinged the renal capacities. Pre-treatment of animals with naringin 60 min preceding glycerol infusion particularly lessened renal brokenness, morphological adjustments, diminished raised TBARS and re-established the exhausted renal antioxidant enzymes.

Prabu *et al*. [76] assessed the remedial adequacy of the consolidated pre-treatment with naringenin (NGN) mix with vitamin C, and E on Cd initiated oxidative nephrotoxicity in rodents. Consolidated pre-treatment of NGN in mix with Vit. C and E in Cd inebriated rodents standardized the serum and pee nephritic markers (urea, uric acid, and creatinine) and brought down the degree of renal oxidative stress markers like LOOH, TBARS, and PC. Moreover, they likewise expanded the degrees of renal non-enzymatic and enzymatic cell reinforcements. Also, their co-administration fundamentally improved the modified histopathological changes in the kidney of Cd inebriated rodents. From the outcomes, it was reasoned that the joined pre-treatment of NGN in a mix with Vit. C and E may be advantageous in treating Cd nephrotoxicity, and this defensive adequacy of these cancer prevention agents against Cd harmfulness is more articulated in their mixes instead of in their therapy routine.

Naringenin

Naringenin is 4',5,7-Trihydroxyflavan-4-one widely found in grapefruits. The impact of naringenin on the intense nephrotoxicity delivered by cisplatin at 7 mg/kg, i.v. was explored in the rodent by Badary *et al*. [77]. Oral permit of Naringenin at 20 mg/kg/day for ten days, beginning five days before cisplatin single i.v. infusion created significant protection of renal function. Naringenin diminished the degree of cisplatin-actuated nephrotoxicity, as proven by a huge decrease in serum urea and creatinine fixations, diminished polyuria, decrease in bodyweight reduction, checked decrease in urinary fragmentary sodium discharge and glutathione S-transferase movement, and expanded creatinine clearance. Cisplatin-prompted changes in renal cortex lipid peroxides and GST action were especially improved by naringenin. Cisplatin-actuated changes in the renal cortex cell reinforcement safeguard framework were extraordinarily forestalled by NAR. In cisplatin- naringenin joined treatment group, cancer prevention agent compounds, specifically SOD, glutathione peroxidase (GSH-Px), and catalase (CAT) were fundamentally expanded contrasted with cisplatin-treated animals. The platinum renal substance was not influenced by naringenin treatment.

Renugadevi and Prabu [78] examined the impacts of naringenin on Cd-prompted harmfulness in the kidney of rodents. In experimental rodents, the oral permit of cadmium chloride at 5 mg/kg/day for about a month essentially instigated renal harm, which was apparent from the expanded degrees of serum urea, uric acid, and creatinine massive decline in creatinine freedom. Cadmium additionally effectively diminished the degrees of urea, uric acid, and creatinine in urine. Notably expanded degrees of lipid peroxidation markers (thiobarbituric acid receptive substances and lipid hydroperoxides) and protein carbonyl substance with a critical abatement in non-enzymatic cell reinforcements (absolute sulfhydryl gatherings, diminished glutathione, nutrient C and nutrient E) and enzymatic cancer prevention agents (SOD, catalase (CAT), glutathione peroxidase (GPx) and glutathione S-transferase (GST)), just as glutathione using catalysts (glutathione reductase (GR) and glutathione-6-phosphate dehydrogenase (G6 PD)), were additionally seen in cadmium-treated rodents. Co-administration of naringenin at 25 and 50mg/kg/day alongside Cd brought about an inversion of Cd-incited biochemical changes in the kidney joined by a huge abatement in lipid peroxidation and an increment in the level of a renal cancer prevention agent protection framework. The histopathological concentrates in the kidney of rodents likewise showed that naringenin at 50mg/kg/day uniquely decreased the poisonousness of Cd and saved the normal histological design of the renal tissue.

Paeonol

Paenol is a phenolic constituent having numerous biological actions like anticancer, anti-inflammatory and antioxidant, etc. To decide the vital impact and action paeonol on intense kidney injury prompted by endotoxin, an intense kidney injury model was set up by Fan *et al.* [79] by intraperitoneal permit of lipopolysaccharide in mice *in vivo* and on LPS-initiated dendritic cells *in vitro*. Treatment of paeonol effectively cuts histopathological scores and weakens the convergences of blood urea nitrogen and serum creatinine as a list of renal injury seriousness. Furthermore, paeonol diminishes favourable inflammatory cytokines and expands calming cytokines invigorated by LPS in a dose-dependent way. Paeonol additionally repressed the declaration of phosphorylated NF-κB p65, IκBα and IKKβ, and controls NF-κB p65 DNA-restricting movement. Paeonol treatment likewise constricted the impacts of LPS on dendritic cells, with the massive hindrance of supportive of incendiary cytokines delivery, and afterward, TLR4 articulation and NF-κB signal pathway have been smothered.

Picroliv

Picroliv is a glucoside and a potent antioxidant extracted from the roots and rhizome of kutki known as *Picrorhiza kurroa*. Lipid peroxidation and receptive oxygen species are related to tissue injury in post-ischemic intense renal disappointment. The viability of picroliv was evaluated in an *in vivo* model of renal ischemia-reperfusion injury (IRI) in rodents at a dose of 12 mg/kg orally for seven days. Expanded lipid peroxidation and apoptotic cell number mirrored the oxidative harm following renal IRI. Picroliv-pretreated rodents showed lower lipid peroxidation, improved cancer prevention agent status, and decreased apoptosis, demonstrating better practicality of renal cells. Furthermore, Immunohistochemical considers uncovered that picroliv pre-treatment weakened the declaration of intercellular attachment particle 1 in the glomerular district. These outcomes proposed that picroliv pretreatment shields rodent kidneys from IRI, maybe by weak of free radical harm [80].

Protein from *Cajanus indicus*

Ghosh and Sil [81] researched the defensive impact of a 43 kDa protein extracted from *Cajanus indicus*, against acetaminophen-prompted hepatic and renal poisonousness. Male albino mice were treated with the protein for four days at 2 mg/kg body wt (i.p.) earlier or post to oral administration of acetaminophen at a dose of 300 mg/kg bw for two days. Levels of various marker proteins (to be specific, glutamate pyruvate transaminase and ALP), creatinine and blood urea nitrogen were estimated in the test sera. Intracellular responsive oxygen species creation and total antioxidant activity were additionally decided from acetaminophen and protein treated hepatocytes. Indices of different antioxidant enzymes (in particular, catalase, SOD, glutathione-S-transferase) just as lipid peroxidation final results of glutathione were resolved in both liver and kidney homogenates. Furthermore, Cytochrome P450 action was additionally estimated from liver microsomes. At last, histopathological tests were performed at liver segments of control, acetaminophen initiated and protein pre-and post-treated mice. Permitting acetaminophen resulted in raised levels of creatinine and other serum biochemical parameters alongside the improvement of hepatic and renal lipid peroxidation. Plus, the use of acetaminophen to hepatocytes expanded receptive oxygen species creation and decreased the total antioxidant capacity of the treated hepatocytes. It likewise diminished the levels of antioxidant enzymes and cellular reserves of glutathione in the liver and kidney. Also, acetaminophen upgraded the cytochrome P450 action of liver microsomes. Treatment with the protein altogether switched these progressions to practically typical. Aside from these, histopathological changes also uncovered the protein's defensive action against acetaminophen incited necrotic harm to the liver tissues. Results recommend that the protein secures hepatic and renal tissue.

Proteins from *Terminalia arjuna*

Mittal *et al*. [82] explained the characterization of the antilithiatic protein fraction from *Terminalia arjuna*. Proteins were separated from the dried bark of *T. arjuna,* and components of that MW> 3 kDa were exposed to anion exchange chromatography and then gel filtration chromatography. Four proteins were recognized, showing inhibitory action against CaOx crystallization. The cytoprotective and hostile to apoptotic adequacy of these decontaminated proteins was also explored on oxalate harmed renal epithelial cells, wherein oxalate was essentially injury weakened and prompted a portion subordinate expansion in the feasibility of these cells. These proteins likewise forestalled the communication of the CaOx precious stones to the cell surface and diminished the number of apoptotic cells. Recognizable proof of these four anionic proteins from the bark of *T. arjuna* was completed by Matrix-helped laser desorption/ionization-time of flight Mass spectrometry (MALDI-TOF MS). This was trailed by data set to hunt with the MASCOT worker, and grouping comparability was found with Nuclear pore anchor, DEAD Box ATP-dependent RNA helicase 45, Lon protease homolog 1, and Heat stun protein 90-3. These tale proteins disconnected from *T. arjuna* can hinder CaOx crystallization and advance cell endurance and in this manner, offer novel roads which should be investigated further for the clinical administration of urolithiasis.

Protein from *Tribulus terrestris*

An antilithic protein having anti-apoptotic activity and molecular weight, ~ 60 kDa was isolated from *Tribulus terrestris*. Aggarwal *et al*. [83] evaluated the *T. terrestris* activity on the nucleation and growth of CaOx crystals and oxalate-initiated cell injury of NRK 52E renal epithelial cells. The experiments were straightforward that extract of *T. terrestris* not only has the potential to inhibit nucleation and growth of the CaOx but also has an antiapoptotic role.

Quercetin

Quercetin is a 3,3',4',5,7-Pentahydroxyflavone found abundantly in nature. Ferric nitrilotriacetate (Fe-NTA), an iron chelate, instigates intense proximal tubular putrefaction as an outcome of lipid peroxidation and oxidative tissue harm that in the end prompts a high frequency of renal adenocarcinomas in rodents. Singh *et al*. [84] researched the impact of quercetin, with antioxidant potential, on Fe-NTA-actuated nephrotoxicity in rodents. One hour after a solitary intraperitoneal (i.p.) infusion of Fe-NTA at 8 mg iron/kg, a checked disintegration of renal structure and renal capacity was noticed. Fe-NTA prompted a huge renal oxidative pressure showed by raised thiobarbituric acid responding substances (TBARS) and a decrease in exercises of renal catalase, SOD, and glutathione reductase. Pre-treatment of animals with quercetin at a dose of 2 mg/kg, i.p.for 30 minutes before Fe-NTA administration notably lessened renal brokenness, morphological changes, decreased raised TBARS, and reestablished the exhausted renal cell reinforcement proteins. These outcomes unmistakably show the job of oxidative pressure and its connection to renal brokenness and propose a defensive impact of quercetin on Fe-NTA-prompted nephrotoxicity in rodents.

Quercetin is an intense antioxidant and a metal chelator. Spirits *et al.* [85] assessed the impact of quercetin on Cd-prompted kidney harm and oxidative stress and action. Wistar rodents were disseminated in four exploratory groups: control rodents, Cd; quercetin, and Cd + quercetin. Renal poisonousness was assessed by estimating urinary discharge of proteins, egg whites, glucose, and catalyst markers of cylindrical putrefaction, just as plasma convergence of creatinine. Plasma TBARS fixation and action of cancer prevention agent proteins in the kidney were likewise estimated. Renal cell harm was evaluated by electron microscopy. Creatures that got both Cd and quercetin showed a preferred renal capacity over those getting Cd alone. Album incited rounded injuries were especially decreased in rodents that additionally got quercetin. Compact disc instigated expansion in plasma TBARS was forestalled by the organization of quercetin. All out plasma cell reinforcements and renal SOD and glutathione reductase exercises were higher in the gathering that got Cd and quercetin than in rodents that got Cd alone. Quercetin administration doesn't alter the renal substance or the urinary discharge of Cd.

Dinnimath *et al.* [10] assessed the antiurolithiatic action of quercetin extracted from *Aerva lanata*. Ethylene glycol at 0.75% v/v actuated urolithiasis model was utilized to contemplate the antiurolithiatic action in male Wistar albino rats. The animals were isolated into five groups having six each. In light of the LD50 of the plant separate at a dose of 2000 mg/kg bw comparable portion was determined from their yield. The disconnected compound quercetin of *A. lanata* was evaluated for antiurolithiatic possibilities in calculi male Wistar rats by managing 2 mg/kg b.w/day orally as a test portion for 28 days. The urine volume was discovered to be altogether expanded in the rodents treated with quercetin. Urine microscopy uncovered a critical decrease in calculi size and altogether improved discharge of calcium, oxalate, phosphate, while the degree of magnesium was expanded. SEM of kidney areas has uncovered a decrease in the calculi in treated creatures. Serum investigation has uncovered a critical reduction in the degree of BUN and creatinine in treated rodents.

Resveratrol

Resveratrol, a 3,5,4′-trihydroxy-trans-stilbene produced by several plants. Silan *et al.* [86] explored the conceivable defensive impact of resveratrol on gentamicin-initiated nephrotoxicity. Tests were done in male Wistar rodents weighing in the range of 200-250 g. Gentamicin sulfate and resveratrol at doses of 80 and 10 mg/kg/day i.p., and gentamicin along with resveratrol were directed for six days. Blood urea level was altogether expanded in the gentamicin-treated animals. The investigation showed brought down degrees of urea and creatinine levels in resveratrol controlled animals when contrasted, and gentamicin managed rodents, and the thing that matters was genuinely critical. It has been resolved that resveratrol caused a measurably huge decline in lipid peroxidation and decreased the degree of catalase. Furthermore, the histopathological assessment showed that resveratrol forestalled halfway gentamicin instigated tubular harm.

Rutin (Also Known as Rutoside, Sophorin and Quercetin-3-O-Rutinoside)

Ghodasara *et al.* [87] examined the impact of rutin at a dose of 20 mg/kg bw p.o for 28 days on calcium and oxalate levels in urine, kidney tissues homogenate, and pathological structure of kidneys of rodents presented to ethylene glycol (EG) at a dose of 0.75% v/v, for 28 days and ammonium chloride (NH_4Cl) at 1% w/v, the initial three days in drinking water. They revealed that calcium and oxalate levels in urine and kidney tissue homogenate of rodents both provided with rutin and drinking water containing EG and NH_4Cl were fundamentally lower than those rodents just treated with EG and NH_4Cl. This is most likely an outcome of the impacts of rutin on repressing the blend of oxalate and expanding the bioavailability of nitric oxide to sequester calcium through the cGMP (3', 5' cyclic guanosine monophosphate) pathway in calculi-prompted rodents [88]. Also, it was uncovered in the histopathological assessment that base tissue harm and less number of CaOx stores in kidneys of creatures both treated with rutin and drinking water containing EG and NH_4Cl when contrasted with those just provided with EG and NH_4Cl. Thus, the specialists conjectured that as a mitigating and cancer prevention agent compound, rutin might meddle with the interaction of epithelial cell harm incited by CaOx precious stones and apply an inhibitory impact on the aggravation [89].

Safranal

Safranal is a 2,6,6-Trimethylcyclohexa-1,3-diene-1-carbaldehyde extracted from *Crocus sativus*. There are significant reports that safranal having antioxidant properties applies a defensive impact against ischemic wounds by specific nephrotoxins, including gentamicin. Boroushaki and Sadeghnia [90] analyzed the defensive effect of safranal against gentamicin-instigated nephrotoxicity in rodents. Animals were arbitrarily isolated into three groups having eight rodents in each. At the very first moment, every animal was put independently in a metabolic cage for collecting24-hour urine tests. On day two, in the wake of gathering urine tests for estimating glucose and protein, the rodents in group 1 got saline 1 ml/kg for six days, those in G-2 got gentamicin at 80 mg/kg/day for six days, and the leftover rodents in G-3 got safranal at a dose of 0.5 ml/kg followed by gentamicin at an amount of 80 mg/kg/day for six days. Blood tests were done *via* cardiovascular cut, and concentration of blood urea, creatinine, and urinary glucose and protein, as the pointers of nephrotoxicity, were estimated. In G-2, the concentration of blood urea nitrogen, urinary glucose, creatinine, and protein were fundamentally expanded contrasted and the control and safranal-treated animals. There was no critical contrast between the control and safranal-treated animals. Safranal applies defensive impacts against gentamicin-actuated nephrotoxicity in rodents.

Saponins from American Ginseng (*Panax quinquefolium* L.)

Mama *et al*. [91] assessed the renoprotective impact of Saponins from *Panax quinquefolius* leaves in a mouse model of cisplatin-prompted intense kidney injury (AKI). The degrees of blood urea nitrogen (BUN) and serum creatinine (CRE) was raised in cisplatin-inebriated mice, which were switched by PQS. Renal oxidative pressure, proven by expanded MDA level and decay of glutathione (GSH) and SOD exercises, was essentially eased by PQS pretreatment. The concealment of inflammatory reaction by PQS was acknowledged through the abatement of the mRNA articulation levels of tumor rot factor-α (TNF-α) and interleukin-1β (IL-1β) in kidney tissues, which were estimated by quantitative ongoing polymerase chain response (qRT-PCR). All the while, the overexpression of cytochrome P450 E1 (CYP2E1) and heme oxygenase-1 (HO-1) were lessened by PQS. Moreover, the impacts of Western smearing showed that PQS organization altogether stifled the protein articulation levels of Nox4, cut Caspase-3, separated Caspase-9, Bax, atomic factor-κB (NF-κB), cyclooxygenase-2 (COX-2), and inducible nitric oxide synthase (iNOS), proposing the restraint of apoptosis and irritation reaction. In general, PQS may have defensive impacts in cisplatin-instigated AKI through concealment of oxidative pressure, aggravation, and apoptosis.

Silibinin (Also Called Silybin)

It is the primary active metabolite of silymarin from the seeds of milk thistle. The flavonoid silibinin showed a protective action in animal models of hepatotoxicity. Gaedeke *et al*. [92] assessed, regardless of whether silibinin can likewise improve changes in renal glomerular and renal tubular capacity and morphology initiated by cisplatin. A permitted supply of cisplatin caused a decrease in kidney work inside a day following treatment. For instance, manifestations noticed the decline in creatinine freedom and expansions in proteinuria, in the urinary movement of the proximal tubular compounds alanine aminopeptidase and N-acetyl-bet--D-glucosaminidase and renal magnesium squandering. The impacts of cisplatin on creatinine leeway and proteinuria were forestalled by pre-treatment of the animals with silibinin. Hindrance of proximal rounded capacity was enhanced, that is enzymuria, and magnesium squandering was less articulated. Silibinin alone didn't influence kidney work. Treatment with silibinin unmistakably lessened morphological changes saw in the S3-section of the proximal tubule four days after cisplatin administration. The impacts of cisplatin on glomerular and proximal cylindrical capacity also as proximal tubular morphology could absolutely or mostly be improved by silibinin.

Silibinin hinders lipid peroxidation on hepatic microsomes and mitochondria of rodents and is likewise ready to decrease the action of different monooxygenases. Cyclosporin-instigated lipid peroxidation and influenced cytochrome P-450 may even add to cyclosporine nephrotoxicity. Zima *et al.* [93] inspected the likelihood that silibinin had a defensive impact because of its radical scavenging properties. Silibinin was given at a dose of 5 mg/kg bw i.p., managed 30 min before cyclosporine application at a dose of 30 mg/kg bw every day i.p. The biochemical boundaries, complete MDA in entire blood and kidney homogenates, and explicit substance of cytochrome P-450 in microsomal liver suspension were assessed. Three animal groups were contemplated: controls (con), cyclosporine alone (CsA), and cyclosporine in addition to silibinin (CsA + Sili). Creatinine was altogether raised following fourteen days in both cyclosporine treated gatherings contrasted with controls (CsA 60.2 +/ - 10.6 versus 45.8 +/ - 10.4 mumol/L; and CsA + Sili 72.0 +/ - 8.3 versus 45.8 +/ - 10.4 mumol/L) and glomerular filtration rate (GFR) was essentially diminished in similar gatherings. Complete MDA was raised distinctly in CsA rodents (2.26 +/ - 0.35 mumol/L, in correlation with controls (1.60 +/ - 0.44 mumol/L) and with rodents treated by CsA + Sili (1.65 +/ - 0.27 mumol/L. The particular substance of cytochrome P-450 in microsomal liver suspension was expanded in bunch CsA + Sili (1.179 +/ - 0.115 nmol/mg prot) contrasted with control animals (0.775 +/ - 0.086 nmol/mg prot.) and furthermore CsA bunch (0.806 +/ - 0.098 nmol/mg prot.). Taking everything into account, silibinin diminished cyclosporine-initiated lipid peroxidation without a defensive impact on GFR. This information demonstrates that this pathway isn't significant in cyclosporine-initiated nephrotoxicity. Administration of the two medications raised the particular substance of cytochrome P-450 in liver microsomes. This proposes that the impact of silibinin on cyclosporine biotransformation in the liver is through cytochrome P-450.

The biochemical impact of flavonolignans from *Silybum marianum* has been tried by Sonnenbichler *et al.* [94] on kidney cells of African green monkeys. Two non-malignant cell lines were chosen, with the focal point of the work on the fibroblast-like Vero line. Multiplication rate, biosynthesis of protein and DNA, and the movement of the enzyme lactate dehydrogenase (as a proportion of the cell metabolic action) were picked as boundaries for the impact of the flavonolignans. Silibinin and silicristin show amazing stimulatory consequences for these boundaries, for the most part in Vero cells; in any case, isosilibinin and silidianin end up being dormant. *In vitro* tries different things with kidney cells harmed by paracetamol, cisplatin, and vincristine exhibited that organization of silibinin previously or after the substance incited injury can decrease or keep away from the nephrotoxic impacts.

Steroidal Constituents of *Solanum Xanthocarpum*

The separated mixtures from the berries of *Solanum xanthocarpum* were assessed by Patel *et al.* [95] for their antiurolithiatic action on a rat. Solasonine, a glycoalkaloid, was given in a dose of 80 mg/kg of body weight in-vehicle water. The subsequent compound was solasodine, a steroidal aglycone at 80 mg/kg bw in a 1% CMC vehicle. Na^+ and K^+ particle fixation in urine was assessed utilizing Flame Photometer. For the secluded compound, solasonine ratio (Vt/Vc) acquired 1.6, and for the subsequent compound, solasodine 1.5, which was one of the measures for antiurolithiatic movement and a critical contrast in Na^+ and K^+ particle fixation was seen in both segregated mixtures, that was demonstrated that solasonine showed great action as natriuretic action contrasted with solasodine.

Taraxasterol (Anthesterin)

Taraxasterol, a triterpene compound extracted from aerial parts of *Taraxacum officinale*. Ghale-Salimi *et al.* [96] researched and analyzed the impacts of taraxasterol, and potassium citrate (PC) on CaOx crystallization *in vitro*. The presence of taraxasterol, concentrate, and PC diminished absorbance in trial tests contrasted with control altogether. The nucleation of stones is repressed by taraxasterol, concentrate, and PC. The quantity of CaOx stones was diminished within sight of taraxasterol, concentrate, and PC in a portion subordinate way. The presence of taraxasterol, concentrate, and PC diminished the quantity of CaC_2O_4 monohydrate, while expanded CaC_2O_4 dihydrate stones altogether. Additionally, the width of CaC_2O_4 dihydrate stones was reduced within sight of taraxasterol, concentrate, and PC, altogether. This exploration showed that taraxasterol and extricate have hostile to crystallization exercises and the viability of the concentrate is more intense than taraxasterol.

Thymol and Carvacrol

El-Sayed *et al.* [97] surveyed the possible defensive impacts of thymol and carvacrol against cisplatin (CP)-actuated nephrotoxicity. A solitary dose of CP at 6 mg/kg i.p. infused to male rodents uncovered a critical rise in serum urea, creatinine, and tumor necrosis factor-alpha levels. It additionally raised kidney substance of MDA and caspase-3 movement with a massive decrease in serum albumin, kidney substance of diminished glutathione just as catalase, and SOD action when contrasted with that of the benchmark group. Interestingly, allowing thymol at a dose of 20 mg/kg, p.o, and carvacrol at a dose of 15 mg/kg, p.o. for 14 days before CP infusion and seven days after CP administration re-established the kidney work and inspected oxidative stress boundaries. Taking everything into account, thymol was more viable nephroprotective than carvacrol. Also, a blend of thymol and carvacrol had a synergistic nephroprotective impact that may be credited to anti-inflammatory, antioxidant, and antiapoptotic exercises.

Thymoquinone

It is a natural compound extracted from *Nigella sativa*. The impacts of thymoquinone (TQ) on cisplatin-initiated nephrotoxicity in mice and rodents were concentrated by Badary *et al*. [98]. Oral supply of thymoquinone at a dose of 50 mg/L in drinking water for five days prior and five days after single infusions of cisplatin at a dose of 5 mg/kg, i.v., in rodents and 7 or 14 mg/kg, i.p., in mice extraordinarily improved cisplatin-incited nephrotoxicity in the two species. In mice, comparative modifications in kidney work were noticed. TQ-initiated enhancement of cisplatin nephrotoxicity was noticeable by critical decreases in serum urea and creatinine and a considerable improvement in polyuria, kidney weight, and creatinine freedom. The defensive impacts of TQ against cisplatin-incited nephrotoxicity in the rodent were additionally affirmed by histopathological assessment.

Dirican *et al*. [99] tested the cisplatin and TQ *in vivo* interactions by estimating creatin, serum cystatin C (cys C), and neutrophil gelatinase-related lipocalin (NGAL) levels and dissecting the articulation status of p53 and NGAL by immunohistochemistry. Examinations were completed in male Wistar rodents. Allowing 40 mg/kg, TQ had no impact on serum kidney boundaries. Serum creatinine level was inconsequential in cisplatin received animals, yet serum Csy C and NGAL levels were altogether raised. All serum creatinine, NGAL, and Cys C levels were raised in co-treatment of cisplatin and TQ. Also, renal tubular harm was found in these groups altogether higher than both control and just cisplatin-treated animals.

Xanthorrhizol

Kim *et al*. [100] explored the impact of xanthorrhizol, extracted from *Curcuma xanthorrhiza* Roxb. (Zingiberaceae), on cisplatin-instigated nephrotoxicity in mice. A solitary dose of cisplatin at 45 mg/kg, i.p. fundamentally raised the degrees of serum creatinine, blood urea nitrogen, and the kidney to body weight proportion; however, the pre-treatment of xanthorrhizol at a dose of 200 mg/kg/day, p.o. for four days essentially constricted the cisplatin-actuated nephrotoxicity. The preventive impact of xanthorrhizol was more valuable than that of curcumin with a similar dose of 200 mg/kg. Nonetheless, this impact appeared not to be connected with the capacity of xanthorrhizol to manage the DNA-restricting exercises of record factors, for example, atomic factor-kappaB (NF-kappaB) and activator protein 1 (AP-1).

Zingerone (Also Known as Vanillylacetone)

Zingerone, a ketonic compound extracted from *Zingiber officinale*, having reported actions of antioxidant and anti-inflammatory. Tune *et al.* [101] explored the restorative impacts of zingerone on lipopolysaccharide (LPS)- initiated Acute Kidney Injury (AKI) in mice. Zingerone was given one hour after LPS challenge. BUN and creatinine were estimated in this investigation. ELISA distinguished the provocative cytokines in serum and kidney tissues. The Western blot technique evaluated the formation of MyD88, Toll-like receptor 4 (TLR4), TRIF, IκB, and NF-κB. The outcomes showed that zingerone smothered LPS-actuated BUN, creatinine, IL-6, inflammatory cytokines TNF-α, and IL-1β levels in a portion subordinate way. Zingerone additionally constricted LPS-initiated kidney histopathological changes. Besides, zingerone was found to repress LPS-actuated MyD88, TLR4, TRIF articulation, and NF-κB initiation. Taking everything into account, this investigation showed that zingerone restrained LPS-initiated AKI by smothering TLR4/NF-κB flagging pathway.

Bioactive Substances from *Carthamus tinctorius*

Lan *et al.* [102] screened nephroprotective bioactive substances from dried florets (Carthami flos) of *C. tinctorius* based on triple-color fluorescence probes. The setup strategy was applied to the screening of 53 constituents of *C.flos*, and three segments C17, C18 and C19 were found to display nephroprotective impacts against doxorubicin hydrochloride initiated injury on HK-2 cells. Eight mixtures include 6-hydroxykaempferol-3-O-rutinoside-6-O-glucoside, hydroxysafflor yellow A, 6-hydroxykaempferol-3, 6-di-O-glucoside or 6-hydroxykaempferol-6, 6-hydroxykaempferol-3-O-glucoside or 6-hydroxykaempferol-7-O-glucoside, 7-di-O-glucoside, 6-hydroxykaempferol-3-O-rutinoside, isoquercetin, rutin, and kaempferol-3-O-rutinoside in constituents C17, C18 and C19 were for starters distinguished by LC-MS. Rutin, isoquercetin, kaempferol-3-O-rutinoside, and hydroxysafflor yellow A were affirmed by contrasting and reference substances. Further examination demonstrated that these four mixtures had moderate nephroprotective impacts, while isoquercetin showed a huge nephroprotective impact in a dose-dependent manner. These outcomes propose that rutin, isoquercetin, hydroxysafflor yellow A, kaempferol-3-O-rutinoside, and maybe the nephroprotective bioactive substances in Carthami flos.

Crataeva magna (Lour.) DC. Phytocompounds

Radha [103] evaluated the antiurolithiatic activity of extracts of different parts of the plant *Crataeva magna*. The study was carried out with leaf, stem, and bark of *Crateva magna in vitro* and *in vivo* animal models to isolate the bioactive compound present in the plant with antiurolithiatic properties. The percent inhibition of turbidity increased with extract concentration, and it was greatest with aqueous extract of bark compared to other extracts. For the extract-treated animals, characteristics such as body weight, kidney weight, urine and serum parameters, and BUN were on par with cystone treated group. Radha [103] isolated and identified the bioactive constituents from *Crataeva magna* responsible for the antiurolithiatic activities. The compound isolated from the aqueous extract of the bark was identified and characterized as 14-hydroxy--2-abietene-7-one. By docking analysis, 14-hydroxy-12-abietene-7-one interacted with Tamm-Horsfal protein, and it may inhibit CaOx stone formation.

Rotula aquatica Phytocompounds

Bioactivity-guided extraction of antiurolithiatic compounds from *Rotula aquatica* roots was studied by Prashanthi *et al.* [104]. The extracted constituents showed marked *in vitro* antiurolithiatic action contrasted with cystone. Components were described as a class of phenolic compounds, including p-coumaric acid and gallic acid. The alleged activities incorporate hydrolysis of calcium phosphate and CaOx within sight of – OH of the extracted constituents.

CONCLUSION

Various plant secondary metabolites like alkaloids, glycosides, tannins, resins, flavonoids, and chalcones are the major classes of phytochemicals. These phytochemicals had scientifically proven physiological actions proper as drugs for treating life-threatening illnesses, including renal system issues. This chapter highlighted the more than 50 different phytochemicals extracted and isolated from various medicinal species having nephroprotective properties in a simple helpful manner for researchers and herbal healers.

REFERENCES

[1]   Makbul SAA, Jahan N, Kalam MA. Bio-active compounds from unani medicinal plants and their application in urolithiasis. 2019.
      [http://dx.doi.org/10.1007/978-981-13-7205-6_16]

[2]   Lobine D, Ahmed S, Aschner M, Khan H, Mirzaei H, Mahomoodally MF. Antiurolithiatic effects of pentacyclic triterpenes: The distance traveled from therapeutic aspects. Drug Dev Res 2020; 81(6): 671-84.
[http://dx.doi.org/10.1002/ddr.21670] [PMID: 32314397]

[3]   Ali BH. Agents ameliorating or augmenting experimental gentamicin nephrotoxicity: some recent research. Food Chem Toxicol 2003; 41(11): 1447-52.
[http://dx.doi.org/10.1016/S0278-6915(03)00186-8] [PMID: 12962996]

[4]   Ridzuan NRA, Rashid NA, Othman F, Budin SB, Hussan F, Teoh SL. Protective role of natural products in cisplatin-induced nephrotoxicity. Mini Rev Med Chem 2019; 19(14): 1134-43.
[http://dx.doi.org/10.2174/1389557519666190320124438] [PMID: 30894108]

[5]   Zeng X, Xi Y, Jiang W. Protective roles of flavonoids and flavonoid-rich plant extracts against urolithiasis: A review. Crit Rev Food Sci Nutr 2019; 59(13): 2125-35.
[http://dx.doi.org/10.1080/10408398.2018.1439880] [PMID: 29432040]

[6]   Abdel-Daim MM, Abushouk AI, Donia T, *et al.* The nephroprotective effects of allicin and ascorbic acid against cisplatin-induced toxicity in rats. Environ Sci Pollut Res Int 2019; 26(13): 13502-9.
[http://dx.doi.org/10.1007/s11356-019-04780-4] [PMID: 30911969]

[7]   Supekar AV, Pagar HJ. Evaluation of nephroprotective activity of andrographolide in experimental animal (gentamicin induced nephrotoxicity). World J Pharm Pharm Sci 2019; 8(10): 921-30.

[8]   Bashir S, Gilani AH. Antiurolithic effect of berberine is mediated through multiple pathways. Eur J Pharmacol 2011; 651(1-3): 168-75.
[http://dx.doi.org/10.1016/j.ejphar.2010.10.076] [PMID: 21114977]

[9]   Domitrović R, Cvijanović O, Pernjak-Pugel E, Skoda M, Mikelić L, Crnčević-Orlić Z. Berberine exerts nephroprotective effect against cisplatin-induced kidney damage through inhibition of oxidative/nitrosative stress, inflammation, autophagy and apoptosis. Food Chem Toxicol 2013; 62: 397-406.
[http://dx.doi.org/10.1016/j.fct.2013.09.003] [PMID: 24025684]

[10]   Dinnimath BM, Jalalpure SS, Patil UK. Antiurolithiatic activity of natural constituents isolated from *Aerva lanata*. J Ayurveda Integr Med 2017; 8(4): 226-32.
[http://dx.doi.org/10.1016/j.jaim.2016.11.006] [PMID: 29169771]

[11]   Shimeda Y, Hirotani Y, Akimoto Y, *et al.* Protective effects of capsaicin against cisplatin-induced nephrotoxicity in rats. Biol Pharm Bull 2005; 28(9): 1635-8.
[http://dx.doi.org/10.1248/bpb.28.1635] [PMID: 16141530]

[12]   Soliman KM, Abdul-Hamid M, Othman AI. Effect of carnosine on gentamicin-induced nephrotoxicity. Med Sci Monit 2007; 13(3): BR73-83.
[PMID: 17325631]

[13]   Itoh Y, Yasui T, Okada A, Tozawa K, Hayashi Y, Kohri K. Preventive effects of green tea on renal stone formation and the role of oxidative stress in nephrolithiasis. J Urol 2005; 173(1): 271-5.
[http://dx.doi.org/10.1097/01.ju.0000141311.51003.87] [PMID: 15592095]

[14]   Kohri K, Nomura S, Kitamura Y, *et al.* Structure and expression of the mRNA encoding urinary stone protein (osteopontin). J Biol Chem 1993; 268(20): 15180-4.
[http://dx.doi.org/10.1016/S0021-9258(18)82453-X] [PMID: 8325891]

[15]   Wu H, Lozano G. NF-kappa B activation of p53. A potential mechanism for suppressing cell growth in response to stress. J Biol Chem 1994; 269(31): 20067-74.
[http://dx.doi.org/10.1016/S0021-9258(17)32128-2] [PMID: 8051093]

[16]   Tardif JC, Côté G, Lespérance J, *et al.* Probucol and multivitamins in the prevention of restenosis after coronary angioplasty. N Engl J Med 1997; 337(6): 365-72.
[http://dx.doi.org/10.1056/NEJM199708073370601] [PMID: 9241125]

[17]   Chopra K, Singh D, Chander V. Nephrotoxicity and its prevention by catechin in ferric nitrilotriacetate promoted oxidative stress in rats. Hum Exp Toxicol 2004; 23(3): 137-43.
[http://dx.doi.org/10.1191/0960327104ht427oa] [PMID: 15119533]

[18]   Zhai W, Zheng J, Yao X, *et al.* Catechin prevents the calcium oxalate monohydrate induced renal calcium crystallization in NRK-52E cells and the ethylene glycol induced renal stone formation in rat. BMC Complement Altern Med 2013; 13(1): 228.
[http://dx.doi.org/10.1186/1472-6882-13-228] [PMID: 24044655]

[19]   Niimi K, Yasui T, Hirose M, *et al.* Mitochondrial permeability transition pore opening induces the initial process of renal calcium crystallization. Free Radic Biol Med 2012; 52(7): 1207-17.
[http://dx.doi.org/10.1016/j.freeradbiomed.2012.01.005] [PMID: 22285391]

[20]   Kawai Y, Nakao T, Kunimura N, Kohda Y, Gemba M. Relationship of intracellular calcium and oxygen radicals to Cisplatin-related renal cell injury. J Pharmacol Sci 2006; 100(1): 65-72.
[http://dx.doi.org/10.1254/jphs.FP0050661] [PMID: 16410676]

[21]   Wongmekiat O, Peerapanyasut W, Kobroob A. Catechin supplementation prevents kidney damage in rats repeatedly exposed to cadmium through mitochondrial protection. Naunyn Schmiedebergs Arch Pharmacol 2018; 391(4): 385-94.
[http://dx.doi.org/10.1007/s00210-018-1468-6] [PMID: 29356841]

[22]   Boran T, Gunaydin A, Jannuzzi AT, Ozcagli E, Alpertunga B. Celastrol pretreatment as a therapeutic option against cisplatin-induced nephrotoxicity. Toxicol Res (Camb) 2019; 8(5): 723-30.
[http://dx.doi.org/10.1039/c9tx00141g] [PMID: 31588349]

[23]   Monika J, Bhandari A, Bhandari A, Patel P. Isolation, characterization and *in vitro* antiurolithiatic activity of cerpegin alkaloid from *Ceropegia bulbosa* var. *lushii* root. Int J Drug Dev & Res 2012; 4(4): 154-60.

[24]   Ye H-Y, Jin J, Jin L-W, Chen Y, Zhou Z-H, Li Z-Y. Chlorogenic acid attenuates lipopolysaccharide-induced acute kidney injury by inhibiting TLR4/NF-κB signal pathway. Inflammation 2017; 40(2): 523-9.
[http://dx.doi.org/10.1007/s10753-016-0498-9] [PMID: 28028753]

[25]   Sultana S, Verma K, Khan R. Nephroprotective efficacy of chrysin against cisplatin-induced toxicity *via* attenuation of oxidative stress. J Pharm Pharmacol 2012; 64(6): 872-81.
[http://dx.doi.org/10.1111/j.2042-7158.2012.01470.x] [PMID: 22571266]

[26]   Yarijani ZM, Najafi H, Hamid Madani S. Protective effect of crocin on gentamicin-induced nephrotoxicity in rats. Iran J Basic Med Sci 2016; 19(3): 337-43.
[PMID: 27114805]

[27]   Venkatesan N, Punithavathi D, Arumugam V. Curcumin prevents adriamycin nephrotoxicity in rats. Br J Pharmacol 2000; 129(2): 231-4.
[http://dx.doi.org/10.1038/sj.bjp.0703067] [PMID: 10694226]

[28]   Antunes LM, Darin JD, Bianchi NdeL. Effects of the antioxidants curcumin or selenium on cisplatin-induced nephrotoxicity and lipid peroxidation in rats. Pharmacol Res 2001; 43(2): 145-50.
[http://dx.doi.org/10.1006/phrs.2000.0724] [PMID: 11243715]

[29]   Ali BH, Al-Wabel N, Mahmoud O, Mousa HM, Hashad M. Curcumin has a palliative action on gentamicin-induced nephrotoxicity in rats. Fundam Clin Pharmacol 2005; 19(4): 473-7.
[http://dx.doi.org/10.1111/j.1472-8206.2005.00343.x] [PMID: 16011735]

[30]   Sharma S, Kulkarni SK, Chopra K. Curcumin, the active principle of turmeric (*Curcuma longa*), ameliorates diabetic nephropathy in rats. Clin Exp Pharmacol Physiol 2006; 33(10): 940-5.
[http://dx.doi.org/10.1111/j.1440-1681.2006.04468.x] [PMID: 17002671]

[31]   He L, Peng X, Zhu J, *et al.* Protective effects of curcumin on acute gentamicin-induced nephrotoxicity in rats. Can J Physiol Pharmacol 2015; 93(4): 275-82.
[http://dx.doi.org/10.1139/cjpp-2014-0459] [PMID: 25730179]

[32]   Hashish EA, Elgaml SA. Hepatoprotective and nephroprotective effect of curcumin against copper toxicity in rats. Indian J Clin Biochem 2016; 31(3): 270-7.
[http://dx.doi.org/10.1007/s12291-015-0527-8] [PMID: 27382197]

[33]   Ismail AFM, Salem AAM. Renoprotective effect of curcumin on acetaminophen-induced nephrotoxicity in rats. J Chem Pharm Res 2016; 8(2): 773-9.

[34]   Alkuraishy HM, Al-Gareeb AI, Rasheed HA. Nephroprotective effect of curcumin (*Curcuma longa*) in acute nephrotoxicity in Sprague-Dawley rats. J Contemp Med Sci 2019; 5(2): 122-4.

[35]   Palipoch S, Punsawad C, Chinnapun D, Suwannalert P. Amelioration of cisplatin-induced nephrotoxicity in rats by curcumin and α-tocopherol. Trop J Pharm Res 2014; 12: 973-9.
[http://dx.doi.org/10.4314/tjpr.v12i6.16]

[36]   Barberán FAT, Gil MI, Tomás F, Ferreres F. Flavonoid aglycones and glycosides from *Teucrium gnaphalodes*. J Nat Prod 1985; 48(5): 859-60.
[http://dx.doi.org/10.1021/np50041a040]

[37]   Prabhu VV, Sathyamurthy D, Ramasamy A, Das S, Anuradha M, Pachiappan S. Evaluation of protective effects of diosmin (a citrus flavonoid) in chemical-induced urolithiasis in experimental rats. Pharm Biol 2016; 54(9): 1513-21.
[http://dx.doi.org/10.3109/13880209.2015.1107105] [PMID: 26799954]

[38]   Satoh M, Kashihara N, Fujimoto S, *et al.* A novel free radical scavenger, edarabone, protects against cisplatin-induced acute renal damage *in vitro* and *in vivo*. J Pharmacol Exp Ther 2003; 305(3): 1183-90.
[http://dx.doi.org/10.1124/jpet.102.047522] [PMID: 12649298]

[39]   Ateşşahín A, Ceríbaşi AO, Yuce A, Bulmus O, Cikim G. Role of ellagic acid against cisplatin-induced nephrotoxicity and oxidative stress in rats. Basic Clin Pharmacol Toxicol 2007; 100(2): 121-6.
[PMID: 17244261]

[40]   Grases F, Prieto RM, Gomila I, Sanchis P, Costa-Bauzá A. Phytotherapy and renal stones: the role of antioxidants. A pilot study in Wistar rats. Urolithiasis 2009; 37(1): 35-40.
[http://dx.doi.org/10.1007/s00240-008-0165-1] [PMID: 19066877]

[41]   Sumathi R, Jayanthi S, Kalpanadevi V, Varalakshmi P. Effect of DL alpha-lipoic acid on tissue lipid peroxidation and antioxidant systems in normal and glycollate treated rats. Pharmacol Res 1993; 27(4): 309-18.
[http://dx.doi.org/10.1006/phrs.1993.1031] [PMID: 8367380]

[42]   Chen D-Z, Chen L-Q, Lin M-X, Gong Y-Q, Ying BY, Wei D-Z. Esculentoside A inhibits LPS-induced acute kidney injury by activating PPAR-γ. Microb Pathog 2017; 110: 208-13.
[http://dx.doi.org/10.1016/j.micpath.2017.06.037] [PMID: 28666844]

[43]   Zhao B, Su B, Zhang H, Liu W, Du Q, Li Y. Antiurolithiatic effect of ferulic acid on ethylene glycol induced renal calculus in experimental rats. Trop J Pharm Res 2019; 18(1): 109-15.
[http://dx.doi.org/10.4314/tjpr.v18i1.16]

[44]   Mir SM, Ravuri HG, Pradhan RK, *et al.* Ferulic acid protects lipopolysaccharide-induced acute kidney injury by suppressing inflammatory events and upregulating antioxidant defenses in Balb/c mice. Biomed Pharmacother 2018; 100: 304-15.
[http://dx.doi.org/10.1016/j.biopha.2018.01.169] [PMID: 29448207]

[45]   Micali A, Pallio G, Irrera N, *et al.* Flavocoxid, a natural antioxidant, protects mouse kidney from cadmium-induced toxicity. Oxid Med Cell Longev 2018; 2018: 9162946.
[http://dx.doi.org/10.1155/2018/9162946] [PMID: 29849925]

[46]   Baek SH, Shin BK, Kim NJ, Chang SY, Park JH. Protective effect of ginsenosides Rk3 and Rh4 on cisplatin-induced acute kidney injury *in vitro* and *in vivo*. J Ginseng Res 2017; 41(3): 233-9.
[http://dx.doi.org/10.1016/j.jgr.2016.03.008] [PMID: 28701862]

[47] Baek SH, Piao XL, Lee UJ, Kim HY, Park JH. Reduction of Cisplatin-induced nephrotoxicity by ginsenosides isolated from processed ginseng in cultured renal tubular cells. Biol Pharm Bull 2006; 29(10): 2051-5.
[http://dx.doi.org/10.1248/bpb.29.2051] [PMID: 17015950]

[48] Park JY, Choi P, Kim T, *et al.* Protective effects of processed Ginseng and its active ginsenosides on cisplatin-induced nephrotoxicity: *in vitro* and *in vivo* studies. J Agric Food Chem 2015; 63(25): 5964-9.
[http://dx.doi.org/10.1021/acs.jafc.5b00782] [PMID: 26050847]

[49] Han M-S, Han I-H, Lee D, *et al.* Beneficial effects of fermented black ginseng and its ginsenoside 20(S)-Rg3 against cisplatin-induced nephrotoxicity in LLC-PK1 cells. J Ginseng Res 2016; 40(2): 135-40.
[http://dx.doi.org/10.1016/j.jgr.2015.06.006] [PMID: 27158234]

[50] Li W, Yan M-H, Liu Y, *et al.* Ginsenoside Rg5 ameliorates cisplatin-induced nephrotoxicity in mice through inhibition of inflammation, oxidative stress, and apoptosis. Nutrients 2016; 8(9): 566.
[http://dx.doi.org/10.3390/nu8090566] [PMID: 27649238]

[51] Vu-Huynh KL, Le THV, Nguyen HT, *et al.* Increase in protective effect of *Panax vietnamensis* by heat processing on cisplatin-induced kidney cell toxicity. Molecules 2019; 24(24): 4627.
[http://dx.doi.org/10.3390/molecules24244627] [PMID: 31861213]

[52] Sohn E-J, Kang D-G, Lee H-S. Protective effects of glycyrrhizin on gentamicin-induced acute renal failure in rats. Pharmacol Toxicol 2003; 93(3): 116-22.
[http://dx.doi.org/10.1034/j.1600-0773.2003.930302.x] [PMID: 12969435]

[53] Zhao H, Zhao M, Wang Y, Li F, Zhang Z. Glycyrrhizic acid attenuates sepsis-induced acute kidney injury by inhibiting NF-κB signaling pathway. Evidence-Based Complem Altern Med 2016.
[http://dx.doi.org/10.1155/2016/8219287]

[54] Perez RM, Vargas R, Perez G, Zavala S, Perz CG. Antiurolithiatic activity of 7-hydroxy-2′,4′,5′-trimethoxyisoflavone and 7-hydroxy-4′- methoxy isoflavone from *Eysenhardtia polystachya*. J Herbs Spices Med Plants 2000; 7: 27-34.
[http://dx.doi.org/10.1300/J044v07n02_03]

[55] Chunzhi G, Zunfeng L, Chengwei Q, Xiangmei B, Jingui Y. Hyperin protects against LPS-induced acute kidney injury by inhibiting TLR4 and NLRP3 signaling pathways. Oncotarget 2016; 7(50): 82602-8.
[http://dx.doi.org/10.18632/oncotarget.13010] [PMID: 27813491]

[56] Langeswaran K, Selvaraj J, Ponnulakshmi R, Mathaiyan M, Vijaypraksh S. Protective effect of kaempferol on biochemical and histopathological changes in mercuric chloride induced nephrotoxicity in experimental rats. J Biolocally Active Products from Nature 2018; 8(2): 125-36.
[http://dx.doi.org/10.1080/22311866.2018.1451386]

[57] Sharma D, Gondaliya P, Tiwari V, Kalia K. Kaempferol attenuates diabetic nephropathy by inhibiting RhoA/Rho-kinase mediated inflammatory signalling. Biomed Pharmacother 2019; 109: 1610-9.
[http://dx.doi.org/10.1016/j.biopha.2018.10.195] [PMID: 30551415]

[58] Ayepola OR, Cerf ME, Brooks NL, Oguntibeju OO. Kolaviron, a biflavonoid complex of *Garcinia kola* seeds modulates apoptosis by suppressing oxidative stress and inflammation in diabetes-induced nephrotoxic rats. Phytomedicine 2014; 21(14): 1785-93.
[http://dx.doi.org/10.1016/j.phymed.2014.09.006] [PMID: 25481391]

[59] Alabi QK, Akomolafe RO, Adefisayo MA, *et al.* Kolaviron attenuates diclofenac-induced nephrotoxicity in male Wistar rats. Appl Physiol Nutr Metab 2018; 43(9): 956-68.
[http://dx.doi.org/10.1139/apnm-2017-0788] [PMID: 29847737]

[60] Alabi QK, Akomolafe RO. Kolaviron diminishes diclofenac-induced liver and kidney toxicity in wistar rats *via* suppressing inflammatory events, upregulating antioxidant defenses, and improving

hematological indices. Dose Response 2020; 18(1): 1559325819899256.
[http://dx.doi.org/10.1177/1559325819899256] [PMID: 32165871]

[61]   Hu J, Liu J. Licochalcone A attenuates lipopolysaccharide-induced acute kidney injury by inhibiting NF-κB activation. Inflammation 2016; 39(2): 569-74.
[http://dx.doi.org/10.1007/s10753-015-0281-3] [PMID: 26552405]

[62]   Malarkodi KP, Balachandar AV, Varalakshmi P. The influence of lipoic acid on adriamycin induced nephrotoxicity in rats. Mol Cell Biochem 2003; 247(1-2): 15-22.
[http://dx.doi.org/10.1023/A:1024118519596] [PMID: 12841626]

[63]   Anand R, Patnaik GK, Kulshreshtha DK, Dhawan BN. Antiurolithiatic activity of lupeol, the active constituent isolated from *Crateva nurvala*. Phytother Res 1994; 8: 417-21.
[http://dx.doi.org/10.1002/ptr.2650080708]

[64]   Malini MM, Baskar R, Varalakshmi P. Effect of lupeol, a pentacyclic triterpene, on urinary enzymes in hyperoxaluric rats. Jpn J Med Sci Biol 1995; 48(5-6): 211-20.
[http://dx.doi.org/10.7883/yoken1952.48.211] [PMID: 8718554]

[65]   Baskar R, Malini MM, Varalakshmi P, Balakrishna K, Bhima Rao R. Effect of lupeol isolated from *Crataeva nurvala* stem bark against free radical-induced toxicity in experimental urolithiasis. Fitoterapia 1996; 67(2): 121-5.

[66]   Sudhahar V, Veena CK, Varalakshmi P. Antiurolithic effect of lupeol and lupeol linoleate in experimental hyperoxaluria. J Nat Prod 2008; 71(9): 1509-12.
[http://dx.doi.org/10.1021/np0703141] [PMID: 18717586]

[67]   Vidya L, Varalakshmi P. Control of urinary risk factors of stones by betulin and lupeol in experimental hyperoxaluria. Fitoterapia 2000; 71(5): 535-43.
[http://dx.doi.org/10.1016/S0367-326X(00)00192-1] [PMID: 11449502]

[68]   Vidya L, Lenin M, Varalakshmi P. Evaluation of the effect of triterpenes on urinary risk factors of stone formation in pyridoxine deficient hyperoxaluric rats. Phytother Res 2002; 16(6): 514-8.
[http://dx.doi.org/10.1002/ptr.940] [PMID: 12237806]

[69]   Domitrović R, Cvijanović O, Pugel EP, Zagorac GB, Mahmutefendić H, Škoda M. Luteolin ameliorates cisplatin-induced nephrotoxicity in mice through inhibition of platinum accumulation, inflammation and apoptosis in the kidney. Toxicology 2013; 310: 115-23.
[http://dx.doi.org/10.1016/j.tox.2013.05.015] [PMID: 23770416]

[70]   Atessahin A, Yilmaz S, Karahan I, Ceribasi AO, Karaoglu A. Effects of lycopene against cisplatin-induced nephrotoxicity and oxidative stress in rats. Toxicology 2005; 212(2-3): 116-23.
[http://dx.doi.org/10.1016/j.tox.2005.04.016] [PMID: 15946783]

[71]   Karahan I, Ateşşahin A, Yilmaz S, Ceribaşi AO, Sakin F. Protective effect of lycopene on gentamicin-induced oxidative stress and nephrotoxicity in rats. Toxicology 2005; 215(3): 198-204.
[http://dx.doi.org/10.1016/j.tox.2005.07.007] [PMID: 16125832]

[72]   Yilmaz S, Atessahin A, Sahna E, Karahan I, Ozer S. Protective effect of lycopene on adriamycin-induced cardiotoxicity and nephrotoxicity. Toxicology 2006; 218(2-3): 164-71.
[http://dx.doi.org/10.1016/j.tox.2005.10.015] [PMID: 16325981]

[73]   Su Z, Ye J, Qin Z, Ding X. Protective effects of madecassoside against Doxorubicin induced nephrotoxicity *in vivo* and *in vitro*. Sci Rep 2015; 5: 18314.
[http://dx.doi.org/10.1038/srep18314] [PMID: 26658818]

[74]   Singh D, Chander V, Chopra K. Protective effect of naringin, a bioflavonoid on ferric nitrilotriacetate-induced oxidative renal damage in rat kidney. Toxicology 2004; 201(1-3): 1-8.
[http://dx.doi.org/10.1016/j.tox.2004.03.028] [PMID: 15297014]

[75]   Singh D, Chander V, Chopra K. Protective effect of naringin, a bioflavonoid on glycerol-induced acute renal failure in rat kidney. Toxicology 2004; 201(1-3): 143-51.
[http://dx.doi.org/10.1016/j.tox.2004.04.018] [PMID: 15297029]

[76] Prabu SM, Shagirtha K, Renugadevi J. Reno-protective effect of naringenin in combination with vitamins C and E on cadmium induced oxidative nephrotoxicity in rats. J Pharm Res 2011; 4(6): 1921-6.

[77] Badary OA, Abdel-Maksoud S, Ahmed WA, Owieda GH. Naringenin attenuates cisplatin nephrotoxicity in rats. Life Sci 2005; 76(18): 2125-35.
[http://dx.doi.org/10.1016/j.lfs.2004.11.005] [PMID: 15826879]

[78] Renugadevi J, Prabhu SM. Naringenin protects cadmium-induced oxidative renal dysfunction in rats. Toxicology 2009; 256(1-1): 128-34.
[http://dx.doi.org/10.1016/j.tox.2008.11.012]

[79] Fan HY, Qi D, Yu C, *et al.* Paeonol protects endotoxin-induced acute kidney injury: potential mechanism of inhibiting TLR4-NF-κB signal pathway. Oncotarget 2016; 7(26): 39497-510.
[http://dx.doi.org/10.18632/oncotarget.8347] [PMID: 27027358]

[80] Seth P, Kumari R, Madhavan S, *et al.* Prevention of renal ischemia-reperfusion-induced injury in rats by picroliv. Biochem Pharmacol 2000; 59(10): 1315-22.
[http://dx.doi.org/10.1016/S0006-2952(00)00268-9] [PMID: 10736432]

[81] Ghosh A, Sil PC. Anti-oxidative effect of a protein from *Cajanus indicus* L against acetaminophen-induced hepato-nephro toxicity. J Biochem Mol Biol 2007; 40(6): 1039-49.
[PMID: 18047802]

[82] Mittal A, Tandon S, Singla SK, Tandon C. Mechanistic insights into the antilithiatic proteins from *Terminalia arjuna:* A proteomic approach in urolithiasis. PLoS One 2016; 11(9): e0162600.
[http://dx.doi.org/10.1371/journal.pone.0162600] [PMID: 27649531]

[83] Aggarwal A, Tandon S, Singla SK, Tandon C. A novel antilithiatic protein from *Tribulus terrestris* having cytoprotective potency. Protein Pept Lett 2012; 19(8): 812-9.
[http://dx.doi.org/10.2174/092986612801619552] [PMID: 22702898]

[84] Singh D, Chander V, Chopra K. Quercetin, a bioflavonoid, attenuates ferric nitrilotriacetate-induced oxidative renal injury in rats. Drug Chem Toxicol 2004; 27(2): 145-56.
[http://dx.doi.org/10.1081/DCT-120030729] [PMID: 15198074]

[85] Morales AI, Vicente-Sánchez C, Sandoval JM, *et al.* Protective effect of quercetin on experimental chronic cadmium nephrotoxicity in rats is based on its antioxidant properties. Food Chem Toxicol 2006; 44(12): 2092-100.
[http://dx.doi.org/10.1016/j.fct.2006.07.012] [PMID: 16962696]

[86] Silan C, Uzun O, Comunoğlu NU, Gökçen S, Bedirhan S, Cengiz M. Gentamicin-induced nephrotoxicity in rats ameliorated and healing effects of resveratrol. Biol Pharm Bull 2007; 30(1): 79-83.
[http://dx.doi.org/10.1248/bpb.30.79] [PMID: 17202664]

[87] Ghodasara J, Pawar A, Deshmukh C, Kuchekar B. Inhibitory effect of rutin and curcumin on experimentally-induced calcium oxalate urolithiasis in rats. Pharmacognosy Res 2010; 2(6): 388-92.
[http://dx.doi.org/10.4103/0974-8490.75462] [PMID: 21713144]

[88] Divakar K, Pawar AT, Chandrasekhar SB, Dighe SB, Divakar G. Protective effect of the hydro-alcoholic extract of *Rubia cordifolia* roots against ethylene glycol induced urolithiasis in rats. Food Chem Toxicol 2010; 48(4): 1013-8.
[http://dx.doi.org/10.1016/j.fct.2010.01.011] [PMID: 20079795]

[89] Thamilselvan S, Khan SR, Menon M. Oxalate and calcium oxalate mediated free radical toxicity in renal epithelial cells: effect of antioxidants. Urol Res 2003; 31(1): 3-9.
[http://dx.doi.org/10.1007/s00240-002-0286-x] [PMID: 12624656]

[90] Boroushaki MT, Sadeghnia HR. Protective effect of safranal against gentamicin-induced nephrotoxicity in rat. Iran J Med Sci 2009; 34: 285-8.

[91]   Ma Z-N, Li Y-Z, Li W, *et al.* Nephroprotective effects of saponins from leaves of *Panax quinquefolius* against cisplatin-induced acute kidney injury. Int J Mol Sci 2017; 18(7): 1407.
[http://dx.doi.org/10.3390/ijms18071407] [PMID: 28703736]

[92]   Gaedeke J, Fels LM, Bokemeyer C, Mengs U, Stolte H, Lentzen H. Cisplatin nephrotoxicity and protection by silibinin. Nephrol Dial Transplant 1996; 11(1): 55-62.
[http://dx.doi.org/10.1093/oxfordjournals.ndt.a027066] [PMID: 8649653]

[93]   Zima T, Kameníková L, Janebová M, Buchar E, Crkovská J, Tesar V. The effect of silibinin on experimental cyclosporine nephrotoxicity. Ren Fail 1998; 20(3): 471-9.
[http://dx.doi.org/10.3109/08860229809045136] [PMID: 9606735]

[94]   Sonnenbichler J, Scalera F, Sonnenbichler I, Weyhenmeyer R. Stimulatory effects of silibinin and silicristin from the milk thistle *Silybum marianum* on kidney cells. J Pharmacol Exp Ther 1999; 290(3): 1375-83.
[PMID: 10454517]

[95]   Patel VB, Rathod IS, Patel JM, Brahmbhatta MR. Anti-urolithiatic and natriuretic activity of steroidal constituents of *Solanum xanthocarpum.* Pharma Chem 2010; 2(1): 173-6.

[96]   Yousefi Ghale-Salimi M, Eidi M, Ghaemi N, Khavari-Nejad RA. Inhibitory effects of taraxasterol and aqueous extract of *Taraxacum officinale* on calcium oxalate crystallization: *in vitro* study. Ren Fail 2018; 40(1): 298-305.
[http://dx.doi.org/10.1080/0886022X.2018.1455595] [PMID: 29619876]

[97]   El-Sayed EM, Abd-Allah AR, Mansour AM, El-Arabey AA. Thymol and carvacrol prevent cisplatin-induced nephrotoxicity by abrogation of oxidative stress, inflammation, and apoptosis in rats. J Biochem Mol Toxicol 2015; 29(4): 165-72.
[http://dx.doi.org/10.1002/jbt.21681] [PMID: 25487789]

[98]   Badary OA, Nagi MN, al-Shabanah OA, al-Sawaf HA, al-Sohaibani MO, al-Bekairi AM. Thymoquinone ameliorates the nephrotoxicity induced by cisplatin in rodents and potentiates its antitumor activity. Can J Physiol Pharmacol 1997; 75(12): 1356-61.
[http://dx.doi.org/10.1139/y97-169] [PMID: 9534946]

[99]   Dirican A, Sahin O, Tasli F, *et al.* Thymoquinone enhances cisplatin-induced neprotoxicity in high dose. J Ocological sci 2016; 1: 17-24.

[100]   Kim SH, Hong KO, Hwang JK, Park KK. Xanthorrhizol has a potential to attenuate the high dose cisplatin-induced nephrotoxicity in mice. Food Chem Toxicol 2005; 43(1): 117-22.
[http://dx.doi.org/10.1016/j.fct.2004.08.018] [PMID: 15582203]

[101]   Song J, Fan H-J, Li H, Ding H, Lv Q, Hou S-K. Zingerone ameliorates lipopolysaccharide-induced acute kidney injury by inhibiting Toll-like receptor 4 signaling pathway. Eur J Pharmacol 2016; 772: 108-14.
[http://dx.doi.org/10.1016/j.ejphar.2015.12.027] [PMID: 26698392]

[102]   Lan XH, Xiao S, Gong W, Wang Y, Zhao XP. [Study of screening nephroprotective bioactive substances based on triple-color fluorescence probes in Carthami flos]. Zhongguo Zhongyao Zazhi 2014; 39(10): 1880-5.
[PMID: 25282899]

[103]   Radha SR. Isolation and identification of bioactive constituent from *Crateva magna* (Lour.) DC. and its effect on urolithiasis PhD thesis, Avinashilingam Deemed University for Women, India 2016.

[104]   Prashanthi P, Anitha S, Shashdhara S. Antiurolithiatic bioactives from *Rotula aquatica* Lour. Res & Rev Herbal Science 2019; 8(1): 1-10.

SUBJECT INDEX

www.ingramcontent.com/pod-product-compliance
Lightning Source LLC
Chambersburg PA
CBHW050802220326
41598CB00006B/93